Pathogenesis and Treatment of Nephrolithiasis

Contributions to Nephrology

Vol. 58

KARGER

Basel · München · Paris · London · New York · New Delhi · Singapore · Tokyo · Sydney

3rd Int. Symp. on Recent Advances in Pathogenesis and Treatment of Nephrolithiasis,
Turin, March 21–22, 1986

Pathogenesis and Treatment of Nephrolithiasis

Volume Editors
F. Linari, M. Marangella, M. Bruno, Turin

84 figures and 67 tables, 1987

KARGER

Basel · München · Paris · London · New York · New Delhi · Singapore · Tokyo · Sydney

Contributions to Nephrology

Library of Congress Cataloging-in-Publication Data
Int. Symp. on Recent Advances in Pathogenesis and
Treatment of Nephrolithiasis (3rd: 1986: Turin, Italy)
Pathogenesis and treatment of nephrolithiasis.
(Contributions to nephrology; vol. 58)
Includes bibliographies and index.
1. Kidneys–Calculi–Congresses. I. Linari, F. (Franco) II. Marangella, M. (Martino)
III. Bruno, M. (Michele) IV. Title. V. Series: Contributions to nephrology; v. 58.
[DNLM: 1. Kidney Calculi–etiology–congresses. 2. Kidney Calculi–therapy–congresses.
W1 C0778UN v. 58 / WJ 356 I616 1986p] RC916.I54 1986 616.6'22 87–3382
ISBN 3–8055–4554–1

Drug Dosage

The authors and the publisher have exerted every effort to ensure that drug selection and dosage set forth in this text are in accord with current recommendations and practice at the time of publication. However, in view of ongoing research, changes in government regulations, and the constant flow of information relating to drug therapy and drug reactions, the reader is urged to check the package insert for each drug for any change in indications and dosage and for added warnings and precautions. This is particularly important when the recommended agent is a new and/or infrequently employed drug.

Printed by Konkordia Druck GmbH, Bühl/Baden (FRG)
ISBN 3–8055–4554–1

Contents

Physical Chemistry and Laboratory Investigation

Calcium and Magnesium Renal Handling and Metabolism

Pathogenesis of Idiopathic Hypercalciuria and Hyperoxaluria

Management of Idiopathic Stone Disease

Urease Inhibitors in Infection-Induced Renal Stones

Surgical and Non-Surgical Treatment of Renal Stone Disease

Preface

It has now been 18 years since the First International Stone Conference was held in Leeds. Since then many attempts have been made to conquer the fortress of stone disease. Thanks to mineralogists and chemists we have learned a lot on the fine mechanisms of crystal formation and crystal growth. Much insight into the pathogenesis, incidence, and role of the diverse metabolic derangements has been gained through the work of nephrologists and endocrinologists. The management of stone disease has become more rational following the efforts of specialists from various branches of medicine.

This Third Symposium, held in Turin, had to engage in its own strife with nephrolithiasis, centering on some updated issues. Our efforts in the organization of the meeting have been rewarded by the constructive multidisciplinary participation of experts in the various aspects of the disease, coming from many different European and overseas countries. Thus a multitude of specialists crowded the congress sessions, debating about the recent progress in the pathogenesis and treatment of nephrolithiasis. Some of the recognized experts in basic and clinical research were among them, including all the pioneer urologists specializing in noninvasive techniques of lithotripsy, who confronted their experiences in this exciting revolutionary approach to urinary calculi.

This book should represent the crowning piece of our enterprise, as it contains the symposium proceedings. The majority of the invited lectures and selected communications have been included. We gratefully acknowledge the contribution of all the authors who supplied their manuscripts.

We are also indebted to all the firms who made this symposium possible and to Regione Piemonte and Ordine Mauriziano which generously supported the publication of this book. We hope that the scientific material presented here will contribute to the particular war we are engaged in.

Turin, March 1986

Franco Linari
Martino Marangella
Michele Bruno

Contr. Nephrol., vol. 58, pp. 1–7 (Karger, Basel 1987)

Comparison of Epidemiological Data between Uric Acid and Calcium Oxalate Stone Formers in the South of Portugal

José Manuel Reis-Santos

Department of Urology, Curry Cabral Hospital, Faculty of Medical Science, Lisbon, Portugal

In Portugal uric acid lithiasis is found in approximately 19% of all patients with renal lithiasis, this being the second highest incidence after calcium lithiasis (oxalate and/or phosphate) which occurs in 65% of the cases [1]. It used to be thought that the principal cause was alterations in the metabolism of purines but this does not seem to be the case [2, 3]. As it is not always possible to find alterations in the metabolism of purines, other epidemiological or metabolic factors must be looked for [4].

In this study we shall attempt to show epidemiological and metabolic data found when comparing a group of patients with uric acid stones with another group with calcium oxalate stones and relating these results to the total lithiasis population.

Material and Methods

Since 1974 a total of 1,452 adult patients with renal calculi have been submitted to epidemiological and metabolic evaluation. The same protocol has been used as a guide for each patient's 'stone history', urological evaluation and metabolic study [5, 6]. The epidemiological study took into account intrinsic and extrinsic risk factors in the formation of calculi in the urinary tract. We followed Pak's protocol, with slight modifications, for the metabolic study, with the patient following his normal daily routine. Before giving any therapeutic advice we took 24-hour urine specimens on at least three different occasions. To avoid any variations in results due to climatic differences patients who have not been living in Lisbon or the South of Portugal for the last 5 years have been excluded from this study. From these patients 1,320 upper urinary stones were collected and analysed by crystallography [1].

Table I. Composition of 1,320 upper urinary stones, neglecting extraneous components of <1%, obtained from adult patients living in the South of Portugal

Phase	Number of stones	Sex		%
		M	F	
WH	78	36	42	5.91
WH + WD	148	79	69	11.21
WH + A	122	81	41	9.24
WH + WD + A	433	259	174	32.80
WD	13	11	2	0.98
WD + A	5	4	1	0.38
UA	160	112	48	12.30
UA + WH	48	30	18	3.94
UA + UAD	10	8	2	0.86
UA + WH + WD	8	6	2	0.67
UA + WD + WH + A	5	4	1	0.38
UA + A + WH	15	8	7	1.14
AAU	1	1		0.08
UAD + AAU	1	1		0.08
AAU + UA	3	3		0.32
AAU + S + A	1		1	0.08
Rest	269	21	248	20.53
Total	1,320	664	656	100.00

WH = Whewellite; WD = weddellite; UA = uric acid; UAD = uric acid dehydrate; AAU = ammonium acid urate; A = apatite; S = struvite.

Table II. Variation of mean age of patients according to sex and stone composition in both groups

Composition	Sex		Mean age	
	M	F	M	F
Whewellite	36	42	43.16	41.80
Whewellite + weddellite	79	69	38.5	31.60
Calcium oxalate + apatite	340	215	43.08	37.62
Weddellite	11	2	44.2	32.42
Weddellite + apatite	4	1	42.26	30.0
Uric acid	112	48	51.78	55.57
Uric acid + others	51	31	51.85	51.6

Table III. Distribution of each group according to occupational grade and social class

Job description	Grade and social class	Total patients (n = 1,452) %	Group I (n = 779) %	Group II (n = 252) %
Higher managerial	A/I	0.6	0.8	0.3
Intermediate managerial	B/II	5.8	8.0	0
Supervisory or clerical junior managerial	C/III	57.2	81.0	29.8
Skilled manual labour	D/IV	20.3	8.1	25.8
Semi- and unskilled manual workers	E/V	11.1	1.9	33.0
Pensioners, widows and unemployed	F/VI	5.0	0.2	13.1

Results

Table I shows the composition of 1,320 stones and their distribution according to the sex of the patients. All extraneous components of less than 1% were neglected.

From here two distinct groups were formed: the first consisting of 799 patients (470 males and 329 females) with predominantly calcium oxalate stones (group I) and the second consisting of 252 patients (173 males and 79 females) with predominantly uric acid stones (group II). The ratio of men to women is 1:0.7 in group I and 1:0.4 in group II. We found a considerable difference in the average age of the patients in each group. In group I the average age was 42.24 years for males and 34.6 years for females. These groups can be subdivided as shown in table II. On the other hand, the average age patients with uric acid stones was found to be 51.8 years for males and 53.3 years for females. A family history of lithiasis was found in 19.8% of all the patients which breaks down to 26.5% in group I and 6.3% in group II.

In group I it was frequently found that patients had spent some time in equatorial areas and that this very often coincided with their first lithiasis episode. This was the case in 15.2% of our patients (20.8% in group I and 8.3% in group II). All patients were classified according to the head of the household's occupations and graded into six categories. The comparative results are shown in table III.

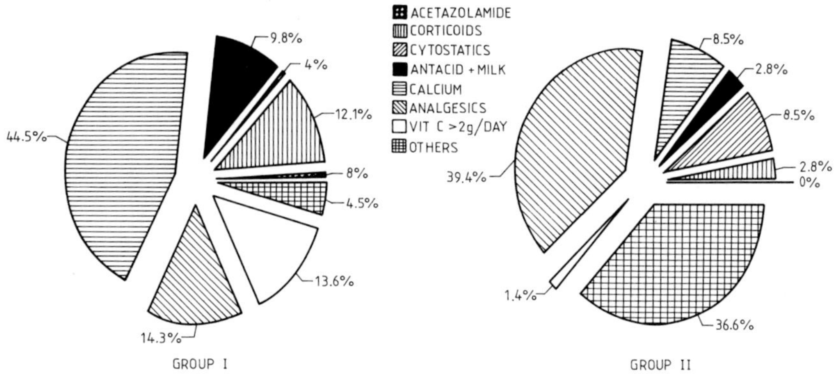

Fig. 1. Comparison of the distribution of drugs, possibly leading to stone formation, in both groups.

The South of Portugal is hot and sunny for most of the year and the local population is not in the habit of drinking much water. As a result many patients on their first visit to our clinic have a total daily urine volume of less than 1,000 ml. The urinary pH was 5.8 ± 0.26 for group I and 5.4 ± 0.18 for group II.

A history of drug ingestion, leading to stone formation, was found in 29.3% of all our patients. This was broken down into 34.0% (265 patients) in group I and 28.1% (71 patients) in group II. Figure 1 compares these results.

A history of disorders known to cause stone formation was found in 58.74% of the patients. Analysing these results for our two groups we have 46.08% (359 patients) and 81.7% (206 patients) in groups I and II, respectively. Figure 2 shows a comparison of these results.

A diet history was studied to evaluate the patients' eating and drinking habits and to determine their total daily caloric intake. We found that 36.2% of the patients had a hypercaloric diet, 4.8% a hypocaloric diet and 59% a normal caloric diet.

A hypercaloric diet was noted in 69.8% of the patients in group II whereas this was only found in 37.6% of the patients in group I. As regards the daily intake of red meat we found no difference between the two groups. As regards the ingestion of liquids each group had its preferences. In group II patients regularly drink alcohol, almost always wine with meals and brandy with coffee afterwards. In group I patients tend to drink more

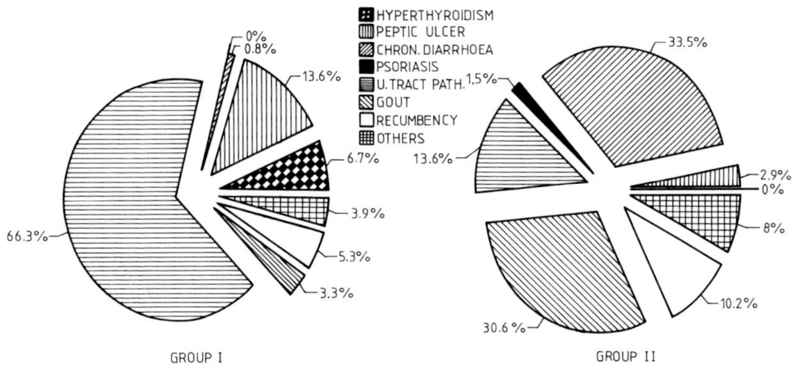

Fig. 2. Comparison of the distribution of disorders and situations predisposing to stone formation in both groups.

bottled or canned beverages and milk. Obesity was found in 28% of the patients in group II but in only 11% of those in group I. Taking into consideration all the patients together (1,452), obesity appeared in 16% of the cases. The biochemical blood values showed no significant differences between the two groups with the exception of the haematocrit, which was higher in group II and which appeared together with the same percentage of obese patients (28%).

The metabolic study showed that 58% of all the patients had hypercalciuria (Ca > 200 mg/day women, > 250 mg/day men). In group I it appeared in 67.9% and in group II in 39.9%. Hyperuricuria (Ua > 600 mg/day in women, > 700 mg/day in men) was found in 62% of the patients on a free diet: 40.8% in group I and 60.3% in group II. Hyperoxaluria was found in 14.2% of the cases in group I and was totally absent in group II. Taking all the patients into account, it appeared in 12%.

Discussion

Naturally, all patients who are sent to any urological department go through some sort of pre-selection. The majority of these patients are candidates for surgery, which would justify the almost equal proportions of males to females in our survey. To confirm this it is sufficient to say that in this series 730 stones were obtained surgically and 590 were passed spontaneously. It is also interesting to note that in 42 patients with anuria, 36 (85.7%) exhibited uric acid lithiasis. Only with this in mind can we begin to interpret the data collected.

In agreement with other surveys we verified that uric acid lithiasis was more common in males. The average age of group I and group II varies; calcium oxalate lithiasis appears earlier in both men and women whereas uric acid lithiasis is more commonly found in older men.

In group I a family history of renal lithiasis was found in about 25% of the patients but only very rarely in group II. Based on previous descriptions, we expected to find an autosomal dominant trait in group II, but this was not so due to the low percentage of patients with a family history of stones in this group [2].

Stays in equatorial regions and the ingestion of small amounts of liquids seem to be favourable to stone formation in both groups. Even when the uric acid content of 24-hour urine is normal, the low urinary pH of patients in group II is an important factor in the formation of calculi. The ingestion of drugs and illnesses or situations conducive to lithiasis in both groups emphasize known data on the aetiology of lithiasis. In group II a hypercaloric diet, obesity and the ingestion of alcohol are important factors. In this group obesity is perhaps the factor which can explain the only biochemical blood values which differed between the two groups – the high haematocrit value in both men and women.

Hypercalciuria was approximately twice as common in group I whereas hyperuricuria was more common in group II. However, hypercalciuria and hyperuricuria were often found side by side in both groups.

Hyperoxaluria (Ox > 40 mg/day) was not found in group II but it does constitute an important potential risk factor for group I even though it was only found in a small percentage of the patients. However, its value was almost always on the upper borderline level of the normal range.

Conclusions

Portugal has a high percentage of uric acid lithiasis (19%), second only to calcium oxalate lithiasis. The comparison of two groups of patients, one with calcium oxalate stones and the other with uric acid stones, showed significant differences. These differences are connected to age, sex, heredity, diet habits, and the ingestion of alcohol as well as the intake of drugs and disorders known to cause lithiasis. As regards ingestion of liquids each group had its preferences, although neither showed any inclination to drink water. In group II patients regularly drink alcohol, almost always wine with meals and brandy with coffee afterwards. In group I patients tend to drink more bottled or canned sugary beverages and milk. Obesity was more predominant in group II and would seem to explain the high haematocrit value found in this group. The urinary pH, hypercalciuria, hyperuricuria and hyperoxaluria show a different distribution in the two groups. Almost all cases of anuria were due to uric acid stones.

With these data we can confirm that these two groups are quite different and the metabolic alteration of the purines in the uric acid group is not enough to explain the aetiology of uric acid stones and, therefore, other factors must be looked for.

References

1 Reis-Santos, J. M.: Composition and frequency of stone minerals in the South of Portugal; in Ryall, Brockis, Marshall, Finlayson, Urinary stone, pp. 309–313 (Churchill-Livingstone, London 1984).

2 De Vries, A.; Frank, M.; Atsmon, A.: Inherited uric acid lithiasis. Am. J. Med. *33:* 880 (1962).

3 Henneman, P. H.; Wallach, S.; Dempey, E. F.: The metabolic defect responsible for uric acid stone formation. J. clin. Invest. *41:* 537 (1962).

4 Zechner, O.; Scheiber, V.: Idiopathic uric acid lithiasis; in Ryall, Brockis, Marshall, Finlayson, Urinary stone, pp. 215–218 (Churchill-Livingstone, London 1984).

5 Reis-Santos, J. M.; Matos-Ferreira, A.: Protocolos de investigação do doente litiásico. 1. História litiásica. Acta med. port. *6:* 45–55 (1985).

6 Reis-Santos, J. M.: Urolithiasis – epidemiological data from the South of Portugal; in Schwille, Smith, Robertson, Vahlensieck, Urolithiasis and related clinical research, pp. 39–42 (Plenum Press, London 1985).

José Manuel Reis-Santos, MD, Universidade Nova de Lisbon,
Faculty of Medical Science, Department of Urology, Curry Cabral Hospital,
P–1000 Lisbon (Portugal)

Contr. Nephrol., vol. 58, pp. 8–15 (Karger, Basel 1987)

Renal Excretion of Calcium, Oxalate and Magnesium between 3 and 16 Years: The Value of Overnight Urine

The Cimitile Study[1]

N. G. De Santo, B. Di Iorio, G. Capodicasa, G. Capasso, C. Paduano, M. Aulisio, F. Russo, L. Fiorino, C. Giordano

Chair of Pediatric Nephrology, Institute of Internal Medicine and Nephrology, 1st Faculty of Medicine, University of Naples, Naples, Italy

In childhood normal urinary calcium excretion is below 4 mg/kg body weight/day [1–13] but all the data with very few exceptions have been collected in hospitalized patients. It is also accepted that oxalate excretion in normal children does not exceed 50 mg/day [14–17]. Such reference data are currently accepted in Italy due to the lack of epidemiological data specific for this age.

The goal of this work is threefold: (1) to evaluate calcium, oxalate and magnesium excretion in children aged 3–16 years; (2) to evaluate the usability of overnight urine [18] for clinical/epidemiological purposes, and (3) to evaluate the incidence of hypercalciuria and hyperoxaluria in children.

Subjects and Methods

The data have been collected in the course of the Cimitile Study [19, 20] designed to collect cardiorenal reference data for ages between 1 and 18 years. We have studied up to now a total of 120 children (66 males) aged 3–16 years (mean 9.9 ± 3.9 years) and weighing 13–83 kg (mean 38.1 ± 16.1 kg). Surface area in this group of subjects ranged between 0.6 and 1.97 m^2. Children distribution by age and sex is presented in figure 1.

Children participating in the study were instructed to collect daily and overnight urine as detailed elsewere [19, 20]. Each of them received two bags (A and B). Bag A was used

[1] Supported by funds of the Ministry of Education made available through programs of local and national interests.

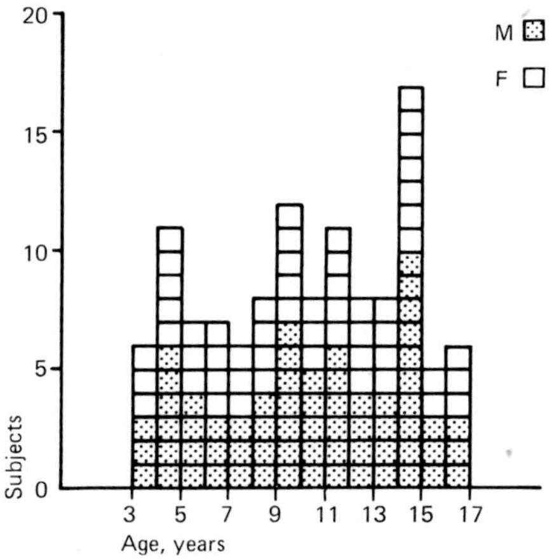

Fig. 1. Distribution by age and sex of 120 children participating in the study.

during daytime (approximately from 7 a.m. to 10 p.m.). Bag B was used for overnight urine (approximately from 10 p.m. to 7 a.m.). Each participant was asked to record the starting time and the finishing time for each period, and thoroughly investigated about the completeness of the collections. The urines in bag A and bag B was measured and analyzed independently. By summing up excretion in bag A plus excretion in bag B the overall (observed) daily excretion was obtained for calcium, magnesium and oxalate.

The duration of overnight urine collection varies from child to child participating in the study. This did not allow the use of excretions during overnight collection as absolute values. For this reason overnight excretion for each studied component had to be extrapolated to 24 h (predicted daily values) as it follows. If the excretion in overnight urine collections (say duration Y min) for component X is known (assume a value of Xo) the predicted 24-hour excretion (duration 1,440 min) for component X (call it Xp) will be calculated according to the equation:

$$\mathrm{Xo} : \mathrm{Y\ min} = \mathrm{Xp} : 1{,}440,$$

that is to say:

$$\mathrm{Xp} = \frac{1{,}440}{\mathrm{Y\ min}} \cdot \mathrm{Xo}.$$

Calcium was measured by the O-cresol-phthalein method [21, 22]; oxalate was measured by the chromotropic acid reaction [23]; magnesium was measured by atomic absorption photometry, and creatinine excretion by Jaffé's reaction [24].

Data are presented as mean ± SD and statistical analysis of differences among means assessed by the Student's t-test.

Table I. Excretions of calcium, oxalate, and magnesium (mg/day) in relation to age

Age, years	n (M + F)	Calcium	Oxalate	Magnesium
3	6	40.25 ± 19.95	12.22 ± 4.97	34.98 ± 11.78
4	11	62.67 ± 34.85	11.13 ± 4.83	43.81 ± 11.88
5	7	77.26 ± 26.47	13.05 ± 4.32	50.37 ± 11.96
6	7	77.12 ± 37.31	10.67 ± 3.11	50.65 ± 8.03
7	6	31.17 ± 17.69	17.56 ± 4.14	78.07 ± 18.02
8	8	106.75 ± 50.39	19.49 ± 6.42	63.49 ± 12.38
9	12	45.65 ± 30.37	18.41 ± 9.86	48.65 ± 19.44
10	8	79.23 ± 50.66	28.81 ± 18.59	67.36 ± 19.60
11	11	86.53 ± 37.84	26.09 ± 11.22	85.63 ± 30.18
12	8	70.78 ± 38.49	23.85 ± 17.17	79.43 ± 26.52
13	8	77.07 ± 41.50	25.04 ± 13.34	98.49 ± 42.74
14	17	114.33 ± 50.42	27.28 ± 11.87	94.33 ± 35.08
15	5	100.91 ± 108.64	17.28 ± 5.59	118.39 ± 32.17
16	6	126.18 ± 88.50	21.07 ± 7.99	93.25 ± 31.96

Results

Table I includes the mean daily excretions of calcium, oxalate and magnesium by age groups. At the age of 3 years calcium excretion was 40.25 ± 19.25 mg/day (mean ± SD), while at the age of 16 it averaged 126.18 ± 88.50 mg/day. A total of 49 children excreted 100–150 mg/day, 1 more than 200 mg/day and 2 more than 300 mg/day (fig. 2). A total of 10 children excreted more than 4 mg/kg (fig. 3). Mean oxalate excretion was 12.22 ± 4.97 mg/day at 3 years of age and increased to 28.81 ± 18.59 mg/day by age of 10 years. No further increase was observed thereafter. A total of 3 patients showed increased urinary oxalate excretion (fig. 4). Magnesium excretion averaged 34.98 ± 11.78 mg/day at 3 years of age and 118.39 ± 32.17 mg/day at the age of 16. A total of 67 subjects showed excretions in the range of 50–100 mg/day (fig. 5). Table II represents a synopsis of the mean urinary excretion for calcium oxalate and magnesium for all ages. Table III reports on various ratios and shows that the mean

2
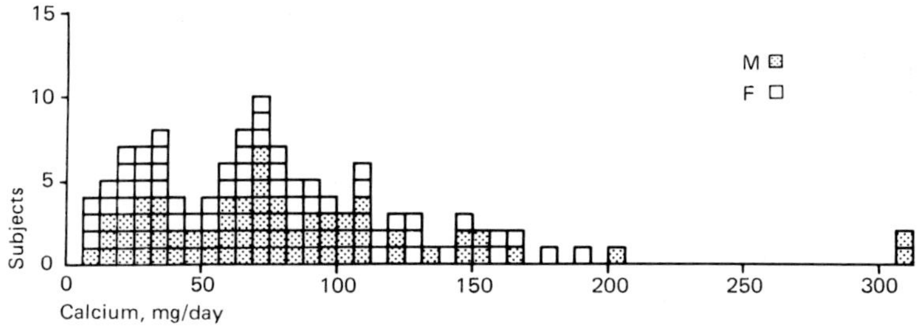

3
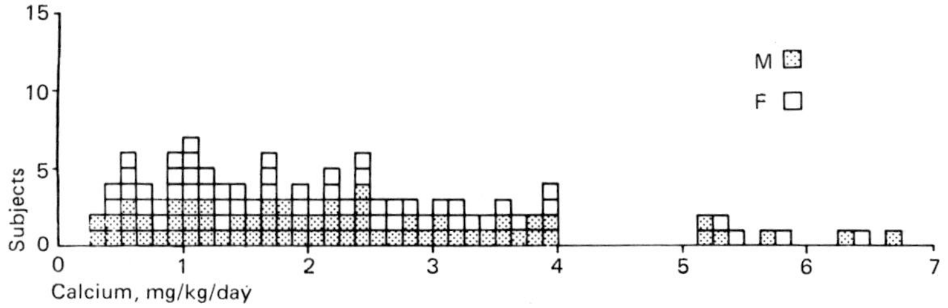

4
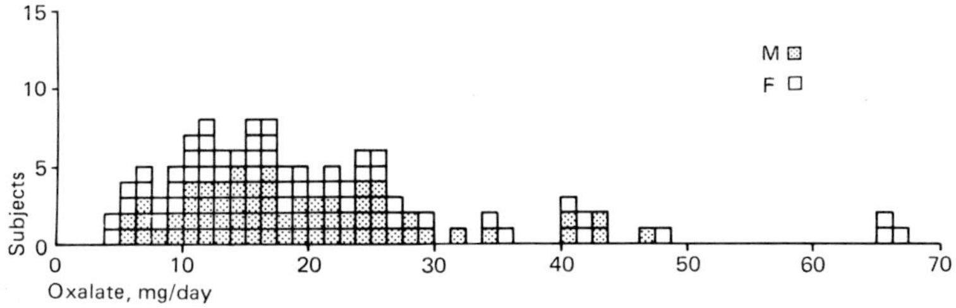

5
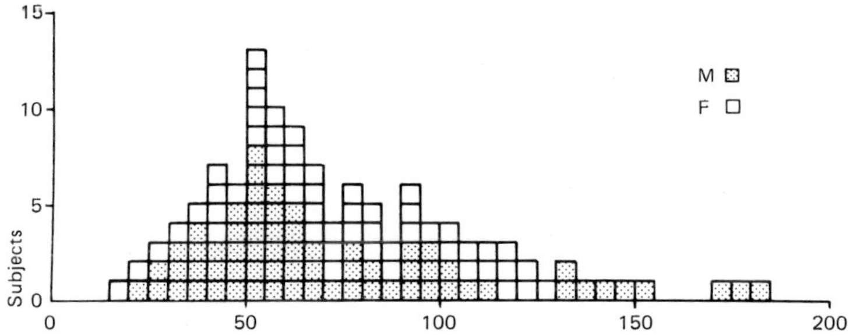

Fig. 2. Urinary calcium excretion (mg/day) in boys and girls.

Fig. 3. Distribution of calcium excretion (mg/kg body weight/day) in boys and girls. A total of 10 children were hypercalciuric.

Fig. 4. Distribution of oxalate urinary excretion (mg/day) in boys and girls. A total of 3 girls was hyperoxaluric.

Fig. 5. Urinary magnesium excretion (mg/day) in boys and girls.

Table II. Daily urinary output of calcium, oxalate, and magnesium in 120 children

	M + F	M	F
Calcium, mg/day	80.58 ± 51.86	82.94 ± 58.10	78.50 ± 49.60
Calcium, mg/kg/day	2.26 ± 1.38	2.25 ± 1.36	2.27 ± 1.32
Oxalate, mg/day	20.62 ± 11.92	20.04 ± 11.20	22.12 ± 13.92
Magnesium, mg/day	73.98 ± 33.86	75.33 ± 38.22	69.62 ± 28.22
Magnesium, mg/kg/day	2.031 ± 0.771	2.037 ± 0.833	2.029 ± 0.693

Table III. Ca/Cr, Mg/Cr, and Mg/Ca ratios in 120 children aged 3–16 years

Ratio	M + F	M	F
Ca/Cr	0.0695 ± 0.0402	0.0698 ± 0.0403	0.0693 ± 0.0400
Mg/Cr	0.066 ± 0.024	0.065 ± 0.021	0.067 ± 0.026
Mg/Ca	1.56 ± 1.22	1.52 ± 1.00	1.59 ± 1.36

Table IV. Mg/Cr and Mg/Ca ratios in 10 hypercalciuric children

Ratio	Normals (n = 110)	Hypercalciurics (n = 10)	p
Mg/Cr	0.066 ± 0.024	0.065 ± 0.027	n.s.
Mg/Ca	1.56 ± 1.22	0.49 ± 0.34	< 0.001

Table V. Comparison of observed excretions of calcium, oxalate, and magnesium with those predicted in overnight urine in 120 children

	Observed, mg/day	Predicted, mg/day	p
Calcium	80.58 ± 51.86	80.96 ± 52.88	n.s.
Oxalate	20.62 ± 11.92	23.04 ± 16.96	n.s.
Magnesium	73.98 ± 33.86	71.88 ± 31.68	n.s.

Ca/Cr ratio was 0.0695 ± 0.0402, and only 10 children (fig. 6) exceeded 0.15.

Mean Mg/Cr ratio was 0.066 ± 0.024 (table III) and no difference was seen when data were analyzed by sex. Table III also reports on the mean Mg/Ca ratio which averaged 1.56 ± 1.22 and was not sex-linked.

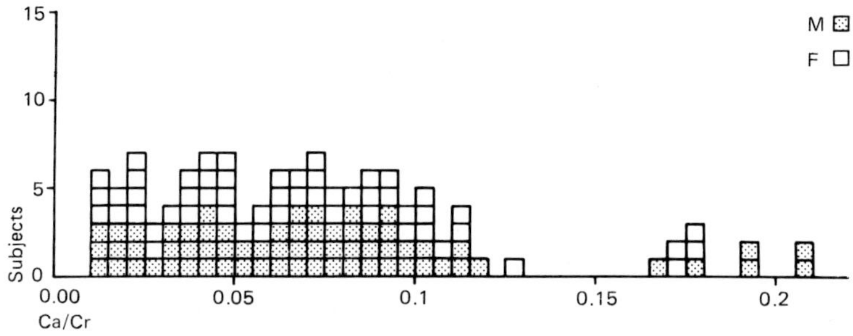

Fig. 6. Urinary Ca/Cr ratio in boys and girls.

The Mg/Cr ratio was not affected by the hypercalciuric status whereas a reduction of the Mg/Ca ratio was seen in hypercalciuric children ($p < 0.001$, table IV). The mean Ca excretion in the study averaged 80.59 ± 51.86 mg/day, a value identical to the daily urinary excretion of calcium predicted by using overnight urine, and the same was true for oxalate and magnesium (table V).

Discussion

The data indicate that the incidence of asymptomatic hypercalciuria is 8.9%. This incidence, which confirms the preliminary trend [19, 20], might present the end effect of dietary/environmental/genetic factors. This high incidence of hypercalciuria in this age group is in poor agreement with the 2.9% incidence reported by Moore et al. [6]. However, one should be aware of the fact that Moore et al. [6] studied children referred to the acute care unit of the Department of Pediatrics at the Michael Reese Hospital in Chicago, 90% of whom were black.

Our mean Ca/Cr ratio is 0.069 so that it is nearly identical to that of Moore et al. [6] but lower than that reported by Ghazali and Barratt [4] and by Bulusu et al. [9]. In our study there was no difference among sexes in the normocalciuric group while Bulusu et al. [9] found increased levels in the female sex.

Calcium excretion in the present study averaged 2.26 ± 1.38 mg/kg while available reports are in the range from more than 2 to more than 9 mg/kg [1, 4, 6, 25]. Our mean Ca excretion is in good keeping with the data by Ghazali and Barratt [4] who mainly reported on hospitalized children. A total of 3 children showed oxalate excretion exceeding 50 mg/day; they were not hypercalciuric. This finding is interesting and deserves further studies. It has to be stressed that the Mg/Ca ratio in normal children averaged 1.56 while it averaged 0.5 in hypercalciuric children. This finding confirms available data [26, 27].

The most striking information in the present work is related to the importance of overnight urine for epidemiological/clinical purposes: this was true for Ca, Mg and oxalate. This possibility, hitherto not explored, deserves further evaluation but the present data confirm the preliminary trend observed at the beginning of the Cimitile Study [19, 20].

References

1 Royer, P.: Exploration biologique du métabolisme calcique chez l'enfant. Helv. paediat. Acta *16:* 320–324 (1961).

2 Massry, S. G.; Coburn, S. W.: The hormonal and non-hormonal control of renal excretion of calcium and magnesium. Nephron *10:* 66–112 (1973).

3 Paunier, L.; Borgeaud, M.; Wyss, M.: Urinary excretion of calcium and magnesium in normal children. Helv. paediat. Acta *25:* 577–579 (1970).

4 Ghazali, S.; Barratt, T. M.: Urinary excretion of calcium and magnesium in children. Archs. Dis. Childh. *49:* 97–101 (1974).

5 Nordin, B. E. C.: Hypercalciuria. Clin. Sci. mol. Med. *52:* 1–5 (1977).

6 Moore, E. S.; Coe, F. L.; McMann, B. J.; et al.: Idiopathic hypercalciuria in children: prevalance and metabolic characteristics. J. Pediat. *92:* 906–910 (1978).

7 Stapleton, F. B.; Noe, F. L.; Jerkins, G.; et al.: Urinary excretion of calcium following an oral calcium loading test in healthy children. Pediatrics, Springfield *69:* 594–596 (1984).

8 Langman, C. B.; Moore, S.: Hypercalciuria in clinical pediatrics. Clin. Pediat. *23:* 135–139 (1984).

9 Bulusu, A.; Hodkinson, A.; Nordin, B. E. C.; Peacock, M.: Urinary excretion of calcium and creatinine in relation to age and body weight in normal subjects and patients with renal calculues. Clin. Sci. *38:* 601–605 (1970).

10 Aladjem, M.; Modan, M.; Lusky, A.: Idiopathic hypercalciuria: a familial generalized renal hypersecretory state. Kidney int. *24:* 549–554 (1983).

11 Stapleton, F. B.; Noe, H. N.; Roy, S.; Jerkins, G.: Hypercalciuria in children with urolithiasis. Am. J. Dis. Child. *136:* 675–678 (1982).

12 Evans, R. A.; Fordes, M. A.; Sutton, R. A. L.; Watson, L.: Urinary excretion of calcium and magnesium in patients with calcium-containing renal stones. Lancet *iv:* 958–961 (1967).

13 Roy, S.; Stapleton, F.; Noe, H. N.; et al.: Hematuria preceding renal calculus formation in children with hypercalciuria. J. Pediat. *99:* 712–719 (1981).

14 Dempsey, E. F.; Forbes, A. P.; Mellick, R. A.: Urinary oxalate excretion. Metab. Clin. Exp. *9:* 52–58 (1960).

15 Gibbs, D. A.; Watts, R. W. E.: The variation of oxalate excretion with age. J. Lab. clin. Med. *73:* 901–908 (1969).

16 Gibbs, D. A.; Xatts, R. W. E.: Biochemical studies on the treatment of primary hyperoxaluria. Archs. Dis. Childh. *42:* 505–508 (1967).

17 Baggio, B.; Gambaro, G.; Favaro, S.; Borsatti, A.: Prevalence of hyperoxaluria in idiopathic calcium oxalate kidney stone disease. Nephron *35:* 11–14 (1983).

18 Liu, K.; Dyer, A. L.; Cooper, R. S.; Stammler, R.; Stammler, J.: Can overnight urine replace 24-hour urine collection to assess salt intake? Hypertension *1:* 529–536 (1979).

19 De Santo, N. G.; Di Iorio, B.; Capasso, G.; Capodicasa, G.; Russo, F.: Escrezione renale di calcio e ossalato tra 8 e 16 anni. Il valore della raccolta overnight. Dati preliminari dello studio Cimitile; in Di Paolo, Sasdelli, Sodi, Litiasi renale, pp. 42–51 (Wichtig, Milano 1985).

20 De Santo, N. G.; Di Iorio, B.; Capodicasa, G.; Russo, F.: Escrezione renale di calcio e ossalato tra 6 e 17 anni. Il valore delle urine overnight per la valutazione dell'escrezione giornaliera di calcio, ossalato, creatinina, sodio, potassio, fosfato. Dati intermedi dello studio Cimitile. G. ital. Nefrol. *3:* 11–15 (1986).

21 Connerty, H. V.; Briggs, A. R.: Determination of serum calcium by means of orthocresolphtalein complex one. Am. J. clin. Path. *45:* 290–298 (1960).

22 Gitelman, H. J.: An improved automated procedure for determination of calcium in biological specimens. Analyt. Biochem. *18:* 520–526 (1967).

23 Hodgkinson, A.; Williams, A.: An improved colorimetric procedure for determination in urine oxalate. Clinica chim. Acta *36:* 127–132 (1972).

24 Bonssnes, R. W.; Taussky, H. H.: On the colorimetric determination of creatinine by Jaffé's reaction. J. biol. Chem. *158:* 581–587 (1951).

25 Knapp, E. L.: Factors influencing the urinary excretion of calcium in normal persons. J. clin. Invest. *26:* 182–185 (1947).

26 Oreopoulos, D. G.; Soxannwo, M. A. O.; McGeown, M. G.: Magnesium calcium ratio in urine of patients with renal stones. Lancet *24:* 420–422 (1968).

27 Evans, R. A.; Fordes, M. A.; Sutton, R. A. L.; Watson, L.: Urinary excretion of calcium and magnesium in patients with calcium-containing renal stones. Lancet *iv:* 458–461 (1967).

N. G. De Santo, MD, Chair of Pediatric Nephrology,
Institute of Internal Medicine, 1st Faculty of Medicine, University of Naples,
I–80131 Naples (Italy)

Contr. Nephrol., vol. 58, pp. 16–20 (Karger, Basel 1987)

Age and Sex as Factors in Oxalic Acid Excretion in Healthy Persons and Calcium Oxalate Stone Patients

A. Hesse, K. Klocke, A. Classen, W. Vahlensieck

Experimentelle Urologie, Urologische Universitätsklinik Bonn, Bonn, FRG

Oxalic acid is the most important determinant of urine saturation with calcium oxalate [3] and its excretion is a better predictor of stone recurrence than other urine constituents [8]. In stone formers the excretion of oxalic acid is found higher than in healthy controls [1, 4–6, 8]. Despite the high significance of oxalic acid there have been only few studies on the dependence of calcium oxalate excretion on age, sex and body weight in groups with a considerable number of stone patients and healthy persons [5].

In healthy persons [7] and in stone formers [4] a higher excretion of oxalic acid in men than in women is reported. It is not clear whether the body weight which has some bearing on the excretion of oxalic acid accounts for this difference. The investigations done by Thind et al. [9] about the effect of sexual hormones on the metabolism of oxalic acid are of some importance in this discussion. Until now there is no proof for the dependency of oxalic acid excretion on age.

In the present study the daily excretion of oxalic acid was determined in 300 healthy persons and 272 recurrent calcium oxalate stone formers. We investigated the extent to which it might be influenced by age and sex.

Subjects and Methods

150 healthy women and 150 healthy men not undergoing any medical treatment were divided into six age groups. 88 female and 184 male stone formers, attending the metabolic ward of the Department of Urology were classified accordingly. All patients were recurrent calcium oxalate stone formers with normal renal function who did not, at the time of investigation, show any sign of urinary infection and did not receive any medical treatment for prevention of stone recurrence.

Table I. Oxalic acid excretion in healthy persons

Age group (years)	Healthy men		p	Healthy women	
	n	mmol/24 h (SEM)		n	mmol/24 h (SEM)
I (19.9)	25	0.421 (0.039)		25	0.346 (0.051)
II (20–29.9)	25	0.404 (0.026)		25	0.353 (0.029)
III (30–39.9)	25	0.451 (0.038)	*	25	0.340 (0.023)
IV (40–49.9)	25	0.498 (0.042)	*	25	0.376 (0.038)
V (50–59.9)	25	0.425 (0.033)	*	25	0.338 (0.021)
VI (60)	25	0.492 (0.033)	***	25	0.299 (0.017)
Total	150	0.448 (0.015)	***	150	0.342 (0.013)

Levels of significance of differences between women and men: * $p < 0.05$; *** $p < 0.001$.

One 24-hour urine sample was collected from each subject at home while patients and controls adhered to their normal diet. Oxalic acid in urine was measured by gas chromatography using the method of Dosch [2] with malonic acid as internal standard that makes it possible to shorten the time required for one analysis by means of back-flushing.

For the evaluation of differences between the groups we used the nonparametric rank sum test of Wilcoxon-Mann-Whitney.

Results

The excretion of oxalic acid in healthy persons is significantly lower ($p < 0.001$) in women (0.342 mmol/day) than in men (0.448 mmol/day). This difference decreases but remains significant ($p < 0.001$) when oxalic acid excretion is related to the body surface of 1.73 m^2.

In order to investigate the influence of age on the excretion of oxalic acid we divided the healthy persons into six age groups of 25 women and 25 men each (table I). We found no difference between the age groups neither in men nor in women. In all age groups men excreted more oxalic acid than women, but only in groups III, IV, V and VI the difference was significant (fig. 1). When excretion values are related to body surface the picture is similar.

Male stone formers show a higher oxalic acid excretion (0.583 mmol/day, $p < 0.001$) than female stone formers (0.453 mmol/day). The mean excretion is higher for men in all age groups, but this is significant only in groups I, III and V (table II, fig. 2).

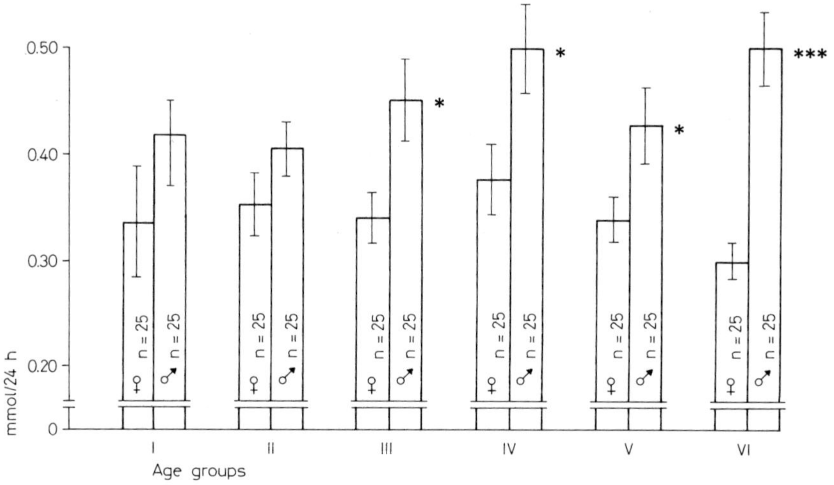

Fig. 1. Daily excretion of oxalic acid. Healthy persons divided into six age groups. For values and significance of differences see table I.

Table II. Oxalic acid excretion in stone patients

Age group (years)	Male stone formers n	mmol/24 h (SEM)	p	Female stone formers n	mmol/24 h (SEM)	p
I (19.9)	9	0.747 (0.164)	* +	5	0.359 (0.082)	
II (20–29.9)	30	0.628 (0.132)		13	0.521 (0.122)	+
III (30–39.9)	26	0.552 (0.051)	**	14	0.342 (0.048)	
IV (40–49.9)	56	0.551 (0.039)		27	0.482 (0.059)	
V (50–59.9)	48	0.545 (0.023)	* ++	19	0.421 (0.035)	+
VI (60)	15	0.697 (0.111)		10	0.546 (0.090)	+++
Total	184	0.583 (0.029)	*** +++	88	0.453 (0.030)	++

Levels of significance of differences between women and men: * $p < 0.05$; ** $p < 0.01$; *** < 0.001.

Levels of significance of differences between healthy persons and stone formers: + $p < 0.05$; ++ $p < 0.01$; +++ $p < 0.001$.

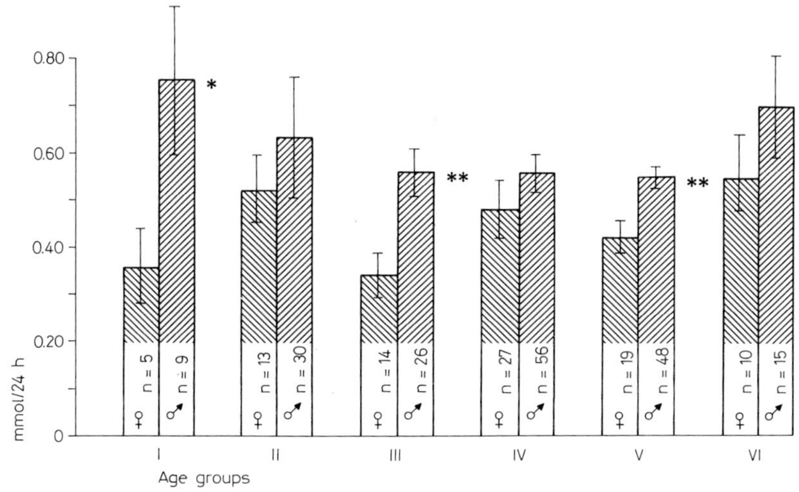

Fig. 2. Daily excretion of oxalic acid. Stone formers divided into six age groups. For values and significance of differences see table II.

Male and female stone formers excrete more oxalic acid than healthy men and women. In women, age groups II, IV, V and VI are chiefly responsible for this difference. This corresponds well with the two peaks of stone incidence in women between 20 and 30 and between 40 and 60 years. In age groups I and III oxalic acid excretion seems to be of minor importance for stone formation in women. In men there are fairly clear differences between controls and stone formers in all age groups. However, only in groups I and V oxalic acid excretion is significantly higher in male calcium oxalate stone formers. The high oxalic acid excretion in age group I suggests a close relation between recurrent calcium stone formation in young men and oxalic acid metabolism.

Conclusion

The daily excretion of oxalic acid was determined in 300 healthy persons and 272 recurrent calcium oxalate stone formers. The mean excretion of oxalic acid was significantly higher in men compared with the women, both in healthy persons and stone formers. The differences could not be accounted for by the distinct mean body surface of men and women. There was no evidence for a relationship between oxalic acid excretion and age.

Both female and male stone formers excreted more oxalic acid than healthy men and women. In men this difference is mainly due to the high oxalic acid excretion of stone formers under 20 and over 50 years of age. In women the stone formers between 20 and 30 years and over 50 years are chiefly responsible for the difference.

We conclude that evaluation of oxalic acid excretion data should be done for men and women separately. No relationship was found between oxalic acid excretion and the age of the subjects, but our results give rise to the conjecture that the contribution of oxalic acid to the risk of forming stones varies between the different age groups both in men and in women.

References

1 Baggio, B.; Gambaro, G.; Favaro, S.; Borsatti, A.: Prevalence of hyperoxaluria in idiopathic calcium oxalate kidney stone disease. Nephron *35:* 11–14 (1983).

2 Dosch, W.: Rapid and direct gas chromatographic determination of oxalic acid in urine. Urol. Res. *7:* 227–234 (1979).

3 Finlayson, B.: Calcium stones: some physical and chemical aspects; in David, Calcium metabolism in renal failure and nephrolithiasis, pp. 337–382 (Wiley & Sons, New York 1977).

4 Hesse, A.; Classen, A.; Klocke, N.; Vahlensieck, W.: The significance of sexual dependency of lithogenic and inhibitory substances in urine; in Schwille, Smith, Robertson, Vahlensieck, Urolithiasis and related clinical research, pp. 25–27 (Plenum Press, New York 1985).

5 Hodgkinson, A.: Relations between oxalic acid, calcium, magnesium and creatinine excretion in normal men and male patients with calcium oxalate kidney stones. Clin. Sci. mol. Med. *46:* 357–367 (1974).

6 Marangella, M.; Daniele, P. G.; Ronzani, M.; Sonego, S.; Linari, F.: Urine saturation with calcium salts in normal subjects and idiopathic calcium stone formers estimated by an improved computer model system. Urol. Res. *13:* 189–193 (1985).

7 Prenen, J. A. C.; Boer, P.; Van Larsum, L.; Oldenburg, S. J.; Endeman, H. J.: Urinary oxalate excretion, as determined by isotope dilution and indirect colorimetry. Clinica chim. Acta *127:* 251–261 (1983).

8 Robertson, W. G.; Peacock, M.; Quimet, D.; Heyburn, P. J.; Rutherford, A.: The main risk factor for calcium oxalate stone disease in man: hypercalciuria or mild hyperoxaluria?; in Smith, Robertson, Finlayson, Urolithiasis, clinical and basic research, pp. 3–12 (Plenum Press, New York 1981).

9 Thind, S. K.; Sharma, V.; Farooqui, S.; Nath, R.: Intestinal absorption of oxalate in gonadectomized rats; in Schwille, Smith, Robertson, Vahlensieck, Urolithiasis and related clinical research, pp. 151–154 (Plenum Press, New York 1985).

PD Dr. A. Hesse, MD, Experimentelle Urologie, Urologische Universitätsklinik Bonn, Sigmund-Freud-Strasse 25, D–5300 Bonn 1 (FRG)

Contr. Nephrol., vol. 58, pp. 21–24 (Karger, Basel 1987)

Urinary Composition in Normal Men on Usual Diet and Life-Style

A Study of 30 Consecutive Days

L. Borghi, G. F. Elia, M. R. Trapassi, F. Barbarese, E. Melloni, F. Amato, A. Guerra, A. Novarini

Istituto di Semeiotica Medica, Università degli Studi di Parma, Parma, Italy

The study of out-patients on a free diet is simpler and more useful because it gives information about dietetic habits and life-style. The main problem is to establish for how many days and in which way we must collect the 24-hour urine samples. The purpose of our study was to measure the variability of the urinary excretion of stone promoters and inhibitors in healty subjects on a usual diet over a long period of time. Moreover, we wanted to verify if even normal men can produce urine containing very high levels of stone promoters and how often it occurs.

Patients and Methods

This study was carried out on 6 healthy subjects (3 M, 3 F; age 27–65 years; weight 50–79 kg; height 160–180 cm). Each of them collected for 30 consecutive days, 24-hour urine samples which they put into two bottles containing hibitane 20%, a small one for a 3-hour urine sample (7–10 a.m.) and a larger one for a 21-hour urine sample (10–7 a.m.). The study was carried out in spring time and within a period of 45 days to minimize the well-known seasonal variations in the excretion of urinary constituents [1]. The subjects followed their ordinary diet and were specifically asked to carry on their normal lives. The variables carried out on the 3- and 21-hour urine samples were the following: creatinine, volume, osmolarity, urea, Na, K, Ca, PO_4, uric acid, oxalic acid, titratable acidity (TA), NH_4, by methods already published [2, 3]. The data of the 24-hour urine samples were obtained by adding together the results of the 3- and 21-hour urine samples. The statistical analysis was carried out by the Mann-Whitney non-parametric test.

Table I. Mean excretion of the urinary constituents expressed as creatinine ratio (osmolarity, mosm/mmol; oxalic acid, μmol/mmol; all the others mmol/mmol)

Values	3-hour fasting urine	24-hour urine	Δ %
Osmolarity	111.4 ± 28.4	109.9 ± 22.0	+ 1.3
Urea	47.5 ± 17.0	43.0 ± 7.3	+ 10.4
Na	15.9 ± 5.3	19.8 ± 4.9	− 19.6
K	5.6 ± 1.3	6.9 ± 1.3	− 18.8
Ca	0.35 ± 0.13	0.43 ± 0.11	− 18.6
PO_4	2.06 ± 0.31	2.37 ± 0.29	− 13.0
Mg	0.44 ± 0.16	0.44 ± 0.11	0.00
Cl	14.6 ± 5.2	19.0 ± 5.0	− 23.1
Uric acid	0.29 ± 0.04	0.34 ± 0.03	− 14.7
Oxalic acid	16.6 ± 3.9	20.6 ± 5.0	− 19.4
Titratable acidity	2.72 ± 1.50	2.55 ± 0.71	+ 6.6
NH_4	4.13 ± 1.06	3.91 ± 0.56	+ 5.6

Results

Mean excretion ± SD (expressed as creatinine ratio) of constituents in the 3- and 24-hour urine samples are shown in table I. There are no differences in the levels of osmolarity and Mg between the two samples; the levels of urea, TA and NH_4 are slightly higher in the fasting urine, while all the other substances are excreted in lower quantities in the morning with percentage variation from 13 to 23%.

We calculated the percentage variations of the standard deviation in relation to their respective averages of each urine constituent of the 3- and 24-hour urine samples. The results indicated that the fluctuation of the various constituents is very high and that in the 3-hour urine sample the fluctuations are not inferior to those of the 24-hour sample.

The substances in which the variability is not different from that of the creatinine (Mann-Whitney test) are: chloride, calcium, oxalic acid, osmolarity, potassium, and TA. The substances in which the variability is statistically higher than that of the creatinine are: magnesium ($p = 0.04$), uric

Table II. Incidence of values exceeding the 'safety limits'

Urinary risk factors and their 'safety limits'	Collection number out of 'safety limits'	%
Volume < 800 ml/day	7	3.9
Osmolarity > 1,000 mosm/l	11	6.1
Ca/creatinine > 0.63 mmol/mmol	17	9.4
Mg/creatinine < 0.20 mmol/mmol	3	1.6
Uric acid/creatinine > 0.40 mmol/mmol	21	11.6
Oxalic acid/creatinine > 0.30 μmol/mmol	26	14.4
pH 3 h < 5, > 7	12	6.6
pH 21 h < 5, > 7	9	5.0

acid ($p = 0.04$), ammonium ($p = 0.03$), phosphate ($p - 0.02$) and volume ($p = 0.01$).

Table II shows the number and relative percentage of the urine samples that were above the 'safety limits' for the most important urinary factors in the evaluation of the lithogenic risk.

Discussion

As we expected this study confirms that the excretion of many urinary substances is lower in the fasting urine sample than in that of the 24-hour urine sample. Calcium, oxalic acid and uric acid, the most important stone promoters, were lower in fasting urine, with percentages respectively equal to 18.6, 19.4 and 14.7%, confirming the results of other literature [4, 5].

The analysis of the standard deviation reveals that on a free diet and in normal conditions of activity the daily excretion of stone promoters is very wide and that the variability is not lower in the fasting urine sample.

Moreover, this demonstrates that the differences in the daily excretion of urinary constituents are not only linked to dietary factors, but they are also connected to more complicated metabolic factors: intestinal absorption, resting, exercise, hormones, stress, perspiration. The constituents with a greater variability were Mg, uric acid, NH_4, PO_4, volume, while Cl, Ca, oxalic acid, osmolarity, K, TA did not have a variability statistically different from that of the creatinine.

Our study demonstrates that even a normal subject may produce a so-called 'stone risk urine' quite frequently. In fact in the 6 subjects who were studied for 30 consecutive days the 'risk' levels for the urinary volume, osmolarity, Ca, Mg, uric acid, oxalic acid and pH were exceeded in 105 out of 1,440 determinations with a percentage equal to 7.3%. If we only examine the data regarding urinary calcium, oxalic acid and uric acid, which are considered to be the most important stone promoters, we note that the percentage of the data above the 'safety limits' is 11.8%. This demonstrates that to classify a subject as normal on a free diet it is incorrect to analyse only one 24-hour urine sample because one runs a high risk of classifying a subject who usually excretes normal urine as hypercalciuric, hyperoxaluric, or hyperuricuric.

In our study the 'risk' data follow on absolutely casual pattern but the averages calculated in 3 consecutive days always resulted within the normal range.

References

1. Robertson, W. G.; Hodgkinson, A.; Marshall, D. H.: Seasonal variation in the composition of urine from normal subjects: a longitudinal study. Clinica chim. Acta *80:* 347–353 (1977).
2. Borghi, L.; Elia, G. F.; Trapassi, M. R.; Barbarese, F.; Manfredi, G.; Montanari, A.; Novarini, A.: Hypocalciuric effect of an antihypertensive drug: indapamide. Min. Met. Res. Italy *5:* 55–57 (1984).
3. Gaetani, E.; Laureri, F.; Vitto, M.; Borghi, L.; Elia, G. F.; Novarini, A.: Determination of oxalate in urine by flow injection analysis. Clinica chim. Acta *156:* 71–76 (1976).
4. Zarembski, P. M.; Hodgkinson, A.: Some factors influencing the urinary excretion of oxalic acid in man. Clinica chim. Acta *25:* 1–10 (1969).
5. Heaton, F. W.; Hodgkinson, A.: External factors affecting diurnal variation in electrolyte excretion with particular reference to calcium and magnesium. Clinica chim. Acta *8:* 246–254 (1963).

L. Borghi, MD, Istituto di Semeiotica Medica, Università degli Studi di Parma,
via Gramsci 14, I–43100 Parma (Italy)

Contr. Nephrol., vol. 58, pp. 25–29 (Karger, Basel 1987)

Drug-Induced Renal Stones: Incidence, Clinical Expression and Stone Analysis

A. Rapado, M. L. Traba, C. Caycho, L. Cifuentes-Delatte

Urolithiasis Laboratory, Department of Medicine and Metabolic Unit, Fundación Jimenez Diaz and Universidad Autónoma, Madrid, Spain

In the last years attention has been focused on the incidence of renal calculi composed totally or partially by drugs. These renal stones present an interesting conceptual and diagnostic challenge [1, 2]. The origin of the pharmacological calculi could be due to: (a) drugs which induce renal stones as alkalis and acetazolamide (calcium phosphates); methoxifluorane, vitamin C and vitamin D (calcium oxalate); uricosuric and antimetabolite drugs (uric acid) and allopurinol (xanthine); (b) drugs which are partial or total components of renal calculi: nitrofurantoin; phenazopyridine; N-acetylsulfadiazine; N-acetylsulfamethoxazole; oxytetracycline; diatrizoate and other urographic contrasts; flumaquine; glifanine; oxypurinol; triamterene or silica [3–5].

This work presents our experience with comments on the incidence, clinical and biochemical expression and stone analysis.

Material and Methods

The last 1,500 urinary stones analyzed in our laboratory from 1981 to 1985 have been reviewed. The protocol carried out to study the patients includes a clinical history; plain abdominal X-ray film; intravenous pyelogram and a metabolic study in blood and 24-hour urine (creatinine clearance, uric acid, phosphorus, calcium, magnesium, oxalate, cystine and acid/base status). Urinary culture with appropriate antibiogram was performed in selected patients.

The renal stone analysis includes: general view on stereoscopic microscope; infrared spectroscopy; polarized light microscopy on thin sections; scanning electron microscopy, energy-dispersive X-ray analysis (EDAX) and element mapping [1].

The following methods were used in triamterene calculi: search of spherules resembling a Maltese cross under polarized light microscopy with crossed nicoles on calculous material suspension; these spherules were also recognized in fresh samples of urine; triamterene characteristic fluorescence under ultraviolet light at 360 nm in urine, serum and stone material suspended in 10% lactic acid; thin-layer chromatography for triamterene metabolite identification [6].

Porphyrins were identified and quantified by thin-layer chromatography after sterification with methanol/sulfuric acid (9/1, v/v) and extraction with chloroform [7, 8].

Results

Twelve (0.8%) of 1,500 analyzed stones were composed of drugs. Three contained silica, 2 sulfamethoxazole and 7 of them triamterene. Three silica stones (obtained by surgery) corresponded to patients with gastroduodenal ulcers and a high intake of magnesium trisilicate antacids for a long time. No abnormalities in the metabolic study were detected.

The analysis of these stones by infrared spectroscopy showed absorbance bands of amorphous silica ($SiO_2\,[H_2O]_n$) at 3,420, 1,625, 1,100, 950, 790 and 470 cm^{-1}. The presence of silica was assessed by EDAX at the central part of the stones while whewellite was prominent in the external layers [4, 9].

Two patients with previous history of recidivant urinary infections and mild renal insufficiency treated for several years with sulfamethoxazole showed calculi composed by N-acetylsulfamethoxazole chlorhydrate. These stones showed absorbance bands at 1,600, 1,310, 1,150 and 660 cm^{-1} by infrared spectroscopy. One of the stones also contained calcium phosphate detected by a wide absorbance band between 1,000 and 1,200 cm^{-1} [10].

Seven calculi composed by triamterene were obtained from 3 patients treated for about 2 years with this diuretic. The clinical history and pathological findings showed an active chronic hepatitis in 2 cases and macronodular hepatic cirrhosis in the third patient. A positive familial history of renal lithiasis was present in 2 patients. In the metabolic study they showed an urinary pH between 6.2 and 6.5. No other abnormalities were detected.

All stones were radiotranslucent on X-ray films except one which presented as a mixed stone composed by whewellite and triamterene. The stones exhibited a dark color suggesting the presence of 'organic' material.

Infrared spectra showed absorbance bands of triamterene at 1,420, 1,330, 820 and 730 cm^{-1} as well as its sulfate ester (1,200 cm^{-1}). The mixed

Table I. Triamterene stones: special stone analysis

	Case 1				Case 2	Case 3	
Stone no.:	4,506	5,149	5,158	5,176	5,685	5,755	5,790
Weight, mg	8	20	12	8	70	–	65
Measure, cm	2 × 1.5	3.5 × 3.0	3.5 × 2.5	2.5 × 1.5	–	3 × 2	11 × 10
Other components	–	–	–	–	–	–	monohydrate oxalate
Porphyrin content, ng/mg							
Coproporphyrin	18.1	6.9	0.7	traces	1.7	16.2	6.0
Uroporphyrin	–	traces	–	–	–	3.8	2.5
Heptacarboxyl-porphyrin	–	–	–	–	–	–	5.6
Hexacarboxyl-porphyrin	–	–	–	–	–	–	traces
Protoporphyrin IX	–	–	–	–	–	–	–

calculus contained in its outer layers triamterene and monohydrate calcium oxalate and it showed an additional band at 1,300 und 770 cm^{-1}. Whewellite was located in the center of the stone [5, 11].

Urine, serum and stone material suspended in 10% lactic acid showed fluorescence under ultraviolet light at 360 nm. Thin-layer chromatography of calculi extracts coeluted with pure triamterene (Rf 6.65). Two small spots at Rf 0.47 and 0.35 correspond to triamterene metabolites (*p*-hydroxitriamterene and triamterene sulfate) [12].

Calculi suspension and fresh urine sediments showed spherules of triamterene under polarized light microscopy and a Maltese cross was observed with crossed nicoles. The calculi demonstrated a spherulitic structure by scanning electronmicroscopy. Porphyrins were assessed in all triamterene stones. Coproporphyrin was predominant (from 0.7 to 16.2 ng/mg of powered calculi) while only two calculi showed the presence of uroporphyrin (octocarboxyl-porphyrin) and heptacarboxyl-porphyrin. Protophyrin IX was not detected in any renal stones (table I).

Discussion

In our experience the incidence of renal calculi composed by drugs is similar (1.0–2.5%) to those described in other series [1, 2]. We stress the importance of an etiological inquiry on drug intake in patients with recidivant renal lithiasis.

Different *individual risk factors* are involved in the development of these stones. Chronic renal failure, liver disease (as in our triamterene patients) or gastrointestinal diseases (in silica stone formers) have been described. A positive familial history of renal lithiasis must not be overlooked [3].

Local risk factors, such as a high excretion of the drug or its metabolites, low drug solubility, changes in urinary volume or pH as well as a long-during treatment with high doses of drugs could play a role either in an increase of saturation or a decrease in inhibitory factors of urinary crystallization [12].

Under scanning electron microscopy silica calculi show organic fibers; some of them were mineralized with silica embedded on its surface as observed by EDAX. These organic fibers are similar to those seen in calcium phosphate stones. It should suggest a similar mineralization mechanism [4].

Beside those aforementioned risk factors several conditions have been described in patients with triamterene stones [13, 14]: different rates of drug intestinal absorption, decreased urinary pH, spontaneous precipitation or active participation of triamterene in the heterogenous nucleation or epitaxial growth in mixed stones.

Although these calculi have been described in patients on high blood pressure treatment and/or prophylactic treatment of renal stones, the presence of hepatic disfunction in our patients as well as a positive familial history of renal lithiasis is relevant.

In the literature [12, 13] a golden tone sometimes colored with several shades of brown has been described in triamterene calculi. This last color was thought to be composed of urinary pigments [12]. In previous work [15, 16] we found several porphyrins as a component of a group of small and 'black' stones.

We have confirmed the presence of porphyrins in all the triamterene stones. The high content of coproporphyrin could be explained due to the high excretion of these porphyrin metabolites in patients with hepatic diseases. These porphyrins could act as a cofactor in the crystalline precipitation of some drugs such as triamterene [16]. There must be different metabolic and local factors which explain the promotion of drug-induced stone formation because in spite of the high drug administration there is a low incidence of stone presentation [2, 17].

References

1 Cifuentes Delatte, L.: Composición y estructura de los càlculos renales, pp. 125–129 (Salvat, Barcelona 1984).

2 Daudon, M.; Reveillaud, R. J.: Drug nephrolithiasis: an unrecognized and underestimated pathology; in Schwille, Smith, Robertson, Vahlensiek, Urolithiasis and related clinical research, pp. 371–378 (Plenum Press, New York 1985).

3 Daudon, M.; Protaly, M. F.; Reveillaud, R. J.: Dépistage et diagnostic des lithiases médicamenteuses. Annls. Biol. clin. *41:* 239–249 (1983).

4 Medina, J. A.; Rodriguez, J.; Santos, M.; Cifuentes, L.: Calculo renal de sílice en un hombre (undécima observación mundial). Rev. clin. esp. *151:* 411–414 (1978).

5 Traba, M. L.; Rapado, A.; Bonet, F.; Cifuentes, L.: Nefrolitiasis por triamterene. Rev. clin. esp. *174:* 127–130 (1984).

6 Sorgel, F.; Hinger, B. E.; Benet, L. Z.: The true composition of kidney stones passed during triamterene therapy. J. Urol. *134:* 871–873 (1985).

7 Enriquez de Salamanca, R.; Peña, M. L.; Chinarro, S.; Olmos, A.; Mingo, D.; Molina, C.; Muñoz, J. J.: Quantitative and qualitative porphyrin excretion in normal subjects. J. Biochem. *14:* 251–253 (1982).

8 Day, R. S.; De Salamanca, R. E.; Eales, L.: Quantification of red cell porphyrins by fluorescence scanning after thin layer chromatography. Clinica chim. Acta *89:* 25–28 (1978).

9 Berg, W.; Bothor, C.; Erler, J.; Lange, P.: Sind Silikate nur Kieselsteine? Z. Urol. Nephrol. *76:* 319–322 (1983).

10 Siegel, W. H.: Unusual complication of therapy with sulfamethoxazole-trimethoprim. J. Urol. *117:* 397–399 (1977).

11 Ettinger, B.; Weil, E.; Mandel, N. S.; Darling, S.: Triamterene-induced nephrolithiasis. Ann. intern. Med. *91:* 745–746 (1979).

12 White, D. J.; Nancollas, G. H.: Triamterene and renal stone formation. J. Urol. *127:* 593–597 (1982).

13 Ettinger, B.; Oldroyd, N. A.; Sorgel, F.: Triamterene nephrolithiasis. J. Am. med. Ass. *244:* 2443–2445 (1980).

14 Dayton, P. G.; Aurley, J.; Pruityt, A. W.: Impairment of *p*-hydroxylation of triamterene in patients with cirrhosis. Pharmacologist *18:* 153–156 (1976).

15 Traba, M. L.; Rapado, A.: Componentes de la sangre en calculos renales de materia orgànica. Arch. esp. Urol. *38:*73–75 (1985).

16 Traba, M. L.; Perpiña, J.; Enriquez de Salamanca, R.: Identificación y cuantificación de diversas porfirinas como componentes en un tipo peculiar de calculo renal. Arch. esp. Urol. *38:* 601–604 (1985).

17 Jick, H.; Dinan, B. J.; Huntor, J. R.: Triamterene and renal stones. J. Urol. *127:* 224–225 (1982).

Aurelio Rapado, MD, Unidad Metabólica/Fundación Jimenez Diaz,
Avenida Reyes Católicos 2, E–28040 Madrid (Spain)

Contr. Nephrol., vol. 58, pp. 30–33 (Karger, Basel 1987)

Recurrence and Family History of Renal Stone Disease

A. Trinchieri, A. Mandressi, P. Luongo, L. Mazza, C. Zaatar, E. Pisani

Istituto di Urologia, Università di Milano, Milano, Italia

Familial patterns have been described in several studies of nephrolithiasis [1–5]. Cystinuria is transmitted as an autosomal recessive trait and isolated hypouricaemia associated with uric acid lithiasis appears to be inherited in an autosomal recessive pattern too. Other hereditary conditions are related to renal stone formation: distal renal tubular acidosis, primary hyperoxaluria, gout, Lesch-Nyhan syndrome, etc. However, the question of a genetic predisposition towards stone formation in primary nephrolithiasis has not been completely explored.

Materials and Methods

We studied 1,039 (569 M, 470 F) patients with renal stone disease (excluding hyperparathyroidism, complete renal tubular acidosis, primary hyperoxaluria, gout, cystinuria and other definite diseases). Out of these 557 had at least 5 years of follow-up from the first occurrence of renal stones.

For all the patients we obtained from our records the family history of stones, the data of the first and of subsequent stones and the composition of stones.

All the patients had a complete metabolic check on a free diet. A 24-hour urine sample and a fasting venous blood sample were analysed by routine methods for calcium, phosphate, sodium, potassium, uric acid, creatinine and oxalate (on urine only). Urinary pH was determined on 2-hour fasting specimens.

A control group of 1,525 subjects (810 M, 715 F) was considered. The controls had no history of renal stones. Data on the occurrence of renal stones in parents, brothers, sisters and offspring were obtained for each subject. It was decided to consider a family history as positive if at least one first-degree relative had suffered from renal stones; more distant relatives were excluded. Statistical evaluation was performed by Student's t-test and by the χ^2-test for frequency analysis.

Table I. Frequencies of renal stones among the relatives of 1,039 stone patients and 1,525 controls

Calcium	48/312	M	(15%)*			
	63/254	F	(25%)***			
	111/566	T	(20%)***			
Infection	17/165	M	(10%)			
	35/179	F	(19%)**			
	52/344	T	(15%)*			
Uric acid	17/65	M	(26%)***	control	86/810	M (11%)
	9/25	F	(36%)***	group	79/715	F (11%)
	26/90	T	(29%)***		165/1,525	T (11%)
UA/CAOX	12/27	M	(44%)***			
	5/12	F	(42%)***			
	17/39	T	(43%)***			
All stones	94/569	M	(16%)**			
	112/470	F	(24%)***			
	206/1,039	T	(20%)***			

M = Males; F = females; T = total.
Significance of differences (χ^2-test) between stone patients and controls: * $p < 0.05$; ** $p < 0.01$; *** $p < 0.001$.

Results

Stone disease is more frequent among relatives of renal stone formers than among control relatives (table I). Clinical records and laboratory findings are shown in table II.

Discussion

The formation of stones depends on many factors, such as urine volume, overexcretion of various urinary substances, presence of inhibitors. So stone disease may be conditioned by various familial factors, which can influence different pathogenetic mechanisms. Moreover, as a fundamental epidemiologic observation, it is well known that stone formers generally begin to form stones after the second decade of life. This suggests the possibility of delayed genetic expression or the accumulation of adverse environmental factors over the childhood years.

Table II. Clinical records and laboratory findings separated with regard to family history and type of stones

		Calcium		Uric acid	UA/CAOX	Infection
		males	females			
CaU, mg/day	+	287 ± 130	200 ± 99	–	309 ± 111	196 ± 130
	–	252 ± 130	221 ± 113	–	247 ± 161	188 ± 110
UaP, mg/dl	+	–	–	5.7 ± 1.5	4.9 ± 1.3	–
	–	–	–	5.4 ± 1.8	5.4 ± 1.7	–
UaU, mg/day	+	641 ± 317	490 ± 165	641 ± 329	753 ± 363	580 ± 363
	–	612 ± 303	551 ± 227*	656 ± 407	706 ± 337	556 ± 296
OxU, mg/day	+	56 ± 19	45 ± 19	–	–	53 ± 27
	–	50 ± 29	46 ± 21	–	–	55 ± 30
Urinary pH	+	5.7 ± 0.6	5.9 ± 0.7	6.0 ± 0.7	5.8 ± 0.7	5.8 ± 0.6
	–	5.6 ± 0.6	5.6 ± 0.6*	5.4 ± 0.6**	5.5 ± 0.5	5.9 ± 0.7
Age onset, years	+	32 ± 13	32 ± 13	39 ± 14	33 ± 43	38 ± 19
	–	36 ± 13	38 ± 14**	47 ± 12*	43 ± 11*	38 ± 14
Recurrence at 5 years, %	+	54		66	50	54
	–	45		73	66	46

Significance of differences between patients with (+) and without (–) family history: * $p < 0.05$; ** $p < 0.01$.

Genetic and environmental factors must operate for some time before they can precipitate stone formation. In this study we were not able to separate the effects of environmental from those of genetic factors; however, our findings support the suggestion that genetic factors play a role in producing the diathesis.

The observed frequency of renal stones among the parents and siblings of renal stone formers exceeded the estimates based on the incidence in control relatives. Particularly among the female stone formers a positive family history was reported by 24% of the patients. Moreover, in the group of female calcium stone formers there appeared a significant association between a family history of stone disease and a high value of urinary pH. Incomplete defects in urinary acidification can be inherited and are common among calcium stone formers (in males and in a still greater proportion in females). A genetic defect in urinary acidification with variable expressivity might be associated with a high frequency of family history of stone formation among female calcium stone formers.

However, among idiopathic calcium stone formers there are no relationships between family history of renal stones and abnormalities of calcium, uric acid and oxalate excretion rates. Uric acid or mixed uric acid/calcium oxalate stone formers seem to have a greater familial predisposition towards stone formation; however, we did not find any association between family history of renal stones and uric acid disorders. Moreover, the patients without a family history of stone disease were older and had lower urinary pH values than the patients with a family history of stone disease. In the large group of patients with a family history studied here, there appears to be no disposition to develop early and frequent recurrences; nevertheless, Ljunghall et al. [5] found that the tendency for familial history of stone formation is associated with higher stone recurrence rates. Indeed the patients with a family history often have an early onset of stone disease.

References

1 McGeown, M.: Heredity in renal stone disease. Clin. Sci. *19:* 465–471 (1960).

2 Resnick, M.; Pridgen, D. B.; Goodman, H. O.: Genetic predisposition to formation of calcium oxalate renal calculi. New Engl. J. Med. *278:* 1313–1318 (1968).

3 Säfwenberg, J.; Backman, U.; Danielson, B. G.; Johansson, G.; Ljunghall, S.: HLA and kidney stone disease. Scand. J. Urol. Nephrol. *12:* 151–154 (1978).

4 Ljunghall, S.: Family history of renal stones in a population study of stone-formers and healthy subjects. Br. J. Urol. *51:* 249–252 (1979).

5 Ljunghall, S.; Danielson, B. G.; Fellström, B.; Holmgren, K.; Johansson, G.; Wikström, B.: Family history of renal stones in recurrent stone patients. Br. J. Urol. *57:* 370–374 (1985).

Alberto Trinchieri, MD, Istituto di Urologia, via Commenda 15, I–20100 Milano (Italy)

Contr. Nephrol., vol. 58, pp. 34–38 (Karger, Basel 1987)

Patterns of Citrate Excretion in Healthy Subjects and Patients with Idiopathic Stone Disease

M. Marangella[a], *O. Bianco*[a], *M. L. Grande*[a], *M. Petrarulo*[a], *D. Valente*[b], *C. Vitale*[a], *F. Linari*[a]

[a]Laboratorio Calcolosi Renale and [b]Servizio di Fisica Sanitaria, Ospedale Mauriziano Umberto I, Torino, Italia

Sound biochemical and physicochemical evidences suggest that urine citrate (uCit) plays an important role as a preventing factor against stone formation in the urinary tract [1–5]. Many authors have searched for derangements of uCit and Cit metabolism in patients with stone disease. Hypocitraturia has been described as a constant feature in case of renal tubular acidosis [6], renal insufficiency [7], infection-induced renal stones [8], and chronic diarrheal syndromes [9]. Some authors have also reported hypocitraturia to frequently occur in patients with idiopathic calcium (ICaSD) or uric acid stone disease (IUASD), but the results so far achieved are not always in agreement [3, 7, 10–13]. Many reasons are invoked to explain the reported differences, including variations of uCit with sex [7, 13], age [14], renal function [7], dietary influences [15], acid-base balance-related factors [16]. In this paper we report data of citraturia from our laboratory concerning a wide series of healthy subjects and patients with ICaSD and IUASD. Patterns of uCit have also been studied in relation to some clinical and biochemical parameters.

Methods and Material

603 subjects have been considered on the whole, none having significant decrease in renal function or urinary tract infection at the time of the study. Three groups have been identified: group A, 66 healthy persons with no history of stone disease; group B, 435 idiopathic calcium stone formers (ICaSF); group C, 92 idiopathic uric acid stone formers (IUASF). All the subjects were investigated while on their usual life-style and dietary habits.

Table I. Citrate excretion in whole series and in each group according to sex

	All	Males	Females
Whole	2.87 ± 1.49 (603)	2.85 ± 1.55 (379)	2.83 ± 1.31 (215)
Group A	3.05 ± 1.13 (66)	2.95 ± 1.29 (33)	3.14 ± 1.22 (33)
Group B	2.81 ± 1.53 (435)	2.81 ± 1.64 (272)	2.81 ± 1.32 (163)
Group C	2.83 ± 1.27 (102)	2.94 ± 1.30 (74)	0.44 ± 1.14* (19)

* $p < 0.05$ vs normal females.

Citrate was determined by an enzymatic method using citrate lyase, according to previous methods [17]. Oxalate, sulfate and phosphate were determined by ion chromatography, using a Dionex-QIC apparatus as described elsewhere [18]. Routine methods were used for the other serum and urine determinations. Results are expressed as mean ± SD. Significance of differences are assessed by the Student's t-test. Linear regression analysis is used for correlations between parameters.

Results

Table I lists the results of uCit in the whole series and in each group. Data have been further subdivided as to sex. Based on the lower values of uCit found in our controls, we have defined as having hypocitraturia (HCit) those patients with uCit less than 1.4 mmol/24 h. Table II shows the prevalence of HCit in the patients when metabolic presentation is taken into account.

uCit is significantly related to both body weight and creatinine clearance ($p < 0.001$). Highly significant correlations have been found also with the main urine cations (K, Na, Ca, Mg in the order) and with some anions such as sulfate and uric acid ($p < 0.001$). No correlations emerge with urine volume, pH and oxalate. uCit is weakly related to age ($p < 0.025$) when the whole series is considered. This relation disappears when males and females are considered separately.

Table II. Prevalence of hypocitraturia in idiopathic stone formers in relation to metabolic presentation

	Total	Hypocitraturia	%	p[1]
Group B				
No metabolic disorder	191	50	26.2	
Hypercalciuria[2]	111	9	8.1	< 0.001
Hyperuricosuria[3]	63	7	11.1	< 0.025
Hyperoxaluria[4]	128	21	16.5	< 0.05
Group C				
No metabolic disorder	31	4	12.9	
Hyperuricosuria	32	3	9.4	n.s.
Low urine pH[5]	41	2	4.9	n.s.

1 Significance of the differences in prevalence of hypocitraturia versus no metabolic disorder patients in each group assessed by the χ^2-test.

2 Urine calcium higher than 0.1 mmol/kg body weight/24 h.

3 Urine uric acid more than 4.5 and 4.0 mmol/24 h in males and females, respectively.

4 Urine oxalate more than 0.5 mmol/24 h.

5 Urine pH less than 5.5.

Discussion

Citrate excretion in man is determined by at least three separate mechanisms which work at various renal sites. In the glomerulus plasma citrate is almost completely and freely filtered; in the proximal tubule the bulk reabsorption of the filtered load occurs; finally citrate is actively taken up by the tubular cells, where it can be metabolized in the mitochondria [16, 19, 20]. The numerous factors which influence uCit can act at several levels, so that the complexity of renal handling, on the one hand, and the multiplicity of influences on diverse renal sites, on the other hand, account for the width of the range of uCit also in normals. Indeed in our controls uCit had means comparable to what so far reported and varied by a factor of 7.5, which is higher than the values of 3.9 and 6.5 found by some authors [14, 21] and lower than the values of 50 found by others [13]. This variability also in healthy persons partly explains the disagreement of the results when uCit of ISF is compared with normals [10–13, 21].

In a preliminary analysis of the raw data as shown in table I, differences in uCit among the three groups seem mild as only female IUASF show lower values than females from group A and B. However, if corrected

Table III. Urine citrate, expressed as mmol/100 ml GFR in whole subjects and in each group subdivided as to sex. ** $p < 0.025$ vs males of the same group

	Males	Females
Whole	2.79 ± 1.57	3.10 ± 1.44**
Group A	2.71 ± 1.19	3.17 ± 1.53
Group B	2.75 ± 1.67	3.13 ± 1.48**
Group C	2.99 ± 1.32	2.78 ± 0.89

for creatinine clearance as shown in table III, uCit is significantly lower in males, namely in ICaSF, and the differences of females from group C disappear. This means that no difference at all can be found when patients and controls are matched as to sex, age and degree of renal function. However, HCit is a rather frequent feature also in our experience, as it occurs in up to 18% of the whole stone patients. Moreover, it seems to have higher incidence in course of ICaSD in those patients who present without metabolic disorders. This suggests that low uCit could represent a causative factor of stone formation in those instances.

Our findings of good correlations of uCit with the most important urine cations are in agreement with previous reports [21], and are generally explained with the reduction of citrate reabsorption caused by complexation. Also the correlations with other parameters (see the section above) have been investigated by other authors [7, 13, 21], but data from the literature about these topics are not always in agreement, and the explanations for the presumed interactions are far from convincing. Thus, based on our current understanding on metabolism and renal handling of citrate, we have no thorough interpretation of the mechanisms which could play an actual role in the physiological regulation of citrate excretion and believe that further studies have to be devoted to these topics.

References

1 Robertson, W.G.: Measurement of ionized calcium in biological fluids. Clinica chim. Acta *24:* 149–157 (1969).

2 Daniele, P.G.; Marangella, M.: Ionic equilibria in urine: a computer model system improved by accurate stability constant values. Annls Chim. *72:* 25–38 (1982).

3 Marangella, M.; Daniele, P.G.; Ronzani, M.; Sonego, S.; Linari, F.: Urine saturation with calcium salts in normal subjects and idiopathic calcium stone formers estimated by an improved computer model system. Urol. Res. *13:* 189–193 (1985).

4 Wagner, M.; Finlayson, B.: The characteristics of absorption of pyrophosphate and citrate onto whewellite. Investve Urol. *15:* 456–458 (1978).
5 Hallson, P. C.; Rose, G. A.; Sulaiman, S.: Raising urinary citrate lowers calcium oxalate and calcium phosphate crystal formation in whole urine. Urol. int. *38:* 179–181 (1983).
6 Norman, M. E.; Feldman, N. I.; Cohn, R. M.; Roth, K. S.; McCurdy, D. K.: Urinary citrate excretion in the diagnosis of distal renal tubular acidosis. J. Pediat. *92:* 394–400 (1978).
7 Hodgkinson, A.: Citric acid excretion in normal adults and patients with renal calculus. Clin. Sci. *23:* 203–212 (1962).
8 Conway, N. S.; Maitland, A. I. L.; Rennie, J. B.: The urinary citrate excretion in patients with renal calculi. Br. J. Urol. *21:* 30–38 (1949).
9 Rudman, D.; Dedonis, J. L.; Fountain, M. T.; Chandler, J. B.; Gerron, G. G.; Fleming, G. A.; Kutner, M. H.: Hypocitraturia in patients with gastrointestinal malabsorption. New Engl. J. Med. *303:* 657–661 (1980).
10 Elliot, J. S.; Ribeiro, M. E.: The urinary excretion of citrate, hippurate and lactic acid in normal adults and in patients with calcium oxalate urinary calculus disease. Investve Urol. *10:* 102–106 (1972).
11 Welshman, S. G.; McGeown, M. G.: Urinary citrate excretion in stone formers and controls. Br. J. Urol. *48:* 7–11 (1976).
12 Tiselius, H. G.: Urinary excretion of citrate in normal subjects and patients with urolithiasis; in Smith, Robertson, Finlayson, Urolithiasis, clinical and basic research, pp. 39–44 (Plenum Press, New York 1981).
13 Schwille, P. O.; Scholz, D.; Schwille, K.; Leutschaft, R.; Goldberg, I.; Sigel, A.: Citrate in urine and serum and associated variables in subgroups of urolithiasis. Results from an outpatient stone clinic. Nephron *31:* 194–202 (1982).
14 Hosking, D. H.; Wilson, J. W. L.; Liedtke, R. R.; Smith, L. H.; Wilson, D. M.: Urinary citrate excretion in normal persons and patients with idiopathic calcium urolithiasis. J. Lab. clin. Med. *106:* 682–689 (1985).
15 Rudman, D.; Kutner, M. H.; Red, S. C.; Waters, W. C.; Gerron, G. G.; Bleier, J.: Hypocitraturia in calcium nephrolithiasis. J. clin. Endocr. Metab. *55:* 1052–1057 (1982).
16 Simpson, D. P.: Citrate excretion: a window on renal metabolism. Am. J. Physiol. *244:* F223–F234 (1983).
17 Welshman, S. G.; McCambridge, H.: The estimation of citrate in serum and urine using a citrate lyase technique. Clinica chim. Acta *46:* 243–246 (1973).
18 Petrarulo, M.; Bianco, O.; Martini, C.; Marangella, M.; Linari, F.: Dosaggio degli ioni solfato e fosfato urinari mediante cromatografia ionica. G. ital. Chim. clin. *10:* 275–279 (1985).
19 Canary, J. J.; Meloni, C. R.; Clive, D.; Grossman, E.: The renal clearance of citrate in man. Metabolism *13:* 21–30 (1964).
20 Nieth, H.; Schollmeyer, P.: Citratstoffwechsel der menschlichen Niere. Verh. dt. Ges. inn. Med. *71:* 693–696 (1965).
21 Nicar, M. J.; Skurla, C.; Sakhaee, K.; Pak, C. Y. C.: Low urinary citrate excretion in nephrolithiasis. Urology *21:* 8–14 (1983).

Martino Marangella, MD, Laboratorio Calcolosi Renale, Largo Turati 62,
I–10128 Torino (Italy)

Contr. Nephrol., vol. 58, pp. 39–40 (Karger, Basel 1987)

Urinary Citrate in Recurrent Stone-Forming Patients

A. Aroldi, N. Soriani, R. Zubani, C. Castelnovo, G. Graziani

Divisione Nefrologia e Dialisi, Ospedale Maggiore, Milano, Italia

Urinary citrate reduces urinary saturation of calcium oxalate and calcium phosphate salts by forming complexes with calcium and retards the nucleation and the growth of calcium salts. Indeed, hypocitraturia seems to represent an important factor in enhancing calcium oxalate stone formation.

In 49 recurrent stone-forming (RSF) patients, 15 of them hypercalciuric, 24-hour urinary citric acid (CA, mg/dl; UV method, Boehringer Mannheim), calcium (Ca, mg/dl), creatinine (Cr, mg/dl), sodium (Na, mEq/l) were determined as previously described [1].

Results are reported in table I.

Positive correlation was found between 24-hour CA and Ca ($p < 0.01$) and Cr ($p < 0.05$) concentration, whereas there was no correlation between CA and Na concentration or urine volume. The 24-hour CA/Cr ratio was positively correlated with the Ca/Cr ratio ($p < 0.001$) ($y = 1.1x + 0.15$).

Table I. 24-hour urinary calcium (UCa), citric acid (UCA) excretion, calcium/creatinine (Ca/Cr) and citric acid/creatinine (CA/Cr) ratios in 49 RSF patients

Patient no.	UCa, mg/24 h	UCA, mg/24 h	Ca/Cr	CA/Cr
49	250 ± 121	445 ± 237	0.17 ± 0.09	0.34 ± 0.20
15	386 ± 69	545 ± 197	0.27 ± 0.08	0.39 ± 0.18
34	175 ± 67	391 ± 243	0.12 ± 0.05	0.32 ± 0.22

In conclusion, we found lower urinary citric acid levels in 34 normocalciuric patients, traditionally considered 'without metabolic disorders', compared to the 15 hypercalciuric patients. Hypocitraturia may represent a disturbance of pathogenetic relevance in patients with normal Ca excretion; furthermore, a low-normal Ca excretion may represent an additional risk factor in enhancing calcium stone formation in hypercalciuric patients.

Reference

1 Aroldi, A.; Graziani, G.; Passerini, P.; Castelnovo, C.; Mandressi, A.; Trinchieri, A.; Colussi, G.; Ponticelli, C.: High fluid intake or pharmacological therapy in recurrent stone former patients?; in Davison, Guillon, Proc. EDTA-ERA, No. 21, pp. 743–746 (Pitman, London 1985).

A. Aroldi, MD, Divisione Nefrologia e Dialisi, Ospedale Maggiore, Policlinico, via della Commenda 15, I–20122 Milano (Italy)

Contr. Nephrol., vol. 58, pp. 41–43 (Karger, Basel 1987)

Calcium Nephrolithiasis and Renal Tubular Hypouricemia

M. E. De Ferrari[a], *G. Colussi*[a], *E. Benazzi*[a], *G. Rombolà*[a], *M. Surian*[c], *F. Malberti*[c], *S. Brenna*[b], *L. Minetti*[a]

[a]Renal Unit and [b] Biochemistry Department, Ospedale Niguarda-Ca'Granda, Milano; [c]Renal Unit, Ospedale Maggiore, Lodi, Italy

Hypouricemia (HU), conventionally defined as serum urate levels of 2 mg/dl or less, is a very rare condition, with an estimated prevalence from 0.72 to 0.98% [1–3]. Primary isolated renal HU (RHU) appears to be an extremely rare condition; assuming that all reported patients without any apparent cause of HU had RHU (which is very unlikely), the prevalence of this disorder can be estimated to be 0.35% [3].

In our series of 1,049 patients with nephrolithiasis we found 7 patients with persistent HU, who eventually were shown to have RHU. We report clinical and laboratory data of these patients in order to clarify the relationship, if any, between this tubular defect and the attendant nephrolithiasis.

Cases and Biochemical Data

The 7 patients were all women, aged 25–61 years; they had formed a total of 15 calculi (1 stone: 1 patient; 2 stones: 5 patients; 4 stones: 1 patient): all but one (which was X-ray-lucent), were calcium stones (CaOx; CaP) or X-ray-opaque. They represent 1.55% of our stone former female population; assuming that the prevalence of RHU in the general female population is 0.35% [3], as previously discussed, the observed prevalence in our series is statistically higher than that expected by chance ($\chi^2 = 10.5$, $p < 0.05$).

Biochemical parameters are shown in table I. HU was persistent throughout a 3-month to 5-year follow-up; it was due to 'renal leak' as shown by elevated fractional excretion of uric acid; known causes of HU (drugs, pregnancy, malignancy, etc.) were all excluded. Uric acid production was normal as suggested by normal daily excretion in all the patients. Urine saturation for monosodium urate was in the lower metastable or undersaturated region for all

Table I. Main biochemical data

Case No.	P_{Ua} mg/dl	FE_{Ua} %	$U_{Ua}V$ mg/day	F_{Ua} spot	mg/l 24 h	RS_{UaNa}	$U_{Ca}V$ mg/kg/day	$U_{Ox}V$ mg/day	RS_{CaOx}	$U_{cit}V$ mg/day	UpH min–max
1	1.3	22	230	220	62	+ 0.03	3.2	25	+ 1.1	–	5.7–5.8
2	2.0	26	630	314	112	– 0.05	3.5	23	+ 0.68	900	5.0–5.5
3	1.4	24	650	349	16	+ 0.12	3.2	60	+ 0.6	–	5.2–6.0
4	1.6	15	629	140	295	+ 0.2	6.6	23	+ 0.92	1,300	5.0–5.8
5	1.8	69	475	90	80	+ 0.3	3.5	60	+ 1.15	520	4.9–6.0
6	1.6	17	525	200	90	– 0.1	6.1	35	+ 0.8	888	4.8–5.4
7	1.7	44	690	60	22	+ 0.3	3.8	57	+ 1.2	600	5.6–6.3
nv[a]	3.7 ± 0.8	7.9 ± 2	439 ± 144					22 ± 6		613 ± 310	

[a] Normal values in 50 healthy women, aged 20–60 years.
P_{Ua} = Lowest plasma urate level; FE_{Ua} = maximal fractional urate excretion; $U_{Ua}V$ = maximal urate excretion; F_{Ua} = maximal 'undissociated' uric acid urine concentration; RS_{UaNa} and RS_{CaOx} = relative supersaturation (Marshall nomograms) for Na urate and CaOx; $U_{Ca}V$ = Ca excretion on 1 g Ca^{++} diet; $U_{Ox}V$ = oxalate excretion; $U_{cit}V$ = citrate excretion.

the patients, while undissociated uric acid was above 300 mg/l (the physicochemical formation product for uric acid) in spot urines in 2 patients and above 160 mg/l (a value considered 'at risk' for crystallization in vivo) [4] in 24-hour urines in a third patient.

Two patients had idiopathic hypercalciuria (> 4 mg/kg body weight/24 h) and 3 patients had mild hyperoxaluria (> 40 mg/24 h); in one of the patients with normal calciuria and oxaluria low urinary daily output was responsible for CaOx supersaturation. Urine citrate excretion was normal in all the patients.

Discussion

The association of calcium nephrolithiasis and RHU has been previously described in one patient [5]; in 3 additional patients [6] stones were of uric acid in 2 and undefined in 1 patient. We report here 7 cases who formed mainly Ca stones. HU in our stone population was confined to female patients, as was observed in one of the published surveys [3]. Since RHU is known to occur also in males [5, 6], the meaning of this sex restriction is unclear. The nephrolithiasis in our patients had a low activity, in none there had been surgical or urological instrumentations: thus, it is unlikely that the nephrolithiasis could be responsible for the tubular defect. The physicochemical basis for stone formation in these patients appears to be heterogeneous: 2 patients had idiopathic hypercalciuria, an association already described [5, 6].

Three other patients had 'mild' hyperoxaluria; an additional case had a supersaturation for CaOx even without 'absolute' hypercalciuria and hyperoxaluria. Only in 3 patients abnormal urine saturation for uric acid might have contributed to CaOx stone formation, by means of heterogeneous nucleation [4]; in one patient this was the only physicochemical abnormality.

In conclusion, RHU prevalence in our stone formers appears to be higher than in the general population, suggesting that this abnormality might represent a risk factor for CaOx stone formation. The physicochemical basis for stone formation appears to be heterogeneous, and apparently unrelated to the uric acid transport defect, in most patients.

References

1 Mikkelsen, W. M.; Dodge, H. J.; Valkenburg, H.: The distribution of serum uric acid values in a population unselected as to gout or hyperuricemia. Am. J. Med. *39:* 242–251 (1965).

2 Ramsdell, C. M.; Kelly, W. N.: The significance of hypouricemia. Ann. intern. Med. *78:* 239–242 (1973).

3 Van Peenen, H. J.: Causes of hypouricemia. Ann. intern. Med. *78:* 977–978 (1973).

4 Millman, S.; Strauss, A. L.; Parks, J. M.; Coe, F. L.: Pathogenesis and clinical course of mixed calcium oxalate and uric acid nephrolithiasis. Kidney int. *22:* 366–370 (1982).

5 Greene, M. L.; Marcus, R.; Aurbach, G. D.; Kazam, E. S.; Seegmiller, J. E.: Hypouricemia due to isolated renal tubular defect. Dalmatian dog mutation in man. Am. J. Med. *53:* 361–367 (1972).

6 Sperling, O.: Urolithiasis in hereditary renal hypouricemia; in Schwille, Smith, Robertson, Vahlensieck, Urolithiasis and related clinical research, pp. 13–16 (Plenum Press, New York 1985).

M. E. De Ferrari, MD, Renal Unit, Ospedale Niguarda-Ca'Granda,
Piazza Ospedale Maggiore 3, I–20162 Milano (Italy)

Contr. Nephrol., vol. 58, pp. 44–48 (Karger, Basel 1987)

Renal Tubular Acidosis in Recurrent Calcium Nephrolithiasis

Maurizio Surian[a], *Fabio Malberti*[a], *Pablo Cosci*[a], *Bruno Corradi*[a], *Giacomo Colussi*[b], *M. Elisabetta De Ferrari*[b], *Maria Poggi*[a], *Aristide Luini*[a], *Luigi Minetti*[b]

Renal Units, [a]Ospedale Maggiore, Lodi; [b]Ospedale Niguarda-Ca'Granda, Milano, Italy

A frequency of renal tubular acidosis (RTA) ranging from 3.7 [1] to 19% [2] has been reported in unselected series of calcium stone formers (CSF). Moreover a very high incidence of RTA has been documented in medullary sponge kidney [3]; therefore, the discordant data on RTA prevalence in CSF may reflect different selections of patients as well as different diagnostic criteria. Recently, Tessitore et al. [4], documenting a very high incidence of proximal RTA (42%) in CSF with renal hypercalciuria without evidence of infection or obstruction of urinary tract, suggested that renal acidification defects might be an aspect of a more complex tubular impairment, involving sodium and phosphate handling, too.

The purpose of our study was to determine the frequency and type of renal acidification defects in our normocalciuric and hypercalciuric idiopathic CSF.

Materials and Methods

Fasting urinary pH (UpH) and blood gas analysis were evaluated in 94 consecutive ambulatory CSF with normal glomerular filtration rate (GFR), no infection or obstruction of urinary tract nor X-ray finding of renal damage. Patients with medullary sponge kidney, urinary tract malformation or nephrectomized were excluded. All patients had normal arterial pH; those with fasting UpH > 5.5 were submitted to acid loading test. Four out of 94 CSF (4.3%) failed to lower UpH (< 5.3), a finding consistent with an incomplete distal RTA.

The last 26 patients of our series were submitted to short NH_4Cl (0.1 g/kg body weight) loading test and to $NaHCO_3$ (3 mEq/min for 180 min) infusion. The ability to achieve a normal U-BpCO_2 gradient during bicarbonate load was taken as index of adequate renal acidification since in our study UpH was alkaline and urinary bicarbonate concentration ($UHCO_3$) was > 50 mEq/l [5]. The 26 CSF were divided into hypercalciuric (IH, n = 11, uCa > 320 mg/day in males or > 280 mg/day in females, on a 1-gram calcium diet) and normocalciuric (NC, n = 15). In 6 (patients 2, 3, 4, 6, 9 and 10) out of 11 IH, calciuria normalized on low (< 400 mg/day) calcium diet (diet-dependent IH).

Results and Comments

Table I summarizes the data of the patients studied; 4 patients (8-NC; 14-NC; 9-IH and 10-IH) had basal plasma bicarbonate levels ($PHCO_3$) reduced; however, blood pH was maintained in the normal range by respiratory compensation. All patients were able to lower their UpH below 5.3 *during acid load* except 2 patients (9-NC and 11-IH), a finding consistent with distal RTA. In every patient the urinary excretion of ammonia (NH_4E) and titratable acidity (TAE) was normal. *During bicarbonate load* 10 of 26 CSF (38.4%: 8, 9, 10 and 14 of NC group and 2, 3, 4, 9, 10 and 11 of IH group) did not achieve a normal U-BpCO_2 gradient: two (9-NC and 11-IH) were unable to lower UpH adequately, the remaining were considered to have distal RTA in spite of normal UpH during acid load, as proposed by Battle et al [6]. Four of 26 CSF (15.3%: 8-NC, 14-NC, 9-IH and 10-IH) had low basal $PHCO_3$ and reduced renal HCO_3 threshold ($TmHCO_3$) with high (> 7%) fractional excretion of HCO_3 at normal $PHCO_3$ levels, a finding consistent with proximal RTA [7]. In these 4 patients UpH during acid load was normal but the incapacity to achieve a normal U-BpCO_2 gradient indicated a distal tubular defect, too.

In conclusion, excluding conditions frequently associated with RTA (medullary sponge kidney, urinary tract obstruction, pyelonephritis), the incidence of RTA in our CSF was 4.3% (in all 94 CSF), 7% (in the last 26 studied), if evaluated on the basis of basal arterial pH and minimum UpH during acid load. However, with bicarbonate infusion test a greater incidence of acidification defects (isolated distal RTA = 23%, associated proximal and distal defects = 15%) was disclosed. In CSF renal acidification defects do not seem to be related to a peculiar metabolic pattern, being found in our series both in normocalciuric and in diet-dependent or diet-independent hypercalciuric CSF.

Table I. Basal acid-base status and renal acidifying capacity in normocalciuric (NC) and hypercalciuric (IH) calcium stone formers

Patient No.	Basal values							Acid load			Bicarbonate load			
	pH^a	HCO_3^a mEq/l	pCO_2^a mm Hg	TCO_2^b mEq/l	UpH	TAE mEq/l	NH_4E GFR	UpH	TAE mEq/l	NH_4E GFR	$UHCO_3$ mEq/l	U-BpCO_2 mm Hg	$TmHCO_3$ mEq/l GFR	$FEHCO_3^c$ %
1-NC	–	–	–	28	5.80	0.10	0.20	5.06	0.15	0.55	83.6	32	25.2	0.1
2-NC	–	–	–	26.5	6.70	0.16	0.24	5.06	0.22	0.53	122	35	–	1.3
3-NC	–	–	–	27	6.70	0.01	0.08	4.80	0.22	0.43	105	33	26.1	0.4
4-NC	–	–	–	24.4	6.12	0.10	0.15	5.10	0.24	0.32	122	30	23.4	0.1
5-NC	–	–	–	25	5.49	–	–	4.89	–	–	136	46	25.5	0.1
6-NC	–	–	–	25.6	5.16	0.06	0.16	4.69	0.16	0.47	88	30	24.1	0.3
7-NC	–	–	–	28.2	6.68	0.04	0.21	4.70	0.26	0.75	57	20	25.2	0.9
8-NC	7.37	19.8	34.4	21.2	5.65	0.13	0.30	4.95	0.30	0.57	118	14	20.3	7.4
9-NC	7.35	22.3	41.2	23.6	5.94	0.14	0.36	5.72	0.25	0.45	71	18	22.3	0.1
10-NC	–	–	–	26.5	5.18	0.18	0.20	4.81	0.48	0.58	80	5	21.9	0.5
11-NC	7.39	21.6	36.6	–	5.80	–	–	4.90	–	–	155	23	22.4	1.4
12-NC	7.43	25.0	37.0	23.3	6.48	0.07	0.41	4.96	0.35	0.35	91	23	–	0.2
13-NC	7.36	23.3	41.4	–	6.05	0.13	0.43	5.17	0.20	0.50	112	29	–	0.4
14-NC	7.35	21.5	39.7	–	5.41	0.15	0.23	4.93	0.25	0.40	61	7	20.6	7.0
15-NC	7.37	23.3	40.7	23.6	5.05	0.15	0.18	4.66	0.27	0.36	140	39	–	0
$\overline{X} \pm SD$	7.37± 0.02	22.4± 1.5	38.7± 2.5	25.3± 1.7	5.94± 0.57	0.11± 0.05	0.24± 0.10	4.95± 0.25	0.25± 0.08	0.48± 0.11	102.6*± 28.8	24.8**± 12.7	23.3± 1.9	1.3± 2.3

1-IH	7.41	24.9	39.0	–	5.91	0.08	0.17	4.70	0.24	0.42	114	36	22.0	0.3
2-IH	–	–	–	28.7	6.38	0.04	0.13	4.90	0.24	0.53	75	16	24.7	0.9
3-IH	7.38	23.4	39.9	25.8	6.58	0.10	0.23	4.65	0.36	0.67	71	16	25.0	0.7
4-IH	–	–	–	26.3	5.24	0.14	0.37	4.91	0.34	0.50	64	18	25.2	0.2
5-IH	–	–	–	26.0	5.50	–	–	4.88	–	–	163	42	24.7	0.1
6-IH	–	–	–	27.0	6.78	0.05	0.16	5.18	0.17	0.39	101	31	28.0	0.1
7-IH	–	–	–	27.3	5.14	0.16	0.13	4.69	0.22	0.38	134	39	27.4	0
8-IH	7.38	22.4	36.3	27.0	6.55	0.07	0.08	4.94	0.32	0.31	61	22	24.5	0.5
9-IH	7.37	21.4	37.0	21.9	6.00	–	–	5.20	–	–	117	10	21.2	9.7
10-IH	7.40	21.4	35.1	22.3	6.48	0.07	0.18	4.80	0.38	0.57	77	5	21.3	14.3
11-IH	7.39	22.2	37.8	24.2	5.88	0.07	0.21	5.37	0.38	0.60	85	10	21.7	3.0
$\bar{X} \pm SD$	7.39± 0.01	22.6± 1.2	37.5± 1.6	25.5± 2.8	5.95± 0.46	0.09± 0.04	0.19± 0.07	4.93± 0.22	0.29± 0.07	0.48± 0.11	96.5*± 30.9	21.6***± 11.4	24.15± 2.2	3.6± 7.1
$\bar{X} \pm SD$	7.38± 0.02	23.0± 0.7	38.8± 1.8	25.8± 1.6	5.59± 0.42	0.13± 0.07	0.20± 0.09	4.79± 0.20	0.29± 0.09	0.46± 0.17	154.5± 64	36± 8	25.4± 2.0	0.4± 0.3

[a] Arterial blood gas analysis.
[b] Total venous carbon dioxide.
[c] Fractional excretion of bicarbonate at normal plasma bicarbonate levels (> 23 mEq/l).
* $p < 0.02$; ** $p < 0.01$; *** $p < 0.001$ vs controls (n = 12).

References

1 Coe, F.L.: Clinical and laboratory assessment of patients with renal stones; in Coe, Nephrolithiasis, pp. 1–26 (Year Book, Chicago 1978).

2 Backman, U.; Danielson, B.G.; Johanson, G.; Ljunghall, S.; Wikstrom, B.: Incidence and clinical importance of renal tubular defects in recurrent renal stone formers. Nephron *25:* 96–101 (1980).

3 Higashihara, E.; Nutahara, K.; Tago, K.; Ueno, A.; Nijima, T.: Medullary sponge kidney and renal acidification defects. Kidney int. *25:* 453–459 (1984).

4 Tessitore, N.; Ortalda, V.; Fabris, A.; D'Angelo, A.; Rugiu, C.; Oldrizzi, L.; Lupo, A.; Valvo, E.; Gammaro, L.; Loschiavio, C.; Panzetta, G.; Panebianco, R.; Bedogna, V.; Maschio, G.: Renal acidification defects in patients with recurrent calcium nephrolithiasis. Nephron *41:* 325–332 (1985).

5 Halperin, M.L.; Goldstein, M.B.; Haig, A.; Johnson, M.; Stinebaugh, B.J.: Studies on the pathogenesis of type I (distal) renal tubular acidosis as revealed by urinary pCO_2 tensions. J. clin. Invest *53:* 669–677 (1974).

6 Battle, D.; Grupp, M.; Gaviria, M.; Kurtzman, N.: Distal renal tubular acidosis with intact capacity to lower urinary pH. Am. J. Med. *72:* 751–758 (1982).

7 Cogan, M.G.; Rector, F.C.; Seldin, D.W.: Acid-base disorders; in Brenner, Rector, The kidney, pp. 841–907 (Saunders, Philadelphia 1981).

M. Surian, MD, Servizio di Dialisi, Ospedale Maggiore, I–20075 Lodi (Italy)

Contr. Nephrol., vol. 58, pp. 49–58 (Karger, Basel 1987)

In vitro System for Calcium Stone Formation: The Constant Composition Model

G. H. Nancollas, R. P. Singh[1]

Chemistry Department, State University of New York at Buffalo, Buffalo, N. Y., USA

Urine is normally supersaturated with respect to calcium oxalates [1, 2], octacalcium phosphate (OCP) and hydroxyapatite (HAP). From time to time, the urine may also be supersaturated with respect to dicalcium phosphate dihydrate (DCPD) [3]. The results of both clinical and non-clinical studies suggest that the likelihood of calcium oxalate renal stone formation can be related more readily to the free ionic concentrations of calcium and oxalate than to the total stoichiometric values. One of the most important problems, therefore, is that of estimating the degree of complexing of calcium and oxalate ions in whole urine in order to be able to estimate the concentrations of free species which participate in the expressions for the thermodynamic solubility products. Chemical methods of estimating the unbound calcium ion in urine involve lengthy techniques and may not distinguish properly between complexed and free fractions. It has therefore usually been necessary to estimate the ionized calcium concentration from the measured stoichiometric total concentrations by correcting for the more important ion pairs and complexes. For this purpose, a number of speciation programs have been developed which take into account up to 30 ion pairs in order to calculate supersaturation levels in urine specimens [4, 5]. However, these computational methods are able to take into ac-

[1] We thank the National Institutes of Arthritis, Diabetes, Digestive and Kidney Diseases, National Institutes of Health, for a grant (AM–19048).

count only those ionic interactions for which stability constant data are available. With the development of the calcium ion selective electrode, it became possible to measure directly the free ion activity. Unfortunately, however, other urinary components tend to poison the electrode membrane so that most mineralization inhibition studies have resorted to the use of highly diluted urine samples. However, this may lead to problems of interpretation [6].

Although it is unclear how large crystals are formed in the kidney, there is little doubt that minute crystalluria is observed in both normal subjects and stone formers. The real problem relates to how the crystals are retained in the case of stone formers and how they develop to macroscopic size. Here, there is little doubt that processes of aggregation and secondary nucleation may be important as well as the morphology of the developing crystals. Thus results to be presented in this paper indicate that during calcium oxalate monohydrate (COM) crystallization, secondary nuclei may form as the reaction proceeds. These secondary nuclei may aggregate to form large crystals which ultimately develop into kidney stones.

One of the principle interests in the in vitro study of the formation of crystalluria is the possibility of using relevant parameters as an assessment of risk factors for the formation of renal stones in vivo. In the fluctuating concentration environment within the kidney, it is clear that both mineralization and demineralization processes may be involved. Studies of crystal growth in voided urine may therefore give direct information about the possibility of concretions forming in the urinary tract. It is for this reason that numerous seeded crystallization studies have been made of both calcium oxalates and calcium phosphates in simulated urines. Although the earlier studies were involved with spontaneous precipitation, complications arising due to the concomitant nucleation and crystal growth made interpretation of these results difficult. The problems involved using these relatively high supersaturations were overcome by the introduction of the seeded crystallization methods which enable mineralization rates to be determined with considerable reproducibility. The rates of reaction were followed by monitoring the decrease in lattice calcium and oxalate ion concentrations as a function of time. However, in these experiments, the concentrations of lattice ions decreased so that the solutions were supersaturated with respect to different phases as the reactions proceeded. Different phases may therefore form and redissolve during the overall reaction, making it difficult to quantify the kinetics. Moreover, as the process approaches equilibrium, changes in lattice ion concentrations are too small to allow reliable estimates of either stoichiometries or the rates of the solid phases formed.

These problems were overcome by using a technique in which the precipitation was studied under conditions of constant activities of ionic species. In this constant composition (CC) method, following the addition of seed crystals to metastable supersaturated solutions of calcium oxalate, the activities of both calcium and oxalate ions were maintained constant by the simultaneous addition of titrant solutions containing calcium chloride and sodium oxalate, from mechanically coupled burettes [7]. It is important to maintain constant the ionic strengths of all the solutions since changes in activity coefficients could also influence the rate of titrant addition which was controlled by a specific calcium ion electrode. In our laboratory, we have developed a protected calcium electrode for studies of the rate of mineralization in whole urine under conditions of constant supersaturation [8]. Since the electrode monitors the activity of free calcium ions, the initial COM supersaturation could be adjusted to preset values by the addition of lattice ions. In this way, the inhibitory activity of urines may be compared directly at the same degree of supersaturation. In order to compute supersaturations, anionic concentrations were measured by high performance chromatographic methods [9].

In the CC method, relatively large amounts of new solid phases can be formed even at very low supersaturation. It is therefore possible to characterize substantial amounts of newly formed solid phases by numerous physical chemical methods such as χ-ray diffraction, infrared spectroscopy, specific surface area, optical and scanning electron microscopy, and particle size distribution. The excellent reproducibility of the method enables investigations to be made not only of the mechanism of mineralization but also the influence of growth inhibitors present in urine upon the rate of mineralization. Another important advantage of the CC method is the possibility of growing crystals at constant supersaturation in order to achieve a greater lattice perfection prior to their use as seed in the inhibitor assay crystallization experiments. In conventional seeded crystallization experiments in which the lattice ions concentrations are allowed to decrease during the reaction, it is not possible to prepare sufficient amounts of new phases for characterization. More importantly, the CC method can be used to study the mechanism and crystallization of calcium oxalates at non-equivalent calcium/oxalate molar ratios typical of those in urines.

Materials and Methods

Solutions of calcium chloride, potassium oxalate, and sodium chloride were prepared from reagent grade chemicals using triply distilled, deionized water which was filtered before use through 0.22 μm Millipore filters. These filters were prewashed in order to remove any residual wetting agents and surfactants which could influence the measured rates of crystallization. Solutions were standardized by an ion exchange method in which the cations were exchanged for hydrogen ion on a Dowex-50 column and the eluted acid was titrated with standardized potassium hydroxide. COM and calcium oxalate dihydrate (COD) seed crystals were prepared as described previously [10] and were characterized by quantitative analysis and by χ-ray powder diffraction (copper Kα radiation, Phillips XRG 3000 diffractometer).

Crystallization experiments were made in a magnetically stirred Pyrex double-walled reaction vessel maintained at 37 ± 0.1 °C. Nitrogen gas, saturated at 37 °C with respect to 0.15 mol l^{-1} sodium chloride, was bubbled continuously through the crystallization cell during the experiments in order to exclude carbon dioxide. The pH of these solutions was monitored with a glass electrode (Corning), and calcium ion activities in the supersaturated solutions were measured using a calcium ion-selective electrode (Radiometer Model F2112). The reference electrode was a thermal electrolytic silver/silver chloride probe separated from the cell by means of a 0.15-mol l^{-1} sodium chloride solution in order to avoid changes in liquid junction potential. During the crystallization experiments, aliquots of reaction mixture were periodically filtered (0.22 μm Millipore filter) and the filtrate analyzed for calcium by atomic absorption spectrophotometry and for oxalate by ion chromatography. The solid phases were also examined by χ-ray diffraction and by scanning electron microscopy (ISI Model II).

Fasting urines, collected from subjects having no prior history of stone disease, were centrifuged (3,500 rpm for 50 min) and stored out of contact with air in a refrigerator. They were analyzed for calcium, magnesium, oxalate, phosphate, sulfate, and chloride. In the preparation of the supersaturated solutions, the calcium-specific ion electrode, protected by means of a dialysis membrane, was used to measure the free ion activity. The desired initial supersaturation of the urine was then achieved by the addition, if necessary, of small volumes of solutions containing calcium and/or oxalate ions. The reactions were initiated by the addition of COM seed crystals and the first drop in calcium activity accompanying crystallization triggered the potentiostat (Metrohm Combititrator 3D, Brinkmann Instrument Company) to add the titrant solutions in order to maintain the calcium activity constant.

Results and Discussion

Concentrations of ionic species in the supersaturated calcium oxalate solutions were calculated from mass balance and electroneutrality expressions as described previously, by taking into account the formation of calcium oxalate and sodium oxalate ion pairs [10, 11]. Activity coefficients of the divalent cation and anion were assumed to be equal and were obtained from the extended form of the Debye-Hückel equation proposed by Davies [12]:

$$-\log y_z = Az^2 [I^{0.5}/(1+I^{0.5})-0.3I].$$

The rate of crystallization of COM has been shown to be considerably slower than that to be expected for a bulk diffusion process indicating a surface-controlled reaction which follows a rate equation:

$$\text{Rate of crystallization} = R_g = k_g \sigma^n, \quad (1)$$

in which k_g is the rate constant for crystal growth and the relative supersaturation, $\sigma = (\pi/\pi_0)^{0.5}-1$ where π is the ionic product [$= (Ca^{2+})\ (Ox^{2-})$] and π_0 is the value at equilibrium. The concentrations of free calcium and oxalate ions were calculated using conditional equilibrium constants valid at the ionic strength (0.15 mol l^{-1}) of the experiments. The kinetics of crystallization of the COM (pregrown) and COD crystals are illustrated in figure 1 in which the rate of reaction is plotted against the square of the relative supersaturation. The linearity of the plot clearly supports the proposed second order spiral growth mechanism. It is important to note that the mechanism of growth of COM does not change with supersaturation. In contrast, dissolution studies at constant composition indicate that a diffusion controlled process at higher driving forces changes to one of surface control with a rate proportional to the square of the undersaturation close to equilibrium [13].

COM is the most important mineral phase involved in renal stone formation. It is usually formed as irregular radial agglomerates by rapid crystallization. However, coffin-shaped crystals are also found in urine which, in vitro, can be prepared either by pregrowing aged seed crystals at constant supersaturation or by allowing COD to undergo transformation into COM under constant composition conditions. Since different types of crystals may have different surface energies and numbers of growth sites, it is especially important to study the mineralization of different crystals under conditions close to those in vivo in order to understand the role of morphology in kidney stone formation. Typical crystallization rate curves are shown in figure 2 for both aged and pregrown COM seed crystals at the same supersaturation. It can be seen that the rate of mineralization per m^2 of aged crystals was 50–60% higher than that for pregrown samples. This suggests that the pregrowth of aged seed crystals during the process of

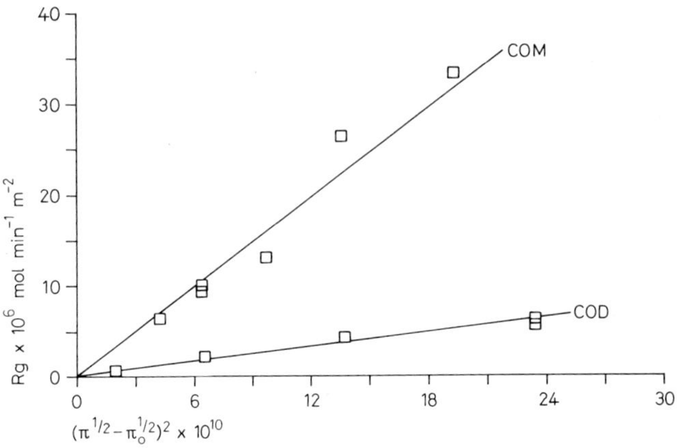

Fig. 1. Mechanism of crystallization of calcium oxalate monohydrate (COM) and calcium oxalate dihydrate (COD). Plots of growth rate against $(\pi^{1/2} - \pi_o^{1/2})^2$.

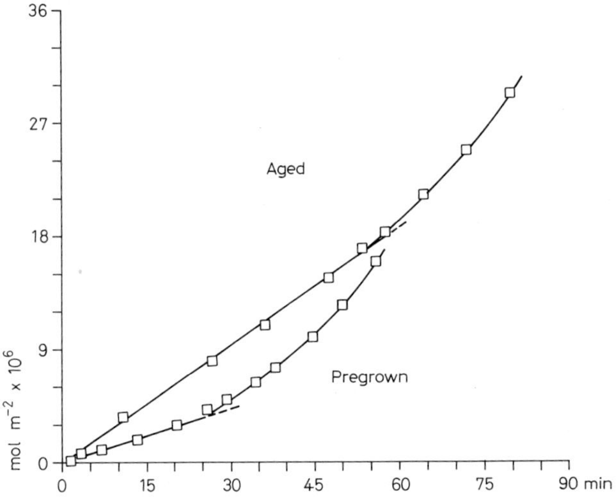

Fig. 2. COM crystallization on different seed preparations at $\sigma = 1.26$.

lattice perfection markedly reduces the density of growth sites on the surface. It has been observed in other crystallizing systems that the initial process of mineralization of aged samples results in lattice perfection due to the rapid outgrowth of fast growing faces [Singh et al., to be published]. Clearly, this process results in a reduction of the growth site density on the

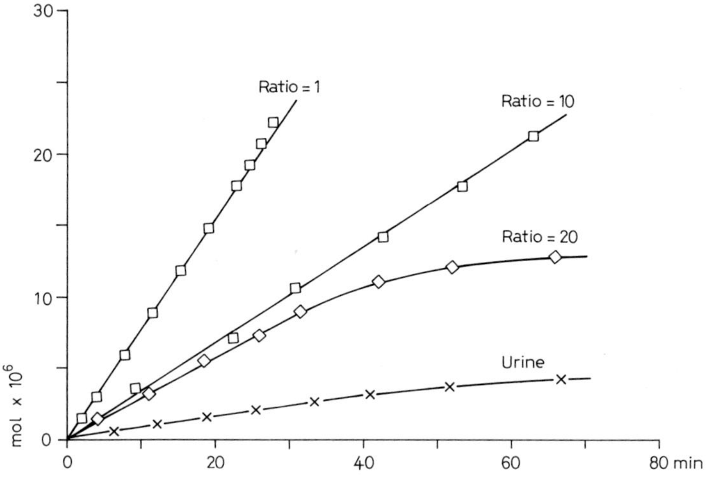

Fig. 3. Crystallization of COM at different molar calcium/oxalate ratios.

crystal surfaces. Another important observation in our CC experiments is that the growth of aged seed crystals beyond approximately 200% with respect to initial seed results in the formation of new particles by a secondary nucleation process. These may form through collision of the growing crystals either with each other or with the walls of the container. It is significant that for pregrown crystals, the secondary nucleation process sets in at lower extents of growth (~ 50–70%) and the overall rate of crystallization rapidly increases (fig. 2). Scanning electron microscopic results and particle size distribution measurements confirm the presence of new secondary nuclei [Singh et al., to be published]. The increasing crystallization rate, at rather well-defined extents of reaction, may be an important factor in the formation of renal stones in vivo. The newly formed secondary nuclei may rapidly aggregate to form large concretions.

An important parameter in the study of the mechanism of crystallization of calcium oxalate concerns the molar ratio of calcium/oxalate; in urine, this ratio may vary from 1 to 50. The constant composition method enables crystallization rates to be investigated under these conditions. Typical results are shown in figure 3 in which it can be seen that the rates of crystallization (represented by the slopes of the curves) are markedly reduced as the calcium/oxalate molar ratios are increased. At a ratio of 10, the rate of crystallization is slower by almost a factor of 2 as compared with

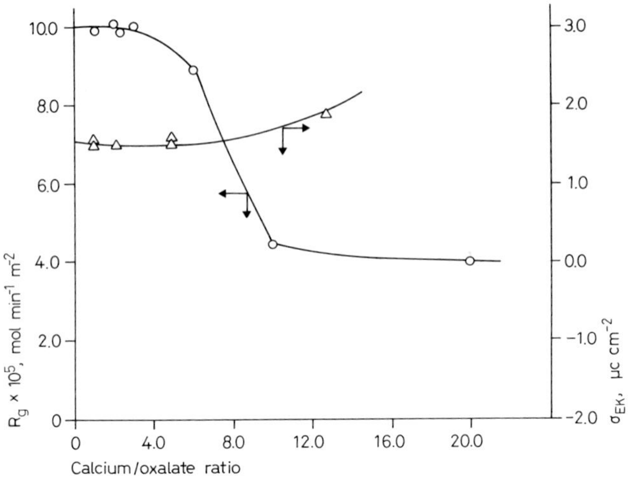

Fig. 4. Plots of COM growth rate and COM surface charge (σ_{EK}) as a function of the Ca/oxalate ratio.

the reaction at equimolar calcium and oxalate concentrations (fig. 4). Moreover, it can be seen in figure 4 that the rate profile at higher calcium/oxalate molar ratios is close to the curve obtained in whole urine. As the ratio is increased from 10 to 20, the initial rate of crystallization undergoes little change but the subsequent reduction in rate increases. This may be interpreted in terms of the marked change in surface potential in the presence of excess lattice cation as can be seen in figure 4.

In order to use the constant composition method as a reliable indicator of urine inhibitory potential, the necessity for insuring reproducible supersaturations cannot be too strongly emphasized. Calcium activity measurements in our laboratory indicate that for the majority of urine specimens, the unbound calcium concentrations increase upon the addition of 0.15 *M* sodium chloride background electrolyte. The release of bound calcium from ion pairs and complexes depends markedly upon the nature and concentration of the complexing ligands in the whole urine. Since the driving force for mineralization depends upon the free ion activity products, speciation elucidation clearly remains one of the most important factors determining the risk of stone formation. Urinary components also influence the nature of the calcium oxalate hydrate which precipitates. Recent work in our laboratory has demonstrated the growth of the thermodynamically less stable COD probably resulting from the more effective inhibition of COM

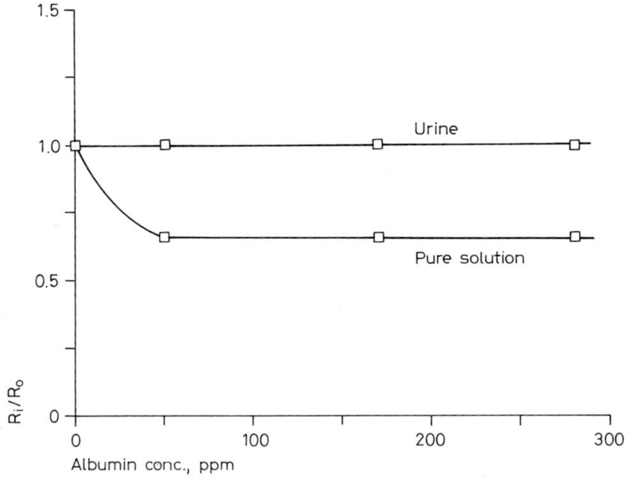

Fig. 5. Effect of human serum albumin (HSA) on COM growth. Plot of R_i (rate in the presence of albumin)/R_0 (in absence of albumin), against albumin concentration.

[Coyle-Rees and Nancollas, to be published]. The degree to which the subsequent transformation reaction COD → COM takes place may therefore also be an important stone risk factor. Moreover, various metastable calcium phosphate phases may behave similarly during their precipitation in whole urines. Recently, it has been found, as shown in figure 5, that the addition of albumin to whole urine in which COM is crystallizing has little influence on the rate of crystallization, suggesting that the inhibitory properties of urinary components may not be simply additive. The possibility of synergistic considerations for the protection of normal subjects from stone formation may be one of the keys to our understanding of the mechanism of urolithiasis. These studies are presently under way in our laboratory.

References

1 Robertson, W.G.; Peacock, M.; Nordin, B.E.C.: Activity products in stone-forming and non-stone-forming urine. Clin. Sci. *34:* 579–594 (1968).

2 Robertson, W.G.; Peacock, M.; Marshall, R.W.; Nordin, B.E.C.: Saturation inhibition index as a measure of the risk of calcium oxalate stone formation in the urinary tract. New Engl. J. Med. *294:* 249–252 (1976).

3 Pak, C.Y.C.: Physiochemical basis for formation of renal stones of calcium phosphate origin: calculation of the degree of saturation of urine with respect to brushite. J. clin. Invest. *48:* 1914–1922 (1969).

4 Robertson, W.G.: Measurement of ionized calcium in biological fluids. Clinica chim. Acta *24:* 149–157 (1969).

5 Werness, P.G.; Brown, C.M.; Smith, L.H.; Finlayson, B.: EQUIL 2: a basic computer program for the calculation of urinary saturation. J. Urol. *134:* 1242–1244 (1985).

6 Robertson, W.G.; Knowles, F.; Peacock, M.: Urinary acid mucopolysaccharide inhibitors of calcium oxalate crystallization; in Fleisch, Robertson, Smith, Vahlensieck, Urolithiasis research, pp. 331 (Plenum Press, New York 1976).

7 Koutsoukos, P.; Amjad, Z.; Tomson, M.B.; Nancollas, G.H.: Crystallization of calcium phosphates. A constant composition study. J. Am. chem. Soc. *102:* 1553–1558 (1980).

8 Gaur, S.S.; Nancollas, G.H.: Kinetics of crystal growth in urine. Kidney int. *26:* 767–768 (1984).

9 Singh, R.P.; Nancollas, G.H.: Determination of urinary citrate by high performance ion chromatography. Kidney int. *28:* 985–987 (1985).

10 Tomazic, B.; Nancollas, G.H.: The kinetics of dissolution of calcium oxalate hydrates. J. Crystal Growth *46:* 355–361 (1979).

11 Nancollas, G.H.: Interactions in electrolyte solutions, pp. 85–90 (Elsevier, Amsterdam 1966).

12 Davies, C.W.: Ion association (Butterworths, London 1962).

13 White, D.J.; Nancollas, G.H.: The kinetics of dissolution of calcium oxalate monohydrate. A constant composition study. J. Crystal Growth *57:* 267–270 (1982).

G.H. Nancollas, DSc, Chemistry Department, State University of New York at Buffalo, Buffalo, NY 14214 (USA)

Contr. Nephrol., vol. 58, pp. 59–64 (Karger, Basel 1987)

Crystallization in Gel Matrices: A New Experimental Model of Calcium Stone Formation[1]

W. Achilles[2]

Universitätsklinikum Marburg, Urologische Klinik (Direktor: Prof. Dr. G. Rodeck), Marburg/Lahn, FRG

Conventional methods for the determination of crystal growth parameters which intend to model urinary stone formation are time-consuming and therefore not suitable to clinical routine measurements [1]. Furthermore, most of them are carried out using high urine dilution thus providing results of questionable physiological relevance.

For these reasons, we have developed an optical micromethod for the kinetic determination of crystal growth parameters of precipitating phases in gel matrices, which represents a new experimental model of urinary stone formation (gel crystallization method, GCM) [2–4]. It may be applied to large-scale measurements of crystal growth kinetics of calcium oxalates and phosphates under urinary conditions, thereby showing a high precision of measuring results.

This study reviews briefly the actual features of the GCM, practical experience from clinical routine measurements, as well as present applications.

Method

Principles

From two ions which are able to form a precipitating solid phase one is dissolved as a soluble compound (e.g. sodium oxalate or calcium chloride) in a gel. The gel is located in multiple wells of a multicuvette (96-well microplate). Solutions containing the counterion

[1] This work has been supported by the Deutsche Forschungsgemeinschaft, Bonn (Ac 52/1-1).

[2] I am indebted to Mrs. E. Krzyzanek and Mr. H. Schmidt for their excellent technical assistance.

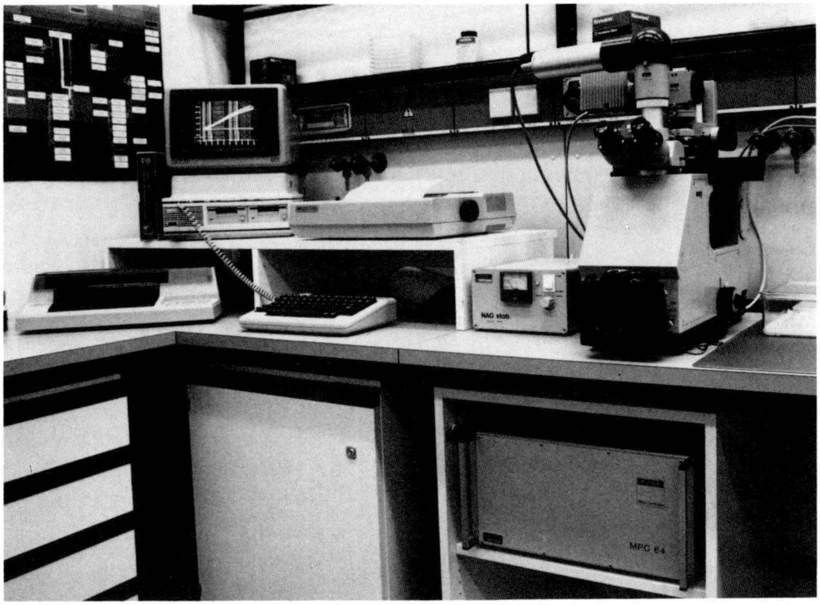

Fig. 1. Microphotometric device (Zeiss, Oberkochen, FRG) for automated multiple determination of crystal growth parameters in gel matrices (gel crystallization method, GCM).

(e.g. Ca^{2+} or phosphate) are pipetted onto the gel. The subsequent crystal formation in the gel matrix is followed by vertical light path photometry as a function of time [2, 3]. High efficiency and precision in measurements is achieved by: (1) multiple sample handling of small volumes; (2) fast sequential photometry in 48–96 positions of the microplate repeating the measuring cycle in prescribed intervals up to 15–30 times, thus collecting time-dependent measuring data; (3) the application of a computer-controlled microphotometer, and (4) current reference to a kinetic standard taking into account blank values [4].

Measuring Device

Automated microphotometric system for transmitted light (Zeiss, Oberkochen, FRG) comprising the following main parts: (1) inverted microscope IM 35 equipped with power-stabilized halogen light source HB 100, rapid (50-μm step) scanning stage for microtitre plates, photometer SFD and camera Contax RTS; (2) electronic control unit MPC 64, and (3) on-line microcomputer HP 9816 S (512 kbyte RAM) with double disk drive HP 9121 D, matrix printer HP 82906 A and plotter HP 7470A for acquisition, processing and display of data (fig. 1). The evaluation of kinetic data has been programmed in HP-BASIC 2.0.

Preparation of Gels and Standard Solutions

Oxalate-Induced Procedure. (1) Dissolution of 0.5 g of dry gel substance (preferably Agar-Agar, high gel strength, Serva) 0.5 g glycerol, 1 mmol/l NaN_3 and 2 mmol/l sodium oxalate in 100 ml of water at 90 °C; (2) generation of seed crystals (or nuclei) by adding 0.5 ml 5 mmol/l $CaCl_2$ at 60 °C, and (3) pipetting of the solution into prewarmed microplates.

Measuring standard solution (total concentrations given in mmol/l): NaCl (80), NH_4Cl (25), KCl (30), Na_2SO_4 (15), KH_2PO_4 (10), $Na_2HPO_4 \cdot 2H_2O$ (10), urea (250), citric acid (2), $MgCl_2$ (3), $CaCl_2$ (4), NaN_3 (1), pH = 6.05.

Calcium-Induced Procedure. Corresponding to oxalate with the following alterations: (1) 20 mmol/l $CaCl_2$ instead of sodium oxalate, and (2) without pre-precipitation of calcium salts.

Measuring standard solution (total concentrations given in mmol/l): NaCl (80), KCl (30), Na_2SO_4 (15), KH_2PO_4 (15), $Na_2HPO_4 \cdot 2H_2O$ (25), urea (250), citric acid (2), $MgCl_2$ (3), NaN_3 (1), pH = 6.65.

The actual features of the GCM which refer to measurements in undiluted urine samples are summarized in table I.

Results and Discussion

The GCM described here provides kinetic data of crystal growth processes of calcium oxalates (a) and phosphates (b) relevant in calcium urolithiasis. While we have only preliminary results with procedure b, oxalate-induced crystallization (a) has been applied in comprehensive measurements.

(1) Using an artificial urine (standard at pH 6.0) as a test system inhibitory activities of different low and high molecular substances could be determined [6]. Because of the very low concentrations of the effectors applied, free Ca^{2+} had not or almost not been changed in this case. The dependence of Vcr (CaOx) on total calcium concentration (Ca_T) in the absence and presence of inhibitors gave further insight into inhibition mechanisms [6].

(2) Varying several parameters in the artificial urine demonstrated their effect on Vcr (CaOx). From these, calcium had the strongest influence followed by citrate, volume, magnesium and pH. The comparison of these experimental kinetic data with corresponding values of normalized supersaturation revealed the overlapping effect of complex formation and kinetic influence on the crystal growth. In particular, citrate could be shown to exert a considerable kinetic effect on Vcr which could not be accounted for by sequestration of calcium [7].

(3) In two groups of recurrent calcium stone formers and normals we determined the crystal growth rate of calcium oxalate and other parameters (Ca_T, Mg_T, Cit_T, Ox_T, pH, volume). The only significant difference we could find between the groups was that for Vcr (CaOx). A highly significant

Table I. Gel crystallization method (GCM): actual features of the determination of kinetic parameters of crystal growth in gel matrices from undiluted urine samples for diagnostic use by automated scanning microphotometry in microtitre plates

	Oxalate induced	Calcium induced
Gel matrix	agar-agar; agarose Na oxalate (2 mmol/l) seed crystals volume: 100 µl	agar-agar; agarose $CaCl_2$ (20 mmol/l) volume: 100 µl
Precipitating phases	$CaOx \cdot H_2O$, $CaOx \cdot 2H_2O$	Ca-phosphates (amorphous?) (not clearly identified up to now)
Measuring solutions	undiluted urine artificial solutions volume: 200 µl	undiluted urine artificial solutions volume: 200 µl
Mode of measurement	(1) dark field (2) polarized light	bright field
Measuring data	increasing light intensity/time	increasing absorption/time
Evaluated kinetic parameter	Vcr (CaOx)	Vcr (CaP)
Definition	$Vcr = \frac{\text{maximal linear slope from test solution}}{\text{maximal linear slope from standard solution}}$ (corrected for blank values)	
Time of measurement (simultaneous determ. of 48 kinetics)	15 min	25 min
Efficiency	150 kinetics/h	100 kinetics/h
Mean unprecision (CV within series)		
Single determin.	2–3%	5–10%
Mean (4-fold determ.)	1–2%	3–5%
Problems	thermodynamic (chemical) instability of urine samples	
Remarks	results from comprehensive measurements in artificial and native urines	preliminary results

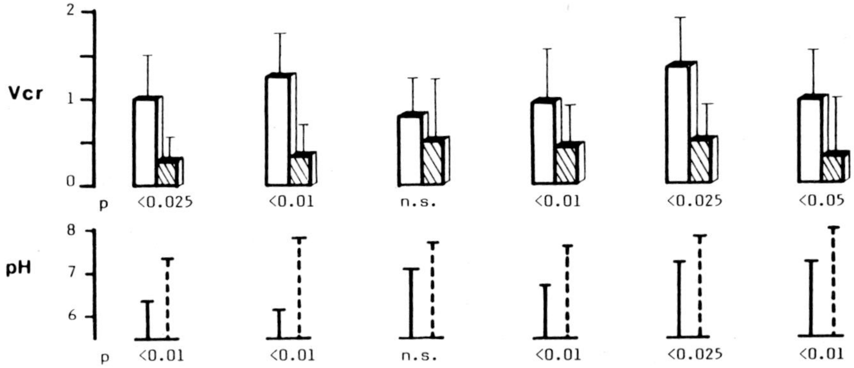

Fig. 2. Mean values of 'relative crystal growth rates' of calcium oxalate (Vcr) and corresponding pH values from 3-hour fractional urine samples in 6 normal persons before (blank columns) and during (hatched columns) therapy with preparation I (Lithurex®).

correlation between total calcium and Vcr ($r = 0.77$; $p < 0.001$) could be shown in the native urines corresponding to the findings in artificial solutions [8].

(4) In a first treatment study we applied a preparation of alkali citrates, magnesium citrate, citric acid and pyridoxine (preparation I: Lithurex®) to 6 normal persons. In 5 of them it resulted in a considerable decrease of CaOx crystal growth rate which could be partially accounted for by increased pH and citrate during therapy (fig. 2). From these results we would conclude that the GCM may be applied as a short-time test to control the effectiveness of prophylactic measures in urolithiasis.

If one compares the GCM with other methods which model urinary stone formation it shows disadvantages and advantages. Nucleation rates of crystal formation, as they may be measured by the constant composition method [9], cannot be determined here. The measuring parameter 'Vcr' is an empirical quantity which has not been related to a clearly defined crystal growth rate in a correct physicochemical sense up to now. On the other side, the high efficiency of the method, the precision of the measuring results and the hitherto proven physiological relevance reveal new capabilities for investigations in urolithiasis and other crystallization processes.They make it suitable to an application in clinical routine measurements as a useful diagnostic mean. Therefore, the model of crystallization in gel matrices in its present form may be regarded as a helpful addition to the models which have been practised up to now.

References

1 Fleisch, H.: Round table discussion on the comparison of models for the study of inhibitory activity in urine; in Schwille, Smith, Robertson, Vahlensieck, Urolithiasis and related clinical research, pp. 903–908 (Plenum Press New York 1985).

2 Achilles, W.; Mergner, C.; Simon, M.: An optical micromethod for the determination of relative crystallization rates of calcium oxalate in gels: method and preliminary results. Urol. Res. *11:* 87–91 (1983).

3 Achilles, W.: Ein optisches Mikroverfahren zur Bestimmung relativer Kristallisationsgeschwindigkeiten (Gelkristallisationsverfahren). Neue Entwicklungen: Kristallisationskinetische Messung durch Mikroskop-Photometrie. Fortschr. Urol. Nephrol. *22:* 377–384 (1984).

4 Achilles, W.: Methodische Neuerungen des kinetischen Gelkristallisationsverfahrens (GKV): Automatisierte Messung des Kalziumoxalat-Kristallwachstums durch Scanning-Mikroskopphotometrie. Fortschr. Urol. Nephrol. *23:* 252–260 (1985).

5 Udich, J. H.; Höft, H.; Börnig, H.: Studies of calcium phosphate formation in artificial matrices. Biomed. Acta *44:* 547–559 (1985).

6 Achilles, W.: Die Wirkung niedermolekularer und hochmolekularer Kristallisationsinhibitoren auf das Wachstum von Kalziumoxalat im Gel. Fortschr. Urol. Nephrol. *23:* 38–44 (1985).

7 Achilles, W.; Ulshöfer, B.: Der Einfluss von Harnparametern auf das "kinetische und thermodynamische Kristallbildungsrisiko" von Kalziumoxalat. Fortschr. Urol. Nephrol. *23:* 341–346 (1985).

8 Achilles, W.; Ulshöfer, B.: Die GKV-Messung relativer Kristallwachstumsgeschwindigkeiten von Kalziumoxalat in 24-Stunden-Sammelurinen von Normalpersonen und Steinträgern mit rezidivierender Kalzium-Urolithiasis. Fortschr. Urol. Nephrol. *23:* 261–266 (1985).

9 Sheehan, M. E.; Nancollas, G. E.: Calcium oxalate crystal growth. A new constant composition method for modelling urinary stone formation. Investve Urol. *17:* 446–450 (1980).

PD Dr. rer. nat. W. Achilles, Universitätsklinikum Marburg,
Urologische Klinik, Baldingerstrasse, D–3550 Marburg/Lahn (FRG)

Contr. Nephrol., vol. 58, pp. 65–72 (Karger, Basel 1987)

Effect of Inhibitors on the Crystal Growth of Calcium Oxalate[1]

C. Minero[a], *P. Maggiorotti*[a], *M. Barbeni*[a], *E. Pelizzetti*[a], *A. Tizzani*[b], *G. Casetta*[b], *P. Piana*[b], *C. Giona*[b]

[a]Dipartimento di Chimica Analitica, [b]Istituto di Nefrologia, Cattedra di Urologia, Università di Torino, Torino, Italia

Calcium oxalate is the most abundant and frequently occurring constituent of upper urinary tract calculi. In normal human subjects calcium and oxalate ions are supersaturated with respect to the salt. The formation in vivo of large crystals and aggregates can be due to many factors, e.g. the increased level of supersaturation with respect to the salt, the increased level of some promoters (such as a heterogeneous nucleator or a promoter for the rate of growth and of sticking crystals together), the low level of inhibitors of crystal growth.

The effect of inhibitors has received particular attention in the past two decades [1], because in vitro experiments can give a knowledge directly related to the in vivo situation, and can be useful for pharmacological applications. Several studies have been carried out on the effect of low molecular weight additives on calcium oxalate monohydrate (COM) [2–5].

This paper reports a systematic investigation on the seeded growth kinetics of COM over a wide range of possible low molecular weight urine inhibitors and of their concentration using the constant composition technique (CCT). The range of relative supersaturation considered (0.2–2.0) is not as high as that found in stone formers' urines, but is crucial in order to elucidate how in normal human subjects urine autoinhibits crystal growth.

[1] Generous support from Regione Piemonte (Progetto Ricerca Sanitaria Finalizzata) is gratefully acknowledged.

Table I. Inhibition properties of low molecular weight components

Compounds	Mean molar concentration in urine, mol l^{-1} [a]	$Q_{0.9}$ [b]	$Q_{0.5}$ [b]
Histamine	1.4×10^{-4}	$> 3 \times 10^{-3}$	
Thiamine (vitamin B_1)	4×10^{-4}	$> 3 \times 10^{-3}$	
Urea	3×10^{-4}	1×10^{-3}	
Pyridoxine	4×10^{-4}	1×10^{-3}	
Glutamic acid	1.4×10^{-3}	$> 2 \times 10^{-3}$	
Nicotinic acid	1.4×10^{-3}	$> 1 \times 10^{-3}$	
p-Aminobenzoic acid	1×10^{-3}	$> 2 \times 10^{-3}$	
L-Ascorbic acid	1×10^{-4}	$> 2 \times 10^{-3}$	
Aspartic acid	6×10^{-5}	8×10^{-4}	
Tartaric acid	–	2×10^{-4}	2×10^{-3}
Citric acid	2.8×10^{-3}	1×10^{-5}	1×10^{-4}
Mg^{++}	3×10^{-3}	1×10^{-4}	1.5×10^{-3}
Pyrophosphate	5×10^{-5} [c]		1×10^{-5} (pH = 6) 3×10^{-6} (pH = 8)

[a] Values taken from Free and Free [13].
[b] See text. Q values estimated in this work. Experimental conditions: calcium and oxalate 5×10^{-4} mol l^{-1}, T = 37 °C, pH = 6.2–6.4, NaCl 0.15 mol l^{-1}, added seeds 50 mg.
[c] Fleisch and Bisaz [14].

Experimental

Calcium chloride and potassium oxalate of PA grade were supplied from Merck. Commercial grade, or RPE grade when available, inhibitors reported in table I were supplied from Carlo Erba. Stock solutions of the lattice ions and of the additives were freshly prepared in doubly distilled water and diluted as required. The solutions for the kinetic measurements were filtered on 0.22-µm Millipore filters. The exact molarity of calcium and oxalate ions was checked using standard analytical methods.

Calcium oxalate seeds were prepared by drop-wise addition of 250 ml of 0.40 *M* calcium chloride and potassium oxalate to 1.5 liters of filtered and well-stirred water at 75 °C. The pH was maintained around 6.2. After aging for 6 h at the same temperature, the seeds were filtered and washed until chloride ions gave a negative test with 0.1 *M* $AgNO_3$. They were left at rest for a month in contact with 200 ml of distilled water, dried at 40 °C for a day and stored. The surface area of the solid material was measured using a BET krypton adsorption (Sorptomatic, Carlo Erba), and estimated to be 2.4 m^2g^{-1}. Differential scanning calorimetry (910 DSC Thermal Analyzer, Dupont Instr.), X-ray analysis (XRG 3000 diffractometer with Co radiation, Phillips), and IR spectra (580 B, Perkin Elmer) confirmed that calcium oxalate was in the monohydrated form.

The crystal growth experiments were performed in a water-thermostated double-walled vessel of 600 ml capacity at 37.0 ± 0.1 °C, under magnetic stirring and flushing of N_2. The supersaturated solution was prepared adding to a 0.15-*M* NaCl the appropriate amount of inhibitor and of potassium oxalate, adjusting the pH at 6.2–6.4 and carefully adding the equivalent amount of $CaCl_2$. In the range of 0.2–1.5 relative supersaturation there is no evidence of crystal formation.

The addition of seeds induces immediate crystal growth. Calcium and oxalate ion activities are maintained constant by the simultaneous automatic addition of reagent solutions containing these ions. In this way the supersaturation is constant during the experiment. The CCT is decribed in detail by Nancollas and co-workers [6, 7].

The apparatus we used is made of two automatic digital burettes electronically coupled (Dosigraph 625, Dosimat 655, Metrohom Herisau), an electronic comparator and a pH meter (Impulsomat 614, digital pH meter 605, Metrohom Herisau). The rate of crystal growth is given directly by the rate of addition of the reagents.

We tested two methods of addition of seeds. In the first case 1.0–5.0 g of seeds were added to 50 ml of water, the suspension was strongly stirred and 1 ml of the slurry was used. In the second case 20–100 mg of seeds were dispersed in 4 ml of water by sonication at low intensity for 3 min (B 15 sonifier, Branson). The whole solution was used. No relevant differences in the absolute rate were detected, but ultrasonically treated seed suspensions gave more reproducible results.

Results and Discussion

Table I lists the presently investigated compounds. The relative rate of growth is defined as the ratio of the observed rate in the presence of inhibitor to the rate in the absence of any additive. In table I the concentration of inhibitor that reduces at 90% the growth rate ($Q_{0.9}$) and at 50% ($Q_{0.5}$) is reported.

It can be noted that organic bases exibit very scarce inhibitor properties, since their effect on the growth rate appears only at very high concentrations in respect to the normal urine values.

Among the organic acids, the more effective inhibitors are aspartic, tartaric and citric acids as shown in figure 1. The effect of citric acid is reported more clearly in figure 2 together with that of magnesium ion. Taking into account their concentration in the urine, these two species show the most efficient inhibitor properties among the compounds considered until now.

The effect of an additive on the crystal growth rate can be due to the complexation capability of the inhibitor towards calcium ion or oxalate, or to a crystal poisoning of the growth sites. In the first case the inhibitor concentration is comparable to that of the precipitating ions, in the second one the additive is effective also at much lower concentration.

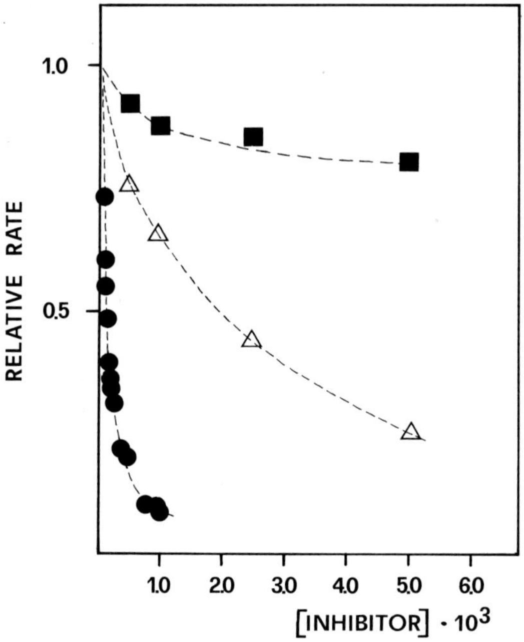
1.0
0.5
RELATIVE RATE
1.0 2.0 3.0 4.0 5.0 6.0
[INHIBITOR] · 10³

1

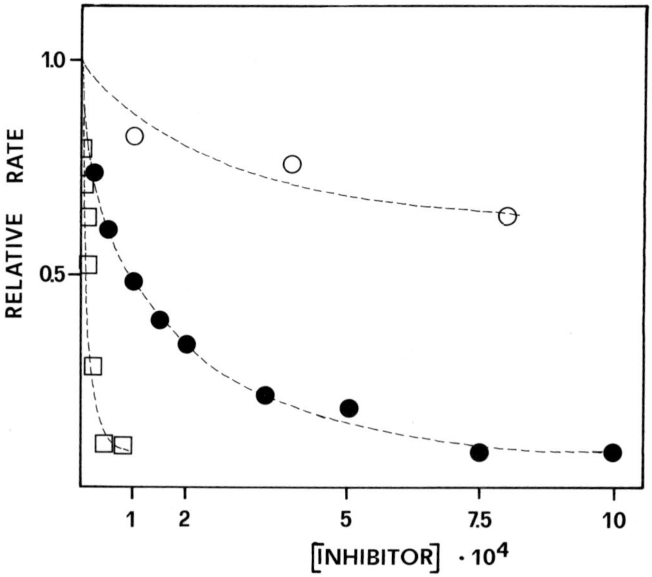
1.0
0.5
RELATIVE RATE
1 2 5 7.5 10
[INHIBITOR] · 10⁴

2

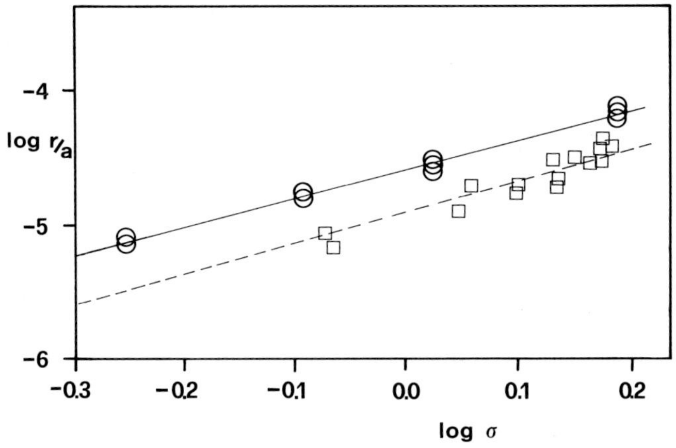

Fig. 3. See text. The data are collected at different total calcium and oxalate concentration, and at different amounts of added seeds, T = 37 °C, pH = 6.2–6.4, NaCl = 0.15 mol l^{-1}. ○ = Without additives; □ = different citrate concentrations added.

The effect of the reported inhibitors can be mainly attributed to the first explanation. In fact the calculation of the concentration of the species in solution, when organic acids or magnesium ions are present, allows one to attribute the decrease in crystal growth rate mainly to the reduction in the activity of free calcium and oxalate ions (with consequent decrease of the supersaturation), due to complexation. The effect of these compounds was already reported in the literature [4], and their use in the therapy is actively under study [8].

The detailed analysis of the data with citric acid has been carried out in order to assess the contribution of calcium complexation and of surface phenomena to the overall inhibition process. Figure 3 shows the data in

---

Fig. 1. Relative growth rate as a function of the molar inhibitor concentration. ■ = Aspartic acid; △ = tartaric acid; ● = citric acid. Experimental conditions: total calcium and oxalate concentration $5 \cdot 10^{-4}$ mol l^{-1}, T = 37 °C, pH = 6.2–6.4, NaCl = 0.15 mol l^{-1}, added seeds 50 mg.

Fig. 2. Relative growth rate as a function of the molar inhibitor concentration. ○ = Magnesium ion; ● = citrate ion; □ = pyrophosphate ion. Experimental conditions as in figure 1.

the presence of citric acid compared with those in the absence of additives for the crystal growth of COM. Plots of log(r/a) as a function of log σ at different concentrations of seeds and of calcium and oxalate ions are reported according to equation 1:

$$r = K_{so}\, k_g a\, \sigma^n, \tag{1}$$

where k_g is the specific growth rate, is the observed rate, a the surface area of seeds, n the order of the reaction, K_{so} the thermodynamic solubility product, and σ the relative supersaturation. For COM:

$$\sigma = ([a_{Ca}\, a_{Ox}]^{1/2} - K_{so}{}^{1/2})/(K_{so}{}^{1/2}). \tag{2}$$

The activities of all the species present in solution are calculated from mass balance and electroneutrality expressions, using the Debye-Huckel equation proposed by Davies [9] and computer-assisted iterative algebraic methods which involve successive approximations to the ionic strength. In the computer program any kind of growth reaction and of additives can be introduced without software changes. The data for the equilibrium constants of formation of the species present in solution, the stoichiometric coefficients for each kind of equilibrium, and the analytical concentrations are introduced in a matrix form. For all calcium and oxalate complexes and ion pairs, the equilibrium constants are taken from Nancollas and co-workers [10, 11].

According to equation 1 the slopes in figure 3 are 2.0–2.1, thus indicating in both cases a surface-controlled mechanism. The intercepts give the specific rate constants k_g of growth for COM, namely 1.1×10^4 and 5.8×10^3 l $mol^{-1}min^{-1}$ m^{-2} in the presence of citrate. The value for COM is slightly different from that reported by White et al. [11]; the discrepancy could be attributed to the slightly different values of the equilibrium stability constants used in the calculation of the relative supersaturation. However, the value of k_g shows that citrate ions have a moderate action of specific inhibition in addition to the most relevant complexation effect.

Figure 4 reports the relative rate observed in the presence of pyrophosphate at two different pHs. Since the effect of inhibition can be observed at a concentration of one hundredth of that of calcium ion, the pyrophosphate is then acting as a crystal poison. It is noteworthy that the concentration of pyrophosphate in the urine is of the same order of magnitude of that reported in figure 4.

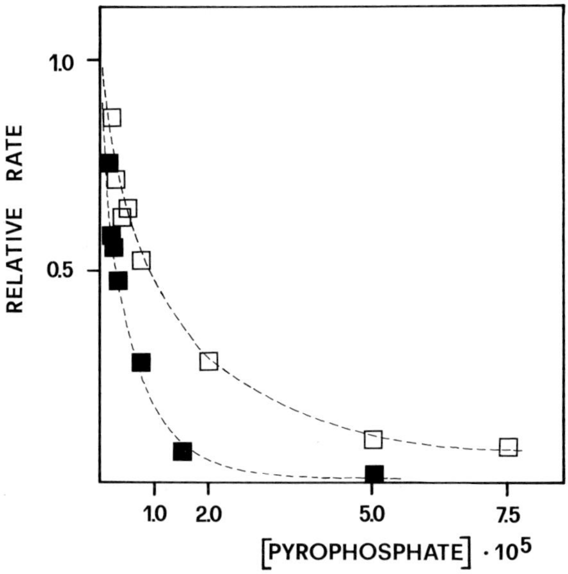

Fig. 4. Relative growth rate as a function of molar concentration of pyrophosphate at two different pH. Other experimental conditions as in figure 1. □ = pH 6.2–6.3; ■ = pH 8.0.

The dependence on pH suggests that the most ionized form of pyrophosphate is responsible for the inhibition. The explanation of the results of figure 4 in terms of a Langmuir adsorption isotherm is not satisfactory, suggesting that other processes, instead of the growth of COM, have to be considered.

A hypothesis could be a relevant inhibition of growth of COM with concomitant growth of the metastable trihydrate form (COT). This suggestion is in agreement with the data reported by Gardner [12], who investigated the nucleation and growth of calcium oxalate crystals by means of another experimental technique. In fact, in the case of COT, the relative supersaturation in the present experimental conditions is much lower than that for COM; as a consequence, according to equation 1 the overall rate is significantly lowered. The same explanation can be given for the difference observed in k_g in the case of citrate inhibition. In that case the growth of the dihydrated metastable phase seems to be the most kinetically favored.

In conclusion, the inhibitor effect of a series of low molecular weight additives on the crystal growth rate of COM has received large attention in the literature. The experimental results obtained with CCT here reported permit one to estimate the efficiency of these compounds as inhibitors, and to formulate some hypothesis about the mechanism of growth.

References

1 Robertson, W. G.; Scurr, D. S.; Bridge, C. M.: Factor influencing the crystallization of calcium oxalate in urine. Critique. J. Crystal Growth *53:* 182–194 (1981).

2 Sutor, D. J.: Growth studies of calcium oxalate in the presence of various ions and compounds. Br. J. Urol. *41:* 171 (1969).

3 Welshman, S. G.; McGeown, M. G.: A quantitative investigation of the effect on the growth of calcium oxalate crystals of potential inhibitors. Br. J. Urol. *44:* 677 (1972).

4 Rodgers, A. L.; Garside, J.: The nucleation and growth kinetics of calcium oxalate in the presence of some synthetic urine constituents. Investve Urol. *18:* 484–489 (1981).

5 Rizkalla, E. M.; Moawad, M. M.: Kinetics of the crystallization of calcium oxalate monohydrated. J. chem. Soc. Faraday Trans. I *80:* 1617–1629 (1984).

6 Sheehan, M. E.; Nancollas, G. H.: Calcium oxalate crystal growth: a new constant composition method for modelling urinary stone formation. Investve Urol. *17:* 446–450 (1980).

7 Lanzalaco, A. C.; Sheehan, M. E.; White, D. J.; Nancollas, G. H.: The mineralization inhibitory potential of urines: a constant composition approach. J. Urol. *128:* 845–849 (1982).

8 Pak, C. Y. C.; Preminger, G. M.; Harvey, Y. A.: Comparative efficacy of specific potassium citrate therapy versus conservative management in nephrolithiasis of mild to moderate severity. J. Urol. *134:* 658–661 (1985).

9 Nancollas, G. H.: Interactions in electrolyte solutions (Elsevier, Amsterdam 1966).

10 Nancollas, G. H.; Gardner, G. L.: Kinetics of crystal growth of calcium oxalate monohydrated. J. Crystal Growth *21:* 267–276 (1974).

11 White, D. J.; Christoffersen, J.; Herman, T. S.; Lanzalaco, A. C.; Nancollas, G. H.: Effect of urine pretreatment on calcium oxalate crystallization inhibition potentials. J. Urol. *129:* 175–179 (1983).

12 Gardner, G. L.: Effect of pyrophosphate and phosphonate anions on the crystal growth kinetics of calcium oxalate hydrates. J. chem. Physiol. *82:* 864–869 (1978).

13 Free, A. H.; Free, H. M.: Urinalysis in clinical laboratory practice (CRC Press, Cleveland 1975).

14 Fleisch, H.; Bisaz, S.: Isolation from urine of pyrophosphate, a calcification inhibitor. Am. J. Physiol. *203:* 671–675 (1962).

Prof. E. Pelizzetti, MD, Dipartimento di Chimica Analitica, via P. Giuria 5, I–10125 Torino (Italy)

Contr. Nephrol., vol. 58, pp. 73–77 (Karger, Basel 1987)

Low Inhibition of Crystal Agglomeration and Citrate Excretion in Recurrent Calcium Oxalate Stone Formers

D. J. Kok, S. E. Papapoulos, O. L. M. Bijvoet[1]

Clinical Investigation Unit, Department of Endocrinology,
University Hospital, Leiden, The Netherlands

It is generally accepted that calcium oxalate renal stone formation is the result of physicochemical processes promoted by abnormal urine composition [1]. Separation, however, of stone formers from healthy persons on the basis of a single physicochemical parameter has been difficult mainly because of lack of methods capable to differentiate between the various processes involved in crystallization. These include solubility, crystal growth and agglomeration. We have developed a method which allows the independent measurement of each one of these processes and we have applied it to the study of renal stone disease. Examination of the urines of a group of calcium oxalate stone formers with high stone production rate revealed loss of the ability to inhibit crystal agglomeration inherent in normal urine. This defect was associated with hypocitraturia and correction of the latter with alkali led to recovery of the ability to inhibit agglomeration.

Patients and Methods

Calcium, phosphate, creatinine, magnesium, oxalate and uric acid were measured by automated techniques and citrate by an enzymatic method [2]. Precautions were taken to prevent bacterial growth which is known to affect urinary citrate measurements and all subjects studied had sterile urine cultures. The separate effects of urines on the crystallization parameters were tested in vitro as previously described [3–5]. Crystal growth inhibition is expressed as the percent reduction of the growth constant derived from a control experiment

[1] We thank Mr. I. Lintang for expert technical assistance. These studies were supported by a generous grant from the Dutch Kidney Foundation.

and solubility and agglomeration are expressed as absolute values. Normal ranges are: growth inhibition 57.4–92%, solubility 0.244–0.429 m*M*, agglomeration inhibition 152–510 min.

Six recurrent calcium oxalate stone formers with a stone production rate between 5 and > 50 stones per year and absence of hypercalciuria or hyperoxaluria were studied. All had normal renal function and could acidify their urine appropriately apart from one patient in whom the lowest pH obtained during a short NH_4Cl loading test was 5.45.

Results

Crystal growth inhibition was found within the normal range in all 6 patients (range 56–82.6%). Solubility was significantly decreased in the stone formers but some overlap with the normal range was observed (range 0.178–0.263 m*M*). A highly significant ($p < 0.001$) difference in agglomeration inhibition between normal subjects and stone formers was found with all patients having abnormally low values (range 59.9–95.1 min).

All patients had normal urinary excretion rates of calcium, phosphate, magnesium, oxalate and uric acid. Urinary citrate excretion, however, was below the lower limit of normal in all (range 1.04–2.06 mmol/24 h; normal range 2.12–8.42 mmol/24 h).

To examine further if there was a physicochemical basis for the relation between citrate and agglomeration inhibition, gradually increasing concentrations of citrate were added in vitro to the urine of one patient. This had a remarkable effect on agglomeration inhibition which became normal concomitantly with the normalization of the citrate concentration (range 90.7–213.3 min). There was no effect on crystal growth inhibition but some increase in solubility was also observed.

The patients were also followed during treatment with alkali (Na/K citrate, sodium or potassium bicarbonate) for periods between 8 and 24 months. Treatment resulted in a significant increase in urinary citrate excretion which became normal in all patients (range 2.20–6.35 mmol/24 h) and had no effect on the other biochemical parameters. The rise in urinary citrate excretion was the same independently of the form of alkali used (fig. 1). Measurement of the crystallization parameters revealed a significant increase ($p < 0.001$) in agglomeration inhibition which became normal in all but one of the patients (fig. 2). No effect on solubility was found and there was some increase in crystal growth inhibition but within the normal range. Urine volume did not change significantly during treatment. The physicochemical and biochemical improvement was associated with a favourable clinical response with complete cessation or reduction of stone production in all patients.

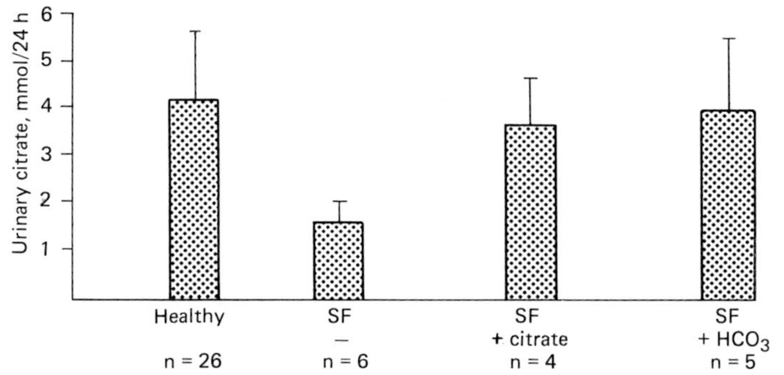

Fig. 1. Urinary citrate excretion (mean ± SD) in healthy subjects and stone formers (SF) before and after treatment with Na/K citrate and sodium or potassium bicarbonate. Four patients were initially treated with citrate and 3 of them continued later with bicarbonate. Two patients received only bicarbonate.

Discussion

Agglomeration of calcium oxalate crystals may be a critical process in renal stone formation. Microscopic examination of an average stone shows clearly an agglomerate structure and it is well known that stone formers excrete more and larger agglomerates than normals for the same degree of crystalluria [6]. However, it has been impossible to investigate the role of agglomeration in the pathogenesis of renal stone disease mainly because of lack of methods for its direct measurement. With the development of the methodology for the independent measurement of the crystallization parameters and its application to clinical practice, we have been able to show that a pronounced loss of the ability to inhibit agglomeration was the main physicochemical abnormality in the urines of a group of recurrent calcium oxalate stone formers [7]. This was associated in all patients with marked hypocitraturia and normalization of the citrate concentrations either in vitro or in vivo led to recovery of the ability to inhibit agglomeration. Thus, our studies strongly suggest that agglomeration inhibition is mainly a citrate-mediated process and provide the link between a disturbed physicochemical parameter and abnormal urine composition in calcium oxalate stone formation.

Restoration of urinary citrate excretion to normal with potassium citrate has been recently shown in large groups of stone formers with hypocitraturia [8]. We have confirmed this and we have also shown that bicarbo-

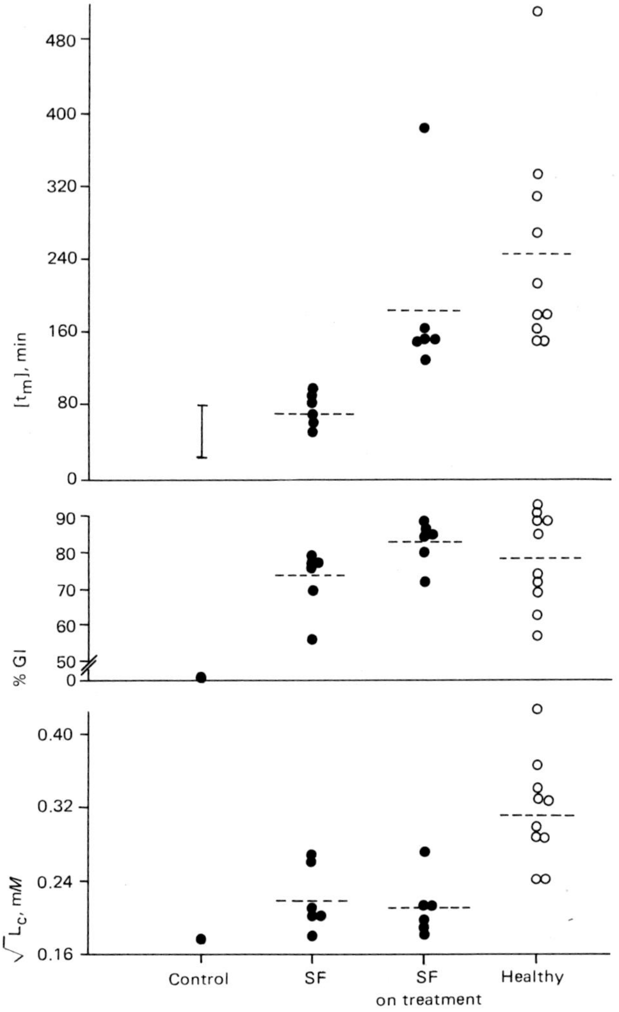

Fig. 2. The effects of alkali therapy on agglomeration inhibition $[t_m]$, growth inhibition (GI) and solubility $\sqrt{L_c}$ of calcium oxalate crystals in 6 calcium oxalate stone formers (SF).

nate is equally effective in correcting hypocitraturia. This suggests that an intrinsic defect in citrate metabolism is unlikely and that other causes for the low citrate excretion must be sought. The alkali-induced increase in urinary citrate is not due to alkalinization of the urine per se as it is known that hypocitraturia occurs even in the presence of alkaline urine when this is associated with systematic acidosis either experimentally produced (acetazolamide) or genetically determined (renal tubular acidosis) [9, for review]. It may be that alkali therapy changes the mitochondrial pH gradient, thus slowing down the mitochondrial uptake of citrate and, therefore, leading to its accumulation in the cytoplasm and reduction of its uptake by the cell. In this way utilization and absorption of citrate are diminished and it appears in the urine. This attractive hypothesis which has been proposed by Simpson [9], however needs confirmation.

Independently of its mode of action, alkali therapy had a favourable physicochemical, biochemical and clinical effect. Stone production rate although clearly decreased did not completely arrest in all patients indicating that there may be other factors which can modulate the effects of citrate on crystal agglomeration. These as well as the factors affecting solubility, which as shown here are probably not citrate-mediated, warrant further investigation. Our methods provide the means for that.

References

1 Blomen, L.J.M.J.; Bijvoet, O.L.M.: Physicochemical considerations in relation to urinary stone formation. Wld J. Urol. *1:* 119–125 (1983).

2 Moellering, H.; Gruber, W.: Determination of citrate with citrate lyase. Analyt. Biochem. *17:* 369–376 (1966).

3 Will, E.J.; Bijvoet, O.L.M.; Blomen, L.J.M.J.; Linden, H. v.d.: Growth kinetics of calcium oxalate monohydrate. I. J. Crystal Growth *64:* 297–305 (1983).

4 Blomen, L.J.M.J.; Will, E.J.; Bijvoet, O.L.M.; Linden, H. v.d.: Growth kinetics of calcium oxalate monohydrate. II. J. Crystal Growth *64:* 306–315 (1983).

5 Bijvoet, O.L.M.; Blomen, L.J.M.J.; Will, E.J.; Linden, H. v.d.: Growth kinetics of calcium oxalate monohydrate. III. J. Crystal Growth *64:* 316–325 (1983).

6 Robertson, W.G.; Peacock, M.; Nordin, B.E.C.: Calcium crystalluria in recurrent renal-stone formers. Lancet *ii:* 21–24 (1969).

7 Kok, D.J.; Papapoulos, S.E.; Bijvoet, O.L.M.: Excessive crystal agglomeration with low citrate excretion in recurrent stone formers. Lancet *i:* 1056–1058 (1986).

8 Pak, C.Y.C.; Fuller, C.; Sakhaee, K.; Preminger, G.M.; Britton, F.: Long-term treatment of calcium nephrolithiasis with potassium citrate. J. Urol. *134:* 11–19 (1985).

9 Simpson, D.P.: Citrate excretion: a window on renal metabolism. Am. J. Physiol. *244* (Renal Fluid Electrolyte Physiol., 13): F223–234 (1983).

S.E. Papapoulos MD, Clinical Investigation Unit, Department of Endocrinology, University Hospital, Rijnsburgerweg 10, NL–2333 AA Leiden (The Netherlands)

Contr. Nephrol., vol. 58, pp. 78–81 (Karger, Basel 1987)

A Study of Crystalluria in Calcium Oxalate Stone Patients Treated with Thiazides

M. Daudon[a], *P. Jungers*[b], *R. J. Reveillaud*[a]

[a]Laboratoire Cristal, Hôpital de Saint-Cloud, Saint-Cloud;
[b]Service de Néphrologie, CHU Necker, Paris, France

Crystalluria is the consequence of supersaturation in one or several solutes exceeding urine inhibitory capacities. Its study has not yet been applied in the exploration and the follow-up of stone patients. This is for a number of reasons: the first being methodological difficulties both in the collecting and preserving of urine, and their examination. The second concerns technical selection due to there being more than one method: evaporation test, membrane filtration, direct examination, whose results and standards cannot be compared. There is also a third reason: the choice of urine sample which varies night and day in composition, volume and supersaturation with subsequent variations of crystalluria.

Having unanimously agreed on a higher frequency of crystalluria in stone patients rather than in normal subjects, we were interested in its study before and after treatment. We selected calcium stone formers treated or not with thiazides in order to determine a criterion of therapeutic efficiency.

Material and Methods

We examined the first morning urine of 136 calcium oxalate (CaOx) stone formers, treated for over 2 months with thiazides (hydrochlorothiazide 25–50 mg/day; TzL) and compared them to 78 urines of the same type of patients untreated by thiazides (ToL).

Fresh urines were examined under a polarizing microscope less than 2 h after collection and kept at room temperature. If crystalluria was present, urine was centrifuged and the dried sediment was analysed by infrared spectroscopy (IR). Furthermore, urines or supernatants were kept at + 4 °C and re-examined 48 h later by the same process.

Table I. Crystalluria phases in fresh urine

%	Wd	Wh	Wd + Wh[a]	Ph Ca	Ur Ac
ToL	32.1	7.7	37.2	19.4	2.8
TzL	28.7	12.5	34.6	12.5	2.9
N	6.25	0	0	6.2	3.1

[a] These results include mixed crystalluria.
Wd = Weddellite; Wh = whewellite; Ph Ca = calcium phosphates; Ur Ac = uric acid and amorphous urates.

Table II. Crystalline phases in urine kept 48 h at 4 °C

%	Wd	Wh	Ph Ca	Ur Ac
ToL	84.6	6.4	17.9	23.1
TzL	76.5	12.5	18.4	17.6
N	34.4	0	3.1	15.6

Results

In urine kept at room temperature crystalluria was observed in 9.4% of 38 normal subjects, 46.2% of ToL patients, and 41.2% of TzL patients. Crystalline phases are given in table I; we observed a slight decrease in CaOx dihydrate (Wd) crystalluria, and a slight increase of CaOx monohydrate (Wh) in TzL patients. We never observed Wh crystalluria in normal subjects. On the whole, oxalic crystalluria in lithiasic patients is significantly higher than in normal subjects; it decreases only slightly in TzL as already published by Rose [1]. We observed 19.6% of Wh in ToL female patients and 3.8% in ToL male patients ($p < 0.05$) as we previously reported concerning CaOx stone composition [2]. Calcium phosphate crystalluria decreased in TzL but remained significantly higher than in normal subjects. Uric acid crystalline phases had no significant variations in this examination of fresh urine. Crystalline phases in urine after 48 h at + 4 °C temperature are given in table II. Crystalluria rose in both groups: 37.5% in normal subjects, 96.1% of ToL and 83.8% of TzL. Crystalline phases increased strikingly for Wd, but was unchanged for calcium phosphates. Uric acid crystalluria increased significantly more in ToL (2.8–23.1%) than in TzL (2.9–17.6%).

Discussion

Our results show in lithiasic patients a higher crystalluria than in normal subjects. They appear to be lower compared to other publications [3, 4]. This may be due to the fact that the urines we examined were without concentration and that very low crystalluria with small crystals was not taken into account. In an attempt to appreciate the different constituents of the supersatured phases, we examined the urine stored at 4 °C for 48 h. It appeared that phosphates and Wh crystallization remained unchanged while Wd and uric acid crystallization increased dramatically and revealed the latent phase of supersaturation. In our experience, oxalate crystallization develops to the advantage of Wd as the Ca/Ox ratio rises progressively. In fact, calcium urine concentration is usually much higher than that of oxalate. Each part of a CaOx crystallized mole induces a proportionately more important reduction in oxalate concentration than in calcium concentration, thus resulting in a progressive increase of the Ca/Ox ratio.

The crystalline phase appears when Ca/Ox < 6 (i.e. with relative hyperoxaluria) is only Wh. If the Ca/Ox ratio is > 14 (i.e. hypercalciuria), the crystalline phase is, in contrast, always Wd.

On the other hand, if we followed the progression of crystalline phases in urine which initially contained a very high oxalate concentration, we observed that the first crystalline phase was Wh. Then the second phase was Wd which represented an ever-increasing proportion of the crystals, in relation with the elevation of the Ca/Ox ratio. We have already reported that Wh was rather oxalate-dependent and Wd calcium-dependent [5].

Under TzL treatment calciuria decreases and in some cases oxaluria increases slightly, which may account for the increased frequency of Wh crystals observed in TzL. Moreover, in 4 °C TzL urine we observed a net decrease of urate crystallization with regard to ToL, approaching the normal range.

TzL efficiency does not seem to be the result of a drop in CaOx crystalluria but rather the result of both decreased urine calcium content and decreased urate supersaturation. Brocks et al. [6] already mentioned a decrease of uric acid excretion in TzL patients.

In conclusion, the study of crystalluria in lithiasic patients allows us to determine the behaviour of the different crystalline phases depending on diet and therapy. Crystalluria under thiazides does not seem markedly decreased in our experience, though it does for other authors. But in any case the crystalline phase identification reveals the state of supersaturation all along the different treatments. Prospective and comparative studies will perhaps enable us to answer the question: Are the best results obtained from drugs which most diminish supersaturation?

References

1 Hallson, P.C.; Rose, G.A.: Crystalluria in normal subjects and in stone formers with and without thiazide and cellulose phosphate treatment. Br. J. Urol. *48:* 515–524 (1976).

2 Daudon, M.; Protat, M.F.; Reveillaud, R.J.; Rouchon, M.: Etude de la cristallurie spontanée par spectroscopie infrarouge. Recherche de correlations entre les cristaux – les calculs – les germes et le sexe des malades. Annls Biol. clin. *41:* 199–207 (1983).

3 Caudarella, R.; Malavolta, N.; Cavallari, E.; Rizzoli, E.; Stefani, F.; D'Antuono, G.: Is crystalluria a screening test for idiopathic calcium lithiasis? Proc. 3rd Int. Symp. on Recent Advances in Pathogenesis and Treatment of Nephrolithiasis, Turin 1986 (in press).

4 Werness, P.G.; Bergert, J.H.; Smith, L.H.: Crystalluria. J. Crystal Growth *53:* 166–181 (1981).

5 Daudon, M.; Reveillaud, R.J.: Typage morphologique des calculs oxalocalciques et données étiopathogeniques. Annls Urol. *19:* 299–308 (1985).

6 Brocks, P.; Christiansen, C.; Dirksen, H.; Transbol, I.; Wolf, H.: Effect of thiazides on the urinary calcium oxalate stone-forming potential in normal males. Scand. J. Urol. Nephrol. *17:* 325–328 (1983).

M. Daudon, MD, Laboratoire Cristal, Hôpital de Saint-Cloud,
F–92211 Saint-Cloud (France)

Contr. Nephrol., vol. 58, pp. 82–84 (Karger, Basel 1987)

Indices of Lithogenic Activity in Patients with Primitive Calcium Oxalate Urolithiasis

A. Cupisti, F. Ciardella, E. Morelli, S. Lupetti, S. Luchi, F. Niosi, A. Fosso, A. Carlini, M. Meola, G. Barsotti

Clinica Medica I, Università degli Studi, Pisa, Italia

The discrimination between recurrent calcium-oxalate stone formers (RSF) and single stone formers (SSF) is of critical value for the prognosis and preventive therapy. In this retrospective study we tried to detect any correlation between the clinical lithogenic activity and the urinary excretion of some inhibitors or promoters of stone formation [1].

Materials and Methods

23 RSF (21 males and 2 females), 23–56 years old, 14 SSF (9 males and 5 females) aging between 28 and 46 years, and 16 normal volunteers (11 males and 5 females), 28–44 years old were studied. In all the patients we evaluated the 24-h urinary excretion of calcium (uCa), uric acid (uU), oxalic acid (uOx), citrate (uCit), magnesium (uMg), glycosaminoglycans (uGAG) and daily urinary volume (uV). In addition, the following indices of lithogenic activity were calculated: uOx/uCit and uOx·uCa/uCit·uGAG.

uOx and uCit were determined by enzymatic assays [2, 3], uGAG by Alcian blue 8GS procedure [4], and the other parameters by routine laboratory methods. The statistical analysis of the results was performed by means of Student's t-test for unpaired data.

Results

The results are shown in figure 1. A significant statistical difference was found between RSF and SSF for uCit (2.13 ± 0.93 vs 3.26 ± 0.88 mmol/day, respectively; $p < 0.001$) and uOx (30.3 ± 8.0 vs 22.9 ± 4.9 mg/day; $p < 0.005$). In normals uCit (3.37 ± 0.02 mmol/day) and uOx

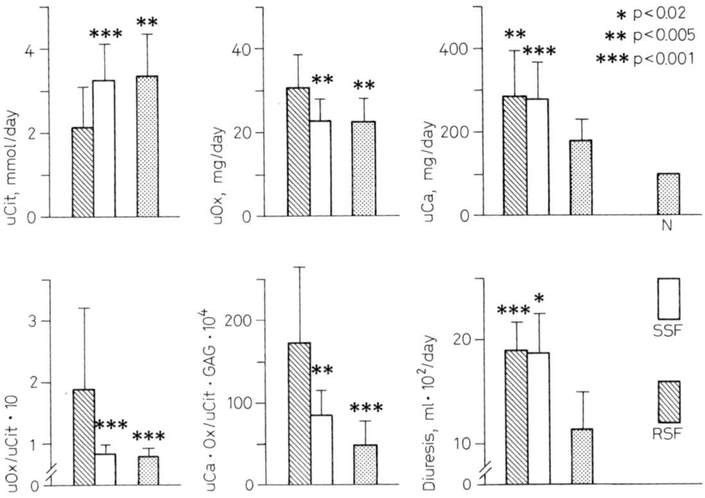

Fig. 1. The behaviour of some urinary risk factors and indices in RSF, SSF and normals (mean ± SD).

(22.7 ± 5.6 mg/day) were similar to SSF, while an evident statistical difference was found versus RSF (fig. 1).

RSF and SSF did not differ for uCa (284.6 ± 109.9 vs 283.7 ± 83.3 mg/day) while both groups showed higher uCa levels than normals (182.2 ± 49.7 mg/day; $p < 0.005$ and $p < 0.001$, respectively); uV also showed a similar behaviour (fig. 1).

uOx/uCit was higher in RSF than either in SSF (1.903 ± 1.303 vs 0.836 ± 0.414; $p < 0.001$) or in normals (0.819 ± 0.256; $p < 0.001$), just like the uCa·uOx/uCit·uGAG ratio (172.8 ± 90.0 vs. 84.6 ± 30.6, $p < 0.005$ and vs 46.6 ± 26.8, $p < 0.001$, respectively). None of the studied groups differed in regard to uU and uMg.

Discussion

These results suggest that hypercalciuria is a less important factor than high levels of uOx or low levels of uCit for the evaluation of lithogenic activity in patients with primitive calcium oxalate stone disease. Furthermore, uOx/uCit and uOx·uCa/uCit·uGAG ratios may be useful to this aim, just pointing out the promoters-inhibitors imbalance that is present in the recurrent calcium oxalate stone disease.

The failure of thiazide preventive therapy in some RSF [5] may be explained by our results. In fact uCit may be lowered by thiazides [6] and uOx is not often modified while the hypocalciuric effect is largely proved [7].

References

1 Fleish, H.: Inhibitors and promoters of stones. Kidney int. *13:* 361–375 (1978).

2 Chiriboga, J.: Some properties of an oxalic oxidase purified from barley seedlings. Biochem. biophys. Res. Commun. *11:* 277–290 (1963).

3 Tompkins, D.; Toffaletti, J.: Enzymic determination of citrate in serum and urine, with use of the Worthington 'Ultrafree' device. Clin. Chem. *28:* 192–196 (1982).

4 Gold, E. W.: A simple spectrophotometric method for estimating glycosaminoglycan concentrations. Analyt. Biochem. *99:* 183–191 (1979).

5 Churchill, D. N.; Taylor, D. W.: Thiazides for patients with recurrent calcium stones: still an open question. J. Urol. *133:* 749–751 (1985).

6 Nicar, M. J.; Peterson, R.; Pak, C. Y. C.: Use of potassium citrate as potassium supplement during thiazide therapy of calcium nephrolithiasis. J. Urol. *131:* 430–433 (1984).

7 Yendt, E. R.; Cohanim, M.: Prevention of calcium stones with thiazides. Kidney int. *13:* 397–409 (1978).

Prof. Giuliano Barsotti, MD, Clinica Medica I, Università degli Studi,
I–56100 Pisa (Italy)

Contr. Nephrol., vol. 58, pp. 85–88 (Karger, Basel 1987)

Enzymatic and Ion Chromatographic Measurement of Urinary Oxalate

A Method Comparison Study

A. Classen, A. Hesse

Urologische Universitätsklinik, Bonn, FRG

Concentration of urinary oxalate is the most powerful predictor of calcium oxalate (CaOx) urolithiasis. Since in 60–70% of all urinary concrements CaOx is a major component, urinary oxalate should be determined routinely in case of stone forming patients. Suppressed ion chromatography is thought to be an excellent method of measuring urinary oxalate. However, this technique needs very expensive technical equipment which is not available in every laboratory. The aim of the present study therefore was to prove whether a recently adapted commercially available enzymatic test kit could be a reliable and suitable alternative.

Material and Methods

Ion Chromatographic Procedure

A system 2000 i (Dionex, FRG) was used which was equipped with a 50-μl sample loop, a NG1 guard column, an AS4 separator column, and an AF1 suppressor column. The sensitivity of the conductivity monitor was set to 1 μS full scale. The eluent used was the standard eluent for anion chromatography, containing 2.8 mmol/l $NaHCO_3$ and 2.2 mmol/l Na_2CO_3. The flow rate was adjusted to 1.6 ml/min with regard to baseline noise. Sample preparation was carried out as suggested by Robertson and Scurr [4].

Enzymatic Procedure

For sample preparation 20 ml of urine were adjusted to pH 1 with HCl, 10 mg EDTA were added, and the samples were heated for 15 min at 80 °C in a water bath. After cooling down to room temperature the pH was adjusted to 5 with NaOH. Ascorbic acid was checked by using a test stick (Behringwerke, Marburg, FRG) since it interferes with the enzymatic assay if its concentration exceeds 0.6 mmol/l. If necessary ascorbate was very easily removed by an ascorbate-oxidase spatula (Boehringer Mannheim, FRG). 0.2 ml of the sample pretreated as described above was analyzed with the enzymatic test kit No. 755 699 (Boehringer Mannheim), which utilizes the coupled reaction of oxalate decarboxylase and formate dehydrogenase.

Method Comparison Experiments

Within-run imprecision was estimated by analyzing 3 urine samples 20 times each, and calculating the coefficient of variation as a measure of imprecision. To estimate total imprecision 3 urine samples were analyzed over a 10-day period by duplicate measurements (a, b). From the b values the coefficient variation was calculated. To estimate absolute accuracy a recovery experiment was carried out. 20 urine samples were spiked with 0.2 mmol/l sodium oxalate, and both the baseline samples and the spiked samples were analyzed in 4 replicates, and the mean values were used to calculate recovery. Relative accuracy was estimated by performing duplicate measurements (a, b) on 80 urine samples by both methods and calculating a regression line using the non-parametric procedure of Passing and Bablock [2, 3].

Results and Discussion

The maximum values for within-run imprecision were 1.9% for the chromatographic and 5.3 for the enzymatic procedure. The corresponding values for total imprecision were 5.3% (chromatography) and 8% (enzymatic assay). In both methods imprecision was found to increase with lower concentrations and it was – probably due to the manual procedure – higher in the enzymatic assay. The recovery of 0.2 mmol/l NaOx was very close to 100% for both methods (table I). The results of the parallel measurements of 80 urine samples show that both methods compare excellently. Neither was the slope of the regression line calculated significantly different from 1 nor was the intercept from 0 (fig. 1). From this it has to be concluded that both methods gave identical results in our experiment.

In our opinion one reason for the good reliability of the enzymatic assay and its agreement with the chromatographic procedure is that separation of oxalate prior to analysis is not necessary and, by this, a main source of error is avoided. Therefore, we think that the assay used here is much more advantageous than another well-known commercially available test kit, which utilizes the enzyme oxalate oxidase, as in the latter oxalate has to be separated before enzymatic analysis [1].

From the results of our experiments we conclude that the enzymatic assay used here is a valuable and reliable alternative if the ion chromatographic technique – for any reason – is not available.

Table I. Recovery experiment

Statistics	Chromatographic	Enzymatic
$\overline{X}$	100.9	98.7
SD	4.54	5.09
CV (%)	4.5	5.2
Minimum value	93.5	90.5
Maximum value	108.5	106.5

$\overline{X}$ = Mean; SD = standard deviation; CV (%) = coefficient of variation in percent.

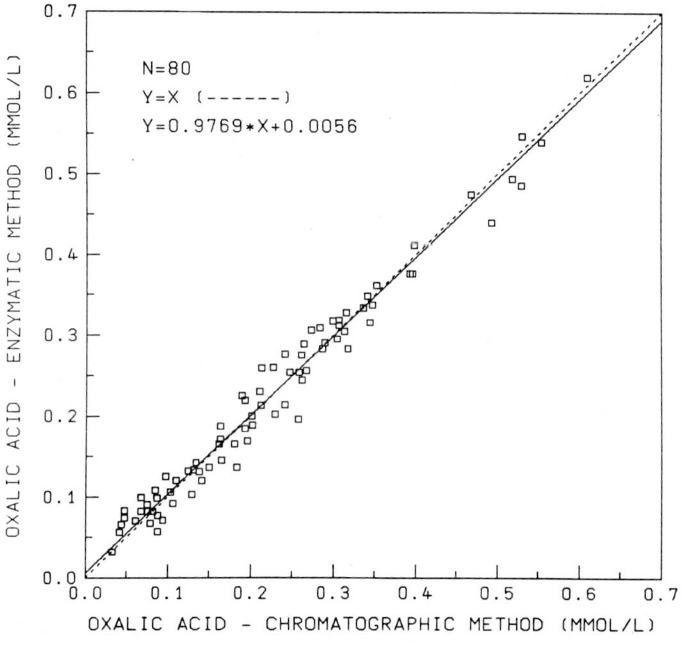

Fig. 1. Comparative analysis of 80 urine samples; identity line (dotted) and regression line.

References

1 Bishop, M.; Freudiger, H.; Largiader, U.; Sallis, J.D.; Felix, R.; Fleisch, H.: Conductivometric determination of urinary oxalate with oxalate decarboxylase. Urol. Res. *10:* 191–194 (1982).

2 Passing, H.; Bablock, W.: A new biometrical procedure for testing the equality of measurements from two different analytical methods. Application of linear regression procedures for method comparison studies in clinical chemistry. Part I. J. clin. Chem. clin. Biochem. *21:* 709–720 (1983).

3 Passing, H.; Bablock, W.: Comparison of several regression procedures for method comparison studies and determination of sample sizes. Application of linear regression procedures for method comparison studies in clinical chemistry. Part II. J. clin. Chem. clin. Biochem. *22:* 431–445 (1984).

4 Robertson, W.G.; Scurr, D.S.: Prevention of ascorbic interference in the measurement of oxalic acid in urine by ion-chromatography. Clinical chim. Acta *140:* 97–99 (1984).

A. Classen, MD, Urologische Universitätsklinik Bonn,
Sigmund-Freud-Strasse 25, D–5300 Bonn 1 (FRG)

Contr. Nephrol., vol. 58, pp. 89–92 (Karger, Basel 1987)

New in vitro Methodological Approaches to GAG Study in Idiopathic Calcium Lithiasis

R. Caudarella[a], *L. Simonelli*[b], *V. Vasi*[b], *E. Rizzoli*[a], *N. Malavolta*[a], *F. Stefani*[a], *R. Cappelletti*[c]

Istituti di [a]Patologia Medica II e [b]Istologia, Università di Bologna, [c]Istituto Patologia Generale, Università Firenze, Italia

Several authors have pointed out that stone formers present a decrease of glycosaminoglycan (GAG) concentration and/or excretion in urine. In previous studies we found similar results in our patients as well as a reduction of GAG excretion below the normal range in about 34% of all cases [1, 2]. In order to evaluate a possible sulphated GAG metabolism impairment a study in vitro was performed on skin fibroblasts derived from patients affected by idiopathic calcium lithiasis and healthy subjects.

Materials and Methods

Our study included 3 normal subjects and 3 patients affected by idiopathic calcium lithiasis with GAG excretion below the normal range. A skin biopsy was performed in both groups.

Cell Culture

The cells cultured in D-MEM (minimal essential medium) supplemented with 10% fetal calf serum and penicillin-streptomycin were kept at 37 °C in a humid atmosphere 5% CO_2 and 95% air. Cultured fibroblasts have been passed less than 10 times since isolation; then they were cultured in Corning's flasks T-70 until a semi-confluent growth occurred. At this step the culture medium was substituted with fresh synthetic medium (without sulphate) supplemented with 5% fetal calf serum and Na_2SO_4 labelled with ^{35}S (4 μCi/ml). To evaluate the uptake of Na_2 ($^{35}SO_4$) pulse fibroblasts were maintained for 70 h under the same conditions previously described. After this period the culture medium labelled with Na_2 ($^{35}SO_4$) was exchanged by fresh D-MEM, containing inorganic sulphate, in order to measure the chase.

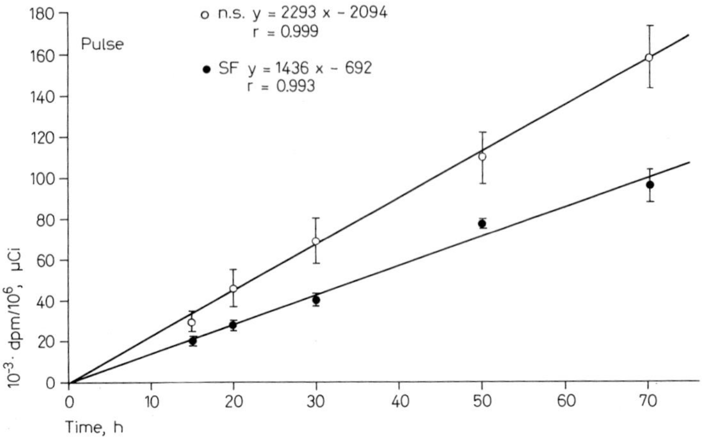

Fig. 1. Na_2 ($^{35}SO_4$) incorporation into normal (○) and stone-forming (●) subjects' fibroblasts.

Analysis of $^{35}SO_4$-Labelled Cell Cultures

The cell layers were removed by an enzymatic procedure (trypsin/EDTA). The fibroblasts, washed three times and centrifuged (10 min at 900 *g*), were suspended in 0.5 ml of 1 *M* NH_3-1% Triton X-100, and finally sonicated for 20 s. The cell pellet extracts were dyalized against 10 *M* NH_3. Determination of radioactivity was performed in a Packard scintillation counter (model 460 CD) employing Instagel as scintillation mixture.

Results

Figure 1 shows the experiments of Na_2 ($^{35}SO_4$) incorporation into fibroblasts of normal and stone-forming subjects. The Na_2 ($^{35}SO_4$) uptake was linear in both groups but normal subjects presented a higher Na_2 ($^{35}SO_4$) incorporation rate as compared to stone formers. Under the same amount of $^{35}SO_4$ the incorporation ratio between normal subjects and stone formers was 1.6. In our cases the behaviour of $^{35}SO_4$ uptake appears more homogeneous in stone formers than in normal subjects (lower value of standard error).

Figure 2 displays the radioactivity decrease in Na_2 ($^{35}SO_4$) labelled fibroblasts of normal and stone-forming subjects. Stone formers showed a higher rate of radioactivity decrease as proved by $^{35}SO_4$ half-time (normal subjects: $T_{1/2}$ = 31 h; stone formers: $T_{1/2}$ = 23 h).

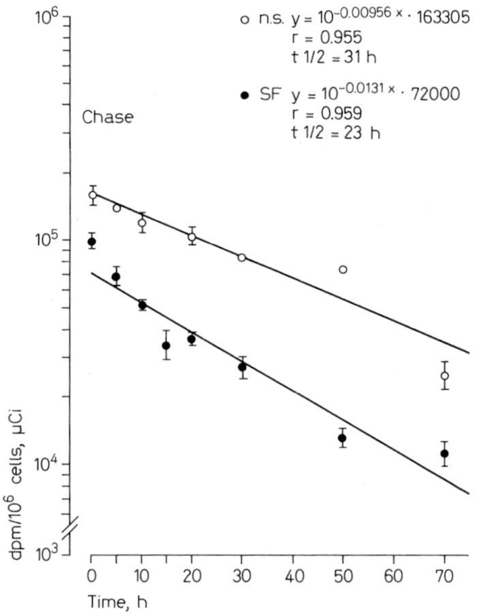

Fig. 2. Radioactivity decrease in Na_2 ($^{35}SO_4$)-labelled fibroblasts of normal (○) and stone-forming (•) subjects.

Conclusions

The metabolic behaviour of stone formers skin fibroblasts seem to present some interesting differences in respect to normal subjects. In fact pulse experiments show a lower Na_2 ($^{35}SO_4$) uptake by skin fibroblasts of stone formers. These results, together with chase data, may be explained by either a smaller GAG intracellular pool or a lower sulphatation degree. Moreover, chase experiments alone point out a faster decrease of radioactivity in stone formers as indicated by $^{35}SO_4$ half-time values in two groups. This data suggests a more rapid turnover of GAG in fibroblasts of these subjects. In conclusion further investigations are necessary for a better understanding of this different metabolic behaviour and for establishing correlations with clinical data.

References

1 Caudarella, R.; Stefani, F.; Rizzoli, E.; Malavolta, N.; D'Antuono, G.: Preliminary results of glycosaminoglycans excretion in normal and stone-forming subjects: relationship with uric acid excretion. J. Urol. *129:* 665–667 (1983).
2 Caudarella, R.; Malavolta, N.; Rizzoli, E.; Stefani, F.; D'Antuono, G.: Studio di alcuni inibitori della cristallizzazione nei pazienti affetti da calcolosi calcica idiopatica; in Aggiornamenti nefrologici della Magna Graecia, pp. 360–362 (Bios, Cosenza 1983).

Prof. Renata Caudarella, MD, Istituto Patologia Medica II,
via Massarenti 9, I–40138 Bologna (Italy)

Contr. Nephrol., vol. 58, pp. 93–100 (Karger, Basel 1987)

Renal Handling of Calcium and Magnesium in Idiopathic Stone Disease

Roger A. L. Sutton

Division of Nephrology, Department of Medicine,
University of British Columbia, Vancouver, B.C., Canada

Numerous investigators have examined idiopathic calcium stone patients, and found that, as a group, they have a significantly elevated urinary calcium excretion when compared with normal control subjects. Robertson and Morgan [1] showed that the frequency distribution of urinary calcium excretions in stone formers had a similar shape to that of normal subjects, but was shifted upwards by an average of 75 mg of calcium per day.

It has been recognized for many years that the increased urinary calcium output of idiopathic stone formers could result either from primary intestinal hyperabsorption of calcium, from obligatory urinary calcium wasting, or from disordered skeletal calcium metabolism. While the controversy remains unresolved, it appears increasingly likely that most 'idiopathic hypercalciuria' does not fulfill the criteria for pure 'absorptive', or pure 'renal' hypercalciuria.

The normal pattern of renal tubular calcium reabsorption in the mammalian nephron, and the influence of various endogenous and exogenous factors upon this reabsorption has recently been reviewed in detail [2]. It is generally believed that calcium transport closely parallels that of sodium in the more proximal portions of the nephron, and that dissociation of calcium from sodium transport, such as would be required to give rise to renal hypercalciuria, most likely would result from a defect in the later portions of the nephron in or beyond the thick ascending limb of Henle's loop. It is therefore of interest that several investigators have published data suggesting the presence of a proximal tubular defect in some idiopathic stone patients. Sutton and Walker [3] examining the responses of unselected calcium stone formers to single oral test doses of various diuretic agents, observed that, by comparison with normal subjects, unselected calcium stone formers showed a significantly exaggerated output of sodium, calcium and magnesium in response to a single oral dose of hydrochlorothiazide. The abnormal response was more marked in those patients who showed hypercalciuria after an overnight fast, who comprised 20 of the 36 unselected stone formers. The natriuretic response to a dose of acetazolamide was significantly blunted in the stone formers compared with the normals. These data were interpreted as being consistent with a defect in proximal bulk reabsorption in the stone formers, leading to increased delivery of ions to the distal nephron, and therefore to an exaggerated response to the diuretic (hydrochlorothiazide) which acts in the distal convoluted tubule. Since that time other data have been published which are consistent with the presence of a proximal tubular defect in idiopathic hypercalciuria. Lau et al. [4] reported an increase in free water clearance (V/GFR) in idiopathic hypercalciuria, which was not corrected by phosphate administration, and was therefore presumably not a consequence of phosphate depletion. Lau and Eby [5] subsequently reported micropuncture studies from genetically hypercalciuric rats which showed a defect in proximal calcium (but not fluid) reabsorption compared with normal rats.

Sakhaee et al. [6] have repeated studies similar to those of Sutton and Walker [3] in small selected subgroups of stone formers, and have reported that the exaggerated natriuretic and calciuric responses to hydrochlorothiazide occur only in the subgroup of patients with 'renal hyperalciuria with secondary hyperparathyroidism'. It is difficult to reconcile this report with that of Sutton and Walker, since the patients of Sutton and Walker with hypercalciuria during fasting, who comprised more than 50% of unselected calcium stone patients, did not have evidence of secondary hyperparathyroidism. Jaeger et al. [7] have suggested that the tubulopathy in nephrolithiasis may be the consequence rather than the cause of the stones. These authors demonstrated increased urinary excretions of lysozyme, γ-GT, glucose, insulin, etc. in a significant number of stone formers, irrespective of type, and apparently related to the presence of large pyelocaliceal stones at the time of study. While the presence of numerous or large stones may well lead to tubular dysfunction, the relevance of this observation to the findings of Sutton and Walker in calcium stone patients, most of whom were stone-free at the time of the study, or in hypercalciuric rats which have not had renal calculi, is uncertain.

If a primary defect in proximal tubular reabsorption is a feature of idiopathic calcium stone disease, the question arises as to what the relationship may be between the proximal defect and the hypercalciuria. As indicated above, an isolated proximal defect would not be expected to cause selective hypercalciuria. It would be necessary to argue that the increased delivery of sodium and other ions to the distal nephron is being reabsorbed, while that of calcium is not, which would seem to imply a coexisting reabsorptive defect for calcium in the distal nephron. An alternative mechanism whereby a proximal defect might cause hypercalciuria involves renal phosphate wasting, leading to hypophosphatemia, stimulation of calcitriol production, and intestinal calcium hyperabsorption [8]. However, hypophosphatemia is an inconsistent manifestation of idiopathic hypercalciuria. Alternatively, the relationship between proximal tubule dysfunction and increased calcitriol production could be more direct, since calcitriol is produced in the presumably abnormal proximal tubules.

Several lines of evidence strongly argue that a primary renal calcium leak is unlikely to be the underlying cause of most idiopathic hypercalciuria. Most investigators have found that few patients show evidence of secondary hyperparathyroidism in the form of increased parathyroid hormone (PTH) levels or an increased urinary adnosine 3′–5′-cyclic phosphate (cyclic AMP) excretion. Indeed, urinary cyclic AMP excretion was reported to be significantly lower in patients with fasting hypercalciuria than in normal subjects or normocalciuric stone formers [9]. Furthermore, Coe et al. [10] showed that, after a prolonged period on a very low calcium intake, although stone patients continued to waste abnormal amounts of calcium into the urine to the extent that they were in substantial net negative calcium balance, their serum calcium levels were significantly higher than those of normal subjects while their serum PTH levels were significantly decreased. These latter data seem best explained by postulating an abnormality in bone turnover in stone patients, such that, faced with dietary calcium deprivation, they mobilize skeletal calcium more readily than normal subjects, maintaining higher serum calcium levels, parathyroid suppression and hypercalciuria. Several other lines of evidence have suggested that bone turnover may be abnormal in patients with renal stones or idiopathic hypercalciuria. Abnormalities of bone density have been reported, as well as abnormalities of calcium radiokinetics [11, 12]. We [13] have recently observed abnormalities in urinary hydroxyproline excretion in calcium stone formers. Whereas normal subjects show a significantly higher urinary hydroxyproline excretion at night, presumably reflecting increased skeletal calcium resorption during fasting, calcium stone patients did not show such a circadian rhythm. In the stone patients, urinary hydroxyproline remained at a relatively high but sustained level throughout the 24 h. This observation would be consistent with the presence of increased bone turnover in the stone patients, which must continue during the day despite the entry of ingested calcium into the extracellular fluid. Since the bone density of recurrent calcium stone patients is usually well maintained, the increased skeletal resorption is presumably accompanied by increased bone formation.

It would be attractive to postulate that increased skeletal resorption might result from elevated calcitriol production in idiopathic calcium stone formers. In a series of elegant studies, Maierhofer et al. [14, 15] have shown that in healthy men given calcitriol to elevate blood levels, if dietary calcium is adequate, increased bone resorption does not occur. However, if dietary calcium is restricted, exogenous calcitriol stimulates bone resorption.

Unfortunately, the data pertaining to circulating calcitriol levels in idiopathic stone patients and idiopathic hypercalciuria are conflicting [16]. Several authors have reported elevated calcitriol levels in idiopathic hypercalciuria, and Broadus et al. [17] have suggested that there may be disordered control of calcitriol production in absorptive hypercalciuria. By contrast, normal calcitriol levels have been reported by several other investigators both in unselected calcium stone patients [16, 18] and in patients with idiopathic hypercalciuria [10, 16].

If calcitriol levels are inappropriately elevated in patients with idiopathic hypercalciuria, they could contribute to the production of the hypercalciuria in several possible ways. There may be intestinal calcium hyperabsorption. If this were the underlying mechanism of most idiopathic hypercalciuria, then patients would be expected to be in overall positive calcium balance, whereas Lemann [19] has shown that this is not the case. An alternative means by which elevated calcitriol levels could contribute to hypercalciuria might be through an influence on the parathyroid set-point [20]. There is increasing evidence that calcitriol lowers the set-point; i.e. in the presence of elevated calcitriol levels, the parathyroids would be more readily suppressed by a given increment in the serum calcium level. In this event, patients with elevated calcitriol levels might show greater parathyroid suppression in response to a given ingested or absorbed calcium load, as a result of which tubular calcium reabsorption would be less avid, and more of the absorbed calcium would be excreted in the urine. In this way, elevated calcitriol levels could contribute to renal calcium wasting. In a much more direct way, Burnatowska et al. [21] have recently shown that under certain circumstances calcitriol can directly antagonize the effect of PTH to promote renal tubular calcium reabsorption. In this manner, elevated calcitriol levels might also contribute to renal calcium wasting. Finally, as discussed above, elevated calcitriol levels might contribute to the increased bone turnover which results in greater skeletal calcium mobilization during fasting.

In summary, the role of abnormal renal calcium handling in idiopathic calcium stone disease remains uncertain. There are numerous possible mechanisms, involving calcium itself, disordered calcitriol production and renal phosphate wasting, through which tubular defects could contribute to idiopathic hypercalciuria and further studies will be required to establish the relative importance of these mechanisms.

By contrast with calcium, the renal handling of magnesium in idiopathic stone disease has been relatively little studied. Some years ago [22], we reported that mean 24-hour urinary magnesium excretions were normal in stone patients with idiopathic hypercalciuria, but tended to be low in normocalciuric calcium stone patients. Since magnesium may act as an inhibitor of stone formation, a reduced urinary magnesium excretion could be of some pathophysiological significance. In the diuretic challenge tests [3] the fasting urinary magnesium/creatinine ratio was not significantly different from normal in any of the groups of stone formers. However, it was higher in the subgroup with hypercalciuria during fasting, and the difference from normals almost reached statistical significance. In response to hydrochlorothiazide, the stone formers with hypercalciuria during fasting showed an exaggerated increment in the urinary magnesium/creatinine ratio, and we interpreted this as being consistent with a defect in reabsorption in the proximal tubule, recognizing, however, that the proximal tubule is a relatively unimportant site of tubular magnesium reabsorption [2]. In subsequent larger studies [23] a group of 32 stone patients with fasting hypercalciuria had a significantly higher magnesium/creatinine ratio than the normal control group (0.064 vs 0.045; $p < 0.05$). Within the whole group of 66 stone formers, there was a highly significant positive correlation between urinary calcium/creatinine and urinary magnesium/creatinine ratios; i.e. those patients with more marked fasting hypercalciuria tended to have higher fasting magnesium excretions. In response to challenge tests with single oral doses of acetazolamide (500 mg), furosemide (60 mg) or hydrochlorothiazide (100 mg), the higher fasting magnesium/creatinine ratio in the patients with fasting hypercalciuria was evident after hydrochlorothiazide but not after furosemide. We interpreted this observation as suggesting that magnesium reabsorption may be impaired in Henle's loop in the hypercalciuric patients. Furthermore, we suggested that such an impairment might be secondary to altered calcium handling, for example it might result from increased calcium delivery to Henle's loop.

In a subsequent study [24], we examined the changes in magnesium metabolism resulting from a 4-day period on a low calcium diet (less than 400 mg/day), together with oral cellulose phosphate (5 g t.i.d.), sufficient to bind about 50 mEq of calcium plus magnesium. The subjects comprised 7 normals and 9 stone formers, of whom 8 showed fasting hypercalciuria. On the free diet, plasma magnesium levels were similar, but in this particular study the stone formers had a significantly higher 24-hour urinary magnesium/creatinine ratio than the normal subjects (0.079 vs 0.056; $p < 0.01$). On the fourth day of the calcium and magnesium restriction, the mean serum magnesium level was unchanged in the normals but had fallen significantly from 2.06 to 1.91 mg/dl ($p < 0.05$) in the stone patients, while the urinary magnesium/creatinine ratio fell to a similar level in both normals and stone formers (to 0.027 vs 0.024, respectively). During the calcium restriction plus cellulose phosphate period, the patients remained significantly hypercalciuric relative to the normals. We interpret the magnesium data, which show a fall in serum magnesium in the stone formers but not in the normals in response to dietary magnesium deprivation (produced by cellulose phosphate), as indicating an impairment of tubular magnesium reabsorption. This apparent tubular magnesium leak may be secondary to the hypercalciuria in the stone formers, or may be a manifestation of an underlying tubule defect.

Other investigators have reported somewhat similar abnormalities in urinary magnesium excretion in stone formers. Coe et al. [10] showed that during severe dietary calcium deprivation, urinary magnesium remained persistently higher in stone patients than in controls. Recently, Martinez et al. [25] have reported higher than normal urinary magnesium levels during fasting in 'renal' hypercalciuria, and higher urinary magnesium levels in both 'renal' and 'absorptive' hypercalciuria under conditions of free and restricted diet.

In conclusion, several subtle abnormalities of renal magnesium handling have been demonstrated in idiopathic stone patients. There is a tendency to higher urinary magnesium outputs, and during dietary magnesium deprivation, serum magnesium levels may fall. These data suggest that there may be a mild impairment of tubular magnesium reabsorption, which is more marked in patients with fasting hypercalciuria. This abnormality in magnesium handling may be secondary to the hypercalciuria, or may be a manifestation of an underlying renal tubular defect. In addition, in a small group of normocalciuric stone formers, urinary magnesium excretion is low, and this could be of some pathophysiological significance since magnesium may act as an inhibitor of stone formation.

References

1 Robertson, W.; Morgan, D.: The distribution of urinary calcium excretions in normal persons and stoneformers. Clinica chim. Acta *27:* 503–508 (1972).

2 Sutton, R.; Dirks, J.: Calcium and magnesium: renal handling and disorders of metabolism; in Brenner, Rector, The kidney, vol. 1, pp. 551–618 (Saunders, Philadelphia 1985).

3 Sutton, R.; Walker, V.: Responses to hydrochlorothiazide and acetazolamide in patients with calcium stones. Evidence suggesting a defect in renal tubular function. New Engl. J. Med. *302:* 709–713 (1980).

4 Lau, K.; Wasserstein, A.; Westby, G.; Bosanac, P.; Grabie, M.; Mitnick, P.; Slatopolsky, E.; Goldfarb, S.; Agus, Z.: Proximal tubular defects in idiopathic hypercalciuria: resistance to phosphate administration. Mineral Electrolyte Metab. *7:* 237–249 (1982).

5 Lau, K.; Eby, B.: Tubular mechanism for the spontaneous hypercalciuria in laboratory rats. J. clin. Invest. *78:* 835–844 (1982).

6 Sakhaee, A.; Nicar, M.; Brater, C.; Pak, C.: Exaggerated natriuretic and calciuric responses to hydrochlorothiazide in renal hypercalciuria but not in absorptive hypercalciuria. J. clin. Endocr. Metab. *61:* 825–829 (1985).

7 Jaeger, P.; Portmann, L.; Jinalski, J.-M.; Jacquet, A.-F.; Temler, F.; Burckhart, P.: Tubulopathy in nephrolithiasis: consequence rather than cause. Kidney int. *29.* 563–571 (1986).

8 Shen, F.; Baylink, D.; Nielsen: Increased serum 1,25-dihydroxy vitamin D in idiopathic hypercalciuria. J. Lab. Med. *19:* 955–962 (1977).

9 Walker, V.; Sutton, R.: Urinary adenosine cyclic 3,5-monophosphate in idiopathic calcium stone formers: response to an oral calcium load. Clin. Sci. *66:* 193–199 (1984).

10 Coe, F.; Favus, M.; Crockett, T.; Strauss, A.; Parks, J.; Porat, A.; Gantt, C.; Sherwood, L.: Effects of low calcium diet on urine calcium excretion, parathyroid function and serum 1,25-OH_2D_3 levels in patients with idiopathic hypercalciuria and in normal subjects. Am. J. Med. *72:* 25–32 (1982).

11 Wilson, D.; Barkin, J.; Strauss, A.: Bone mineral content in calcium urolithiasis. Urol. Res. *12:* 37 (1984).

12 Liberman, U.; Sperling, O.; Atsmon, A.: Metabolic and calcium kinetic studies in idiopathic hypercalciuria. J. clin. Invest. *47:* 2580–2590 (1969).

13 Sutton, R.; Walker, V.: Bone resorption and hypercalciuria in calcium stone formers. Metabolism *35:* 485–488 (1986).

14 Maierhofer, W.; Gray, R.; Cheung, H.; Lemann, J., Jr.: Bone resorption stimulated by elevated serum 1,25-OH_2 vitamin D concentrations in healthy men. Kidney int. *24:* 555–560 (1983).

15 Maierhofer, W.; Lemann, J., Jr.; Gray, R.; Cheung, H.: Dietary calcium and serum 1,25-OH_2 vitamin D concentrations as determinants of calcium balance in healthy men. Kidney int. *26:* 752–759 (1984).

16 Netelenbos, J.; Jongen, M.; Vijgh, W. van der; Lips, P.; Ginkel, F. van: Vitamin D status in urinary calcium stone formation. Archs intern. Med. *145:* 681–684 (1985).

17 Broadus, A.; Insogna, K.; Lang, R.; Ellison, A.; Dreyer, B.: Evidence for disordered control of 1,25-dihydroxy vitamin D production in absorptive hypercalciuria. New Engl. J. Med. *311:* 73–80 (1984).

18 Sutton, R.; Walker, V.; Black, J.: Effect of dietary calcium on plasma 1,25-OH_2D levels in normal subjects and renal calcium stone formers; in Norman, Schaefer, von Harrath, Vitamin D: chemical, biochemical and clinical endocrinology of calcium metabolism, pp. 977–979 (deGruyter, New York 1982).

19 Lemann, J., Jr.: Idiopathic hypercalciuria; in Coe, Brenner, Stein, Nephrolithiasis, pp. 86–115 (Churchill-Livingstone, New York 1980).

20 Silver, J.; Naveh, T.; Meyer, H.; Schmelzer, H.; Popovtzer, M.: Regulation by 1,25-dihydroxy vitamin D_3 of pre-proparathyroid hormone mRNA in vivo. 18th Annu. Meet., Am. Soc. Nephrol., New Orleans 1985, abstr. 23A.

21 Burnatowska, M.; Harris, C.; Sutton, R.; Seely, J.: The effects of vitamin D on renal handling of calcium, magnesium and phosphate in the hamster. Kidney int. *27:* 864–870 (1985).

22 Evans, R.; Forbes, M.; Sutton, R.; Watson, L.: Urinary excretion of calcium and magnesium in patients with calcium containing renal stones. Lancet *ii:* 958 (1967).

23 Sutton, R.; Walker, V.: Renal magnesium handling in calcium stone formers. 8th Int. Congr. Nephrol., Athens, 1981, abstr. 117.

24 Walker, V.; Sutton, R.: Renal magnesium wasting in calcium stone formers. Clin. Invest. Med. *5:* 40B (1982).

25 Martinez, M.; Salinas, M.; Miguel, J.; Herrero, E.; Gomez, P.; Garcia, J.; Sanchez-Sicilia, L.; Montero, A.: Magnesium excretion in idiopathic hypercalciuria. Nephron *40:* 446–450 (1985).

Roger A. L. Sutton, DM, Division of Nephrology, Department of Medicine, 910 West 10th Avenue, Vancouver, B. C., V5Z IM9 (Canada)

Contr. Nephrol., vol. 58, pp. 101–105 (Karger, Basel 1987)

Altered Calcium Handling in Idiopathic Hypercalciuria

V. Nunziata, R. Giannattasio, G. di Giovanni, M.F. Corrado, M. Riccio

Institute of Internal Medicine and Metabolic Diseases,
University of Naples, Naples, Italy

Increased intestinal calcium absorption has been documented in a large proportion of people with hypercalciuria and kidney stones [1–3]. However, calcium renal tubular leak has been also reported in those who excrete high urine calcium on very low calcium intake or on fasting state [4]. Moreover, radiocalcium kinetic studies have shown in hypercalciuric stone formers an enlarged miscible pool size of calcium, increased turnover ratio as well as elevated bone formation and reabsorption [1]. In order to evaluate the role of each of these pathophysiologic disturbances of calcium handling we have examined a group of hypercalciuric patients with kidney calculi diagnosed as absorptives (AH) or renals (RH) according to Pak [3]. In all of them the status of calcium gut absorption has been estimated by assaying 1,25-dihydroxycholecalciferol (1,25-D) serum levels, whereas renal calcium excretion and bone turnover have been assessed by a kinetic analysis of an intravenous calcium infusion test.

Patients and Methods

Sixty-five hypercalciurics, 41 men, mean age 38 years, were studied. Hypercalciuria was defined on the basis of urine calcium exceeding 10 mEq/24 h on 400 mg calcium diet [5]. Among these 44 were classified as AH and 21 as RH whether fasting urine calcium was lesser or greater than 0.11 mg/dl GFR [6]. Forty-four normocalciuric stone formers (NC) with no biochemical abnormalities as well as 23 normal controls, comparable for sex and age, were also tested. In all subjects a fasting blood sample was taken for 1,25-D assay at the end of low calcium diet containing 400 mg calcium, 1,000 mg sodium, 900 mg phosphate, 90 g proteins, 70 g lipids and 300 g carbohydrates. Blood sampling was performed within 2 months (March–April) 1985. 1,25-D was determined according to Eismann et al. [7]. At the end of the above diet the calcium infusion test was performed in 12 hypercalciurics, 6 AH and 6 RH as well as in 7 controls. A venous blood sample was taken for basal serum ionized calcium and an intravenous Ca infusion was then started and continued for 2 h at the constant rate of 0.1 mmol Ca/kg body weight/h as Ca-gluconate. Serum-ionized Ca concentration was determined during the infusion, at 60 and 120 min and later on at 140, 160, 180, 200, 220, 240, 300 and 360 min from the start, to investigate the elimination phase of Ca load. In all subjects three separate urine collections were obtained from zero to 120, 120 to 240 and 240 to 360 min to measure calcium excretion. Ionized Ca was determined by Ca-specific electrode (Orion SS 20), urinary Ca by AA spectrometry (Unicam). Renal Ca clearance was calculated as the ratio of the urinary Ca excretion rate (mmol/min) to the serum ionized Ca concentration measured at the midpoint of urine collection. Total body clearance ($ml \cdot min^{-1} \cdot kg$ body $weight^{-1}$) of the Ca load was estimated by taking the administered dose (0.2 mmol/kg body weight) and the area under the curve (AUC) of serum-ionized Ca concentration. The AUC 'incremental' was calculated by trapezoidal rule [8]. Because of the non-linear decline of serum ionized Ca during the elimination phase the slope for AUC extrapolation to the infinity was calculated by logarithmic least squares regression from the last three time points of the curve (240, 300 and 360 min). Statistical analysis of results was performed by two-tailed Student's t-test [9].

Results

Mean serum 1,25-D value (± SD, pg/ml) was 34 ± 9, 36 ± 9, 34 ± 8 and 43 ± 6 in absorptives, renals, normocalciurics and normal controls, respectively. Therefore, the active metabolite of vitamin D appears significantly reduced in all calcium stone formers independently from the presence of high urine calcium excretion ($p < 0.001$). In figure 1 mean delta ionized calcium of hypercalciurics and controls is presented. During the infusion serum ionized calcium rose almost linearly in all subjects, but at a lower rate in hypercalciurics. In fact mean serum ionized calcium increment (delta) was significantly lower at the end of the test in renals and absorptives compared to normals ($p < 0.001$ and $p < 0.01$, respectively). Fasting renal calcium clearance (ml/min) is increased in renals (4.77 ± 0.41) in comparison to normals (1.72 ± 0.26) and to absorptives (3.24 ± 0.19) but it is also higher in absorptives than in normals ($p < 0.001$). Calcium renal clearance calculated from time zero to 360 min results increased in renals (12.95 ± 1.20) and in absorptives (12.16 ± 0.64)

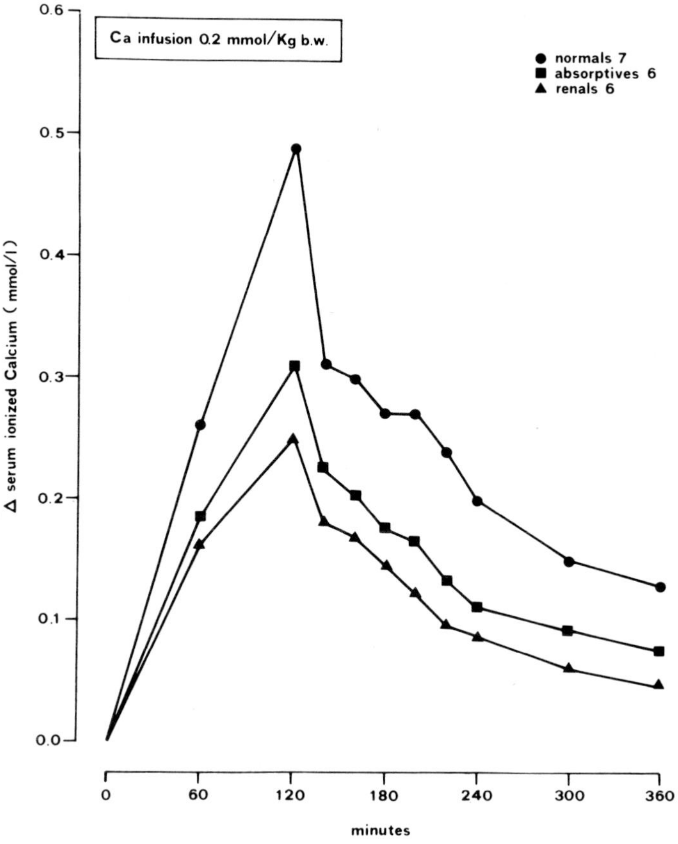

Fig. 1. Δ serum ionized calcium in absorptive and renal hypercalciurics and in normals.

compared to normals (8.14 ± 0.76, $p < 0.01$) whereas no differences are registered between renals and absorptives (p = n.s.). Total body calcium clearance (ml min^{-1} kg body $weight^{-1}$) is higher in renals (3.90 ± 0.10) and in absorptives (2.52 ± 0.11) compared to normals (1.74 ± 0.27) either when calculated to the infinity ($p < 0.01$) as well as to 360 min ($p < 0.001$). Renal clearance represents a small fraction of total body calcium clearance that results higher in both hypercalciuric groups also after subtracting the formers (HR vs controls, $p < 0.001$; HR vs HA, $p < 0.001$; HA vs controls, $p < 0.01$). In fact calcium renal clearance expressed as percent of total body clearance results lower in the hypercalciuric population compared to normals (4.5 in HR, 5.0 in HA, 7.7 in controls).

Discussion

The results of this study indicate that the well-documented calcium gut hyperabsorption in idiopathic hypercalciuria [1–3] is independent of 1,25-D. Therefore, a primary epithelial hyperabsorption of calcium may be postulated causing some reduction of parathyroid activity and consequently of 1,25-D levels. These data agree with those of Coe et al. [10] who have referred decreased serum parathormone and cyclic AMP in hypercalciuric stone formers but their patients were showing normal 1,25-D levels. On the contrary, Broadus et al. [11] have found high 1,25-D concentration due to increased production rate of this hormone [12] but Netelenbos et al. [13] in a large population of hypercalciuric and normocalciuric stone formers studied on constant diet have reported normal 1,25-D serum concentrations. The results of kinetic data of calcium infusion demonstrate a gross abnormality in the control of extracellular calcium concentration in idiopathic hypercalciuria that is not evident in the basal state. However, the most impressive difference between hypercalciurics and normals appears the total body clearance of infused calcium that is increased by a factor of 1.5 and 2.0 in absorptives and in renals, respectively. This increase is independent of the enhanced renal clearance because the latter is a very small fraction of the former. This indicates that in idiopathic hypercalciuria there is a profound alteration of the distribution of body calcium. In fact the primary epithelial calcium hyperabsorption per se does not predict that urine calcium will exceed dietary calcium and, therefore, an extra calcium must come either from the extracellular fluid or from bone. The renal tubular leak of calcium may be partially dependent on a reduced parathyroid activity but it does not explain why some hypercalciurics continue to lose calcium in the fasting state when there are no reasons for parathyroid suppression. Therefore, hypercalciuria must come from both disorders, such as epithelial gut primary hyperabsorption and tubular renal leak. Between these a profound alteration of body calcium turnover exists, acting as a great reservoir of calcium which may be more or less consistently involved depending whether the defect of calcium handling is more or less severe as in renal or absorptive hypercalciuria, respectively.

References

1 Liberman, U. A.; Sperling, O.; Atsmon, A.; Frank, M.; Modan, M.; DeVries, A.: A metabolic and calcium kinetic studies in idiopathic hypercalciuria. J. clin. Invest. *47:* 2580–2590 (1968).
2 Lemann, J.: Idiopathic hypercalciuria; in Coe, Brenner, Stein, Contemporary issues in nephrology, No. 5, pp. 86–115 (Churchill-Livingstone, Edinburgh 1980).
3 Pak, C. Y. C.: Physiological basis for absorptive and renal hypercalciurias. Am. J. Physiol. *237:* F415–423 (1979).
4 Edwards, N. A.; Hodgkinson, A.: Studies of renal function in patients with idiopathic hypercalciuria. Clin. Sci. *29:* 327–334 (1965).
5 Pak, C. Y. C.; Kaplan, R. A.; Bone, H.; Townsend, J.; Waters, O.: A simple test for the diagnosis of absorptive, resorptive and renal hypercalciurias. New Engl. J. Med. *292:* 497–500 (1975).
6 Pak, C. Y. C.; Britton, F.; Peterson, R.; Ward, D.; Northcutt, C.; Breslau, N. A.; McGuire, J.; Sakhaee, K.; Bush, S.; Nicar, M.; Norman, D. A.; Peters, P.: Ambulatory evaluation of nephrolithiasis; classification, clinical presentation and diagnostic criteria. Am. J. Med. *69:* 19–30 (1980).
7 Eisman, J. A.; Hamstra, A. J.; Kream, B. E.; De Luca, H. F.: 1,25-Dihydroxyvitamin D in biological fluids: a simplified and sensitive assay. Science *193:* 1021–1023 (1976).
8 Gibaldi, M.; Perrier, D.: Pharmacokinetics; in Swarbrick (Dekker, New York 1976).
9 Moroney, M. J.: Facts from figures (Penguin, Hardmondsworth 1953).
10 Coe, F. L.; Favus, M. J.; Crockett, A. L.; Strauss, J. H.; Parks, J. H.; Porat, A.; Gantt, C. L.; Sherwood, L. M.: Effects of low calcium diet on urine excretion, parathyroid function and serum $1{,}25(OH)_2D_3$ levels in patients with idiopathic hypercalciuria and in normal subjects. Am. J. Med. *72:* 25–31 (1982).
11 Broadus, A. E.; Insogna, K. L.; Lang, R. L.; Mallette, L. E.; Oren, D. A.; Gertner, J. M.; Kliger, A. S.; Ellison, A. F.: A consideration of the hormonal basis and phosphate-leak hypothesis of absorptive hypercalciuria. J. clin. Endocr. Metab. *58:* 161–169 (1984).
12 Insogna, K. L.; Broadus, A. E.; Dreyer, B. E.; Ellison, A. F.; Gertner, J. M.: Elevated production rate of 1,25-dihydroxyvitamin D in patients with absorptive hypercalciuria. J. clin. Endocr. Metab. *61:* 490–495 (1985).
13 Netelenbos, J. C.; Jongen, M. J. M.; Vijgh, W. J. F. van der; Lips, P.; Gimkel, F. C. van: Vitamin D status in urinary calcium stone formation. Archs intern. Med. *145:* 681–684 (1985).

Prof. V. Nunziata, MD, Istituto di Medicina Interna e Malattie Dismetaboliche, Nuovo Policlinico dell' Università, via Sergio Pansini 5, I–80131 Napoli (Italy)

Contr. Nephrol., vol. 58, pp. 106–110 (Karger, Basel 1987)

About a Primitive Osseous Origin of the So-Called 'Renal Hypercalciuria'

P. Messa[a], *G. Mioni*[a], *D. Montanaro*[a], *M. Adorati*[a], *F. Antonucci*[a], *A. Favazza*[a], *M. Messa*[a], *G. Enzmann*[a], *L. Paganin*[b], *R. Nardini*[c]

Divisions of [a]Nephrology and [b]Urology, Ospedale Civile di Udine;
[c]Health Institute, Udine, Italy

An increase in the fasting urinary excretion of calcium is commonly regarded as the most reliable index of idiopathic hypercalciuria secondary to renal Ca leak. It has also been argued that this chronic loss of Ca by the kidney leads to a condition of secondary hyperparathyroidism (SHP) [1, 2]. However increasing evidences have questioned the finding of the SHP of the so-called renal hypercalciuria and, as a consequence, have challenged the tubular Ca leak hypothesis [3–6]. In order to gain further insights into this controversy, we studied a population of stone formers, with and without hypercalciuria, and firstly challenged the renal Ca leak hypothesis then other possible explanations for fasting hypercalciuria were considered.

Patients and Methods

The study was carried out in 120 idiopathic calcium stone formers (69 M, 51 F; aged 18–62 years), with creatinine clearance above 80 ml/min. Seventy-six patients were hypercalciuric (uCa > 300 mg/day); 52 of them had fasting Ca/Cr ratio higher than 0.11 and were defined as fasting hypercalciuric (FH), the other 24 normalized Ca excretion after fasting and were defined as not fasting hypercalciuric (NFH); the 44 stone formers with normocalciuria, both on a free diet and during fasting, were defined as not hypercalciuric (NH). All individuals were maintained on a diet which provided 400 mg of Ca per day for at least a week, then after an overnight fast, 2-hour urines were collected and a blood sample was taken at the midpoint. Then a standard 1-gram oral Ca load was administered and urine was collected for a 4-hour period and a blood sample was again taken at the midpoint. Urine and blood were analysed for calcium (atomic absorption spectrophotometry), inorganic phosphate (green malachite micromethod), urinary cyclic AMP (by the kit of INC), s PTH (carboxy-terminal fragment by the kit of DPC), total urinary hydroxyproline (resin-catalysed hydrolysis), alkaline phosphatase (by autoanalyzer). In 50 patients (25 FH, 13 NFH, 12 NH) the following parameters were also measured: percentage of intestinal Ca absorption and exchange (% int. Ca abs. and exch.), pool of Ca at the 24th hour, according to previously described methods [7]. Furthermore, 15 FH patients and 5 NH were kept on a very low Ca diet (140 mg) for at least 10 days and the following parameters were evaluated: sCa and uCa, sPTH, ucAMP, % int. Ca. abs., net bone flux of Ca (calculated as: NBF = [diet Ca] × [% int. Ca. abs.] – [daily uCa]). Urinary Ca and OHP were expressed as a ratio with uCr; tubular threshold of phosphate (TTP) was calculated according to Bijvoet [8]; ucAMP was expressed as nmol/dl GFR. All data are expressed as mean ± SD. Statistics were performed by variance analysis and by linear regression analysis.

Results

Table I shows the values of the urinary and blood parameters evaluated in the 3 groups of stone formers after a week on a diet containing 400 mg of Ca. It is evident that no statistically significant difference resulted as regards the signs of SHP (sPTH, ucAMP, TTP). Urinary cAMP showed a trend towards an inverse correlation with fasting Ca/Cr values, but it did not reach a statistically significant level ($r = -0.204$; for a p value of 0.05 $r = 0.254$). No significant correlation was found between % int. Ca abs. and either fasting Ca/Cr ($r = 0.004$) or ucAMP ($r = 0.024$). FH patients did show uOHP levels significantly higher than both NFH and NH stone formers. Furthermore, a good correlation was found between fasting Ca/Cr and uOHP/Cr (Ca/Cr = 0.074 + 1.79 [OHP/Cr]; $r = 0.445$, $p < 0.01$). In NH patients the Ca-restricted diet (140 mg) resulted in a significant reduction of sCa (8.9 ± 0.06 vs 9.6 ± 0.16 mg/dl, $p < 0.05$), with an increase (but not significant) of sPTH (0.89 ± 0.33 vs. 0.77 ± 0.27 ng/ml, p = n.s.) and ucAMP (4.1 ± 1.1 vs 3.5 ± 1.8 nmol/dl GFR, p = n.s.), whereas no variation resulted in sCa (9.7 ± 0.31 vs 9.6 ± 0.44 mg/dl, p = n.s.), sPTH (0.73 ± 0.33 vs 0.74 ± 0.26 ng/ml, p = n.s.) or ucAMP (3.5 ± 1.2 vs 3.4 ± 0.9 nmol/dl GFR, p = n.s.) in FH patients. Moreover, during a Ca-restricted diet NBF resulted well-correlated with both fasting Ca/Cr (Ca/Cr = 0.076 + 4.82 [NBF], $r = 0.723$, $p < 0.01$) and OHP/Cr values ($OHP/Cr = 16.8\ e^{2.73\ NBF}$, $r = 0.563$, $p < 0.05$) (fig. 1).

Table I. Values of urinary and blood parameters in idiopathic stone formers after 1 week on a diet with 400 mg of calcium (mean ± SD)

	sCa mg/dl	24 h uCa mg/day	Fasting Ca/Cr mg/mg	TTP mg/dl	sPTH ng/ml	Fasting ucAMP nmol/dl GFR	Al. ph. U/l	OHP/Cr mg/g	int. Ca abs. %	Ca pool l
FH	9.61 ±0.39	232.5 ± 73.8	0.157 ±0.036	3.28 ±0.58	0.74 ±0.46	3.41 ±1.3	108.8 ± 20.3	28.0 ±13.2	60.7 ±19.4	48.3 ±22.9
NFH	9.4 ±0.28	226.5 ± 55.4	0.082 ±0.015	3.25 ±0.56	0.79 ±0.36	3.4 ±1.1	94.0 ± 18.2	19.8 ± 8.6	59.8 ±20.2	56.3 ±31.5
NH	9.48 ±0.38	121.5 ± 45.4	0.066 ±0.020	3.26 ±0.78	0.78 ±0.30	3.62 ±1.37	96.5 ± 17.4	20.2 ± 7.4	47.8 ±14.4	42.0 ±17.0
p		°°° §§§	°°° § ***					°°° ***	° §	

Significant differences between FH and NH = ° < 0.05, °°° < 0.001; between NFH and NH = § < 0.05, §§§ < 0.001; between FH and NFH = *** < 0.001.

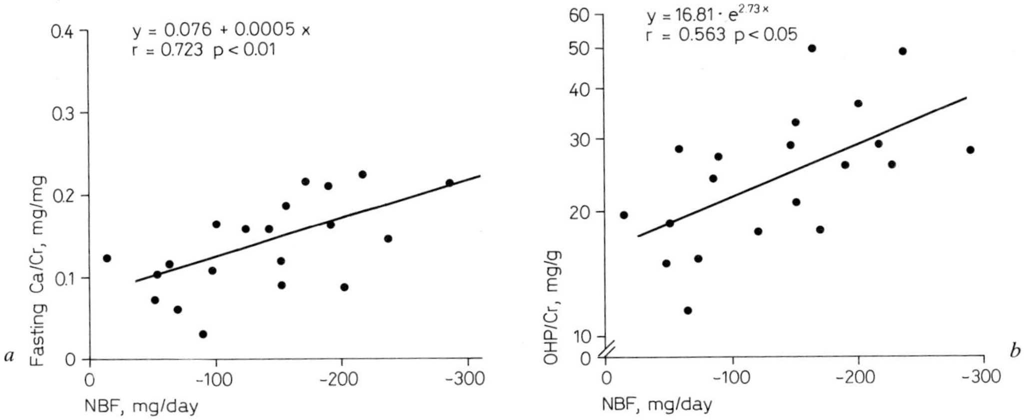

Fig. 1. The net bone flux of Ca, measured after 10 days on a diet with 140 mg of Ca, was well correlated with both fasting urinary Ca excretion (*a*) and OHP excretion (*b*).

Discussion

An increased fasting urinary excretion of Ca, together with biochemical signs of SHP, has been generally regarded as an index of renal Ca leak in stone formers with idiopathic hypercalciuria [1, 2]. However, a lot of studies failed to support the presence of SHP in association with FH [3–6]. Indeed, recent data have shown a trend towards normal-low activity of parathyroid glands in FH [9, 10]. Our data also support the finding of a normal secretion rate of PTH in FH and question the Ca leak theory: indeed if a primary Ca loss was involved, then indices of parathyroid hyperfunction would be expected. Moreover, the Ca-restricted diet did not result in any reduction of sCa or in any stimulation of PTH, as one would expect if a renal leak of Ca was involved. Other authors have recently suggested that FH may be secondary to a great increase in int. Ca abs. with a SHP causing a reduced tubular reabsorption of Ca [10]. If so we would expect to find a direct correlation between the levels of int. Ca abs. and the degree of fasting urinary Ca excretion: in the patients we studied we were not able to find any correlation between these two parameters and high fasting Ca/Cr values were found also in patients with normal levels of int. Ca abs. Furthermore, no inverse correlation was found between int. Ca abs. and the indices of parathyroid function (i.e. ucAMP). Our data did show an increased excretion of OHP in urine of FH patients when compared with the other groups of stone formers, and the levels of the OHP excretion were well correlated with the degree of FH. Moreover, we found that net bone flux of Ca, measured when a steady state was attained during Ca restriction, resulted significantly correlated with both fasting urinary excretion of Ca and OHP. In conclusion, in agreement with recent data [11], our study seems to support the hypothesis of a primary role of bone in the pathogenesis of FH.

References

1 Coe, F.L.; Canterbury, J.M.; Firpo, J.J.; Reiss, E.: Evidence for secondary hyperparathyroidism in idiopathic hypercalciuria. J. clin. Invest. *52:* 134 (1973).
2 Broadus, A.E.; Dominguez, M.; Bartter, F.C.: Pathophysiologic studies in hypocalciuria: use of an oral calcium tolerance test to characterize distinctive hypercalciuric subgroups. J. clin. Endocr. Metab. *47:* 751 (1978).
3 Burckhardt, P.; Jaeger, P.: Secondary hyperparathyroidism in idiopathic renal hypercalciuria: fact or theory? J. clin. Endocr. Metab. *53:* 550 (1981).
4 Lilienfeld-Toal,V.H.; Bach, D.; Hesse, A.; Frank, H.; Issa, S.: Parathyroid hormone is normal in renal stone patients with idiopathic hypercalciuria and high fasting urinary calcium. Urol. Res. *10:* 205 (1982).
5 Messa, P.; Sommariva, E.; Cattalini, M.; Antonucci, F.; Montanaro, D.; Adorati, M.; Mioni, G.: Analisi discriminante fra l'ipercalciuria renale e l'iperparatiroidismo primitivo; in Nefrologia, dialisi, trapianto '83, p. 133 (1983).
6 Messa, P.; Mioni, G.: L'ipercalciuria a digiuno: teorie e mode. G. ital. Nefrol. *2:* 147 (1985).
7 Messa, P.; Mioni, G.; Favazza, A.; Montanaro, D.; Antonucci, F.; Messa, M.: Acetazolamide and intestinal Ca absorption in nephrotic syndrome; in Puschett, Diuretics, p. 491 (1984).
8 Bijvoet, O.L.M.: Relation of plasma phosphate concentration to renal tubular reabsorption of phosphate. Clin. Sci. *37:* 23 (1969).
9 Coe, F.L.; Favus, M.J.; Crockett, T.: Effects of low calcium diet on urine Ca excretion, parathyroid function and serum 1,25$(OH)_2D_3$ levels in patients with idiopathic hypercalciuria and in normal subjects. Am. J. Med. *72:* 25 (1982).
10 Broadus, A.E.; Karl, L.J.; Lang, R.: A consideration of the hormonal basis and phosphate leak hypothesis of absorptive hypercalciuria. J. clin. Endocr. Metab. *58:* 161 (1984).
11 Barkin, J.; Wilson, D.R.; Manuel, M.A.; Bayley, A.; Murray, T.; Harrison, J.: Bone mineral content in idiopathic calcium nephrolithiasis. Mineral Electrolyte Metab. *11:* 19 (1985).

Piergiorgio Messa, MD, Nefrologia e Dialisi, Ospedale Civile di Udine,
I–33100 Udine (Italy)

Contr. Nephrol., vol. 58, pp. 111–114 (Karger, Basel 1987)

Evidence for a Reduced Urinary Magnesium/Creatinine Ratio in Patients with Calcium Urolithiasis

G. Vagelli, A. Mazzotta, V. Ferraris, G. Pratesi, G. Calabrese, M. Gonella

Servizio di Nefrologia e Dialisi, Divisione di Urologia, Ente Ospedaliero, Casale Monferrato, Italia

Magnesium is an important in vitro inhibitor of calcium-oxalate (Ca-Ox) crystal formation and accounts for about 20% of the total inhibitory activity of the urine, by forming complexes with Ox and avoiding its precipitation by Ca [1, 2]. Data concerning urinary daily Mg excretion (uMg) in Ca stone formers are conflicting because it has been found to be normal [3, 4], decreased [5] and even increased [6, 7]. Since these discrepancies could be due to sex and age differences between normals and stone formers, uMg/urinary creatinine ratio (uMg/Cr) was investigated in both groups in order to correct uMg for the lean body mass.

Patients and Methods

65 Ca stone formers (52 males and 13 females), mean age 43 years (range 18–69) and 31 normal subjects (17 males and 14 females), mean age 44 years (range 18–80) were examined for uMg, uCa and uCr on one day individual diet and no drugs administration. Patients suffering from primary hyperparathyroidism or from other causes of hypercalcemia were excluded from this study.

Mg and Ca were measured by atomic absorption spectrophotometry, Cr by autoanalyzer method. The results were compared by the Student's t-test for unpaired data. The linear correlation coefficient was used to assess the dependency between two variables. All data were expressed as mean values ± SD.

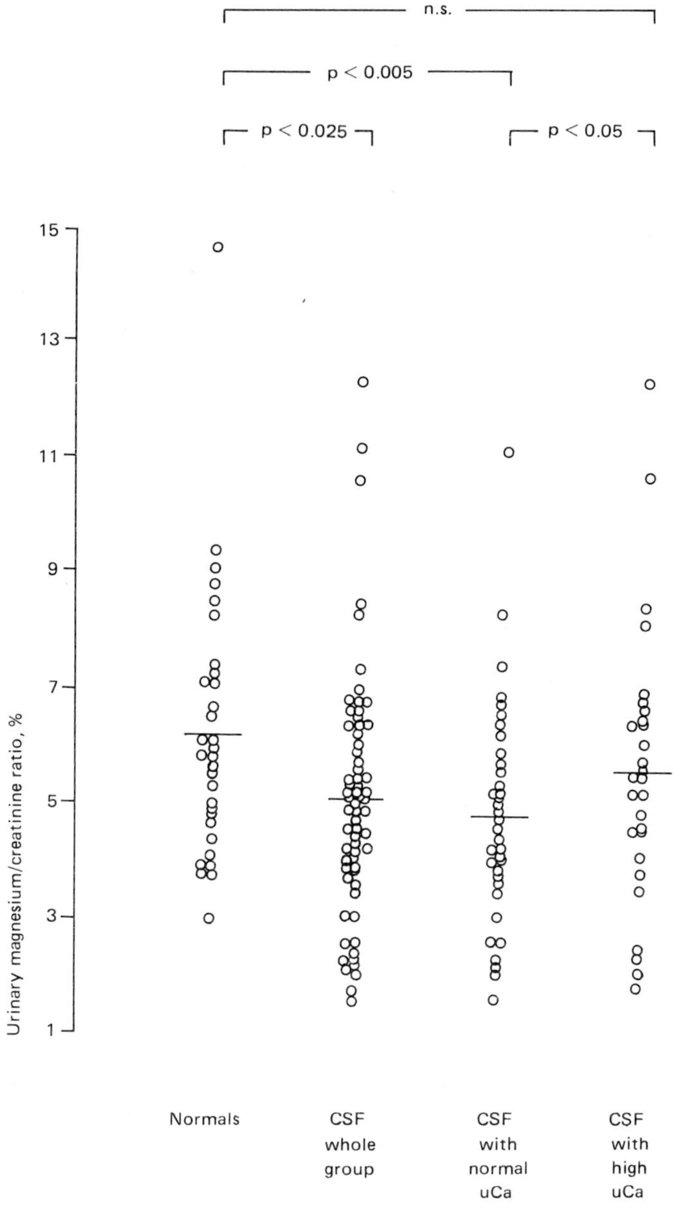

Fig. 1. Values of uMg/Cr in the examined groups. The values were compared among the different groups by the Student t-test for unpaired data.

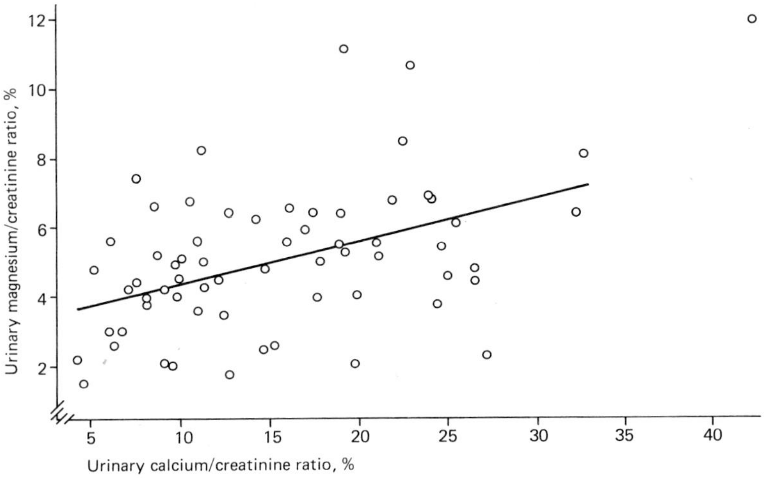

Fig. 2. Direct correlation between uMg and uCa in the whole group of stone formers ($r = 0.46$, $p < 0.001$).

Results

Among the studied patients, 28 stone formers (43%) showed hypercalciuria (uCa > 4 mg/kg/day) and 37 (57%) were normocalciuric. uMg/Cr was significantly higher in normals (6.2 ± 2.3%) than both in stone formers as a whole group (5.1 ± 2.2%) ($p < 0.025$) and in normocalciuric patients (4.8 ± 1.9%) ($p < 0.005$), whereas it was not significantly different if only hypercalciuric patients were considered (5.6 ± 2.3%); uMg/Cr significantly lower in normocalciuric than in hypercalciuric patients ($p < 0.05$) (fig. 1). Furthermore, a direct correlation was detected between uMg and uCa in the whole group of stone formers (fig. 2) but not in the normals.

Discussion

The distribution of the above-considered stone formers with respect to uCa was similar to that reported in the literature [8]. The investigation of uMg related to uCr and, furthermore, the comparison of this ratio between selected groups concerning uCa could explain the uMg discrepancies found in previous patients [3–7]. In fact uMg/Cr resulted to be significantly lower in the whole group of stone formers and even lower in the normocalciuric ones than in healthy persons, whose uMg/Cr, on the other hand, was not significantly different from that of the hypercalciuric patients.

In conclusion, these findings support the role of a low uMg as a possible risk factor in favoring urolithiasis especially in normocalciuric patients, and, therefore, Mg supplements are suggested as a therapeutical approach in preventing stone relapses.

References

1 Desmars, J.F.; Tawashi, R.: Dissolution and growth of calcium oxalate monohydrate: effect of magnesium and pH. Biochim. biophys. Acta *313:* 256–267 (1973).

2 Hallson, P.C.; Rose, G.A.; Sulaiman, S.: Magnesium reduces calcium oxalate crystal formation in human whole urine. Clin. Sci. *62:* 17–19 (1982).

3 Bach, D.; Hesse, A.; Strange, A.; Vahlensieck, W.: Magnesium excretion in urine on condition of individual as well as standard diet in healthy controls and calcium oxalate stone formers; in Smith, Robertson, Finlayson, Urolithiasis, clinical and basic research, pp. 45–49 (Plenum Press, New York 1981).

4 Vagelli, G.; Cristofano, C.; Lupetti, S.; Pratesi, G.; Gonella, M.; Barsotti, G.: Magnesium excretion in patients with calcium urolithiasis (Abstract). Bari Semin. Nephrol., pp. 90 (1984).

5 Johansson, G.: Magnesium metabolism. Studies in health, primary hyperparathyroidism and renal stone disease. Scand. J. Urol. Nephrol., suppl. 51, pp. 4–47 (1979).

6 Bataille, P.; Pruna, A.; Finet, I.; Seflon, P.; Makdassi, R.; Galay, C.; Fievet, P.; Fournier, A.: Magnesium renal wasting in calcium stone-formers with idiopathic hypercalciuria contrasting with lower magnesium/calcium urinary ratio. Proc. Eur. Dial. Transpl. Ass. *21:* 747–750 (1984).

7 Martinez, M.E.; Salinas, M.; Miguel, J.L.; Herrero, E.; Gomez, P.; Garcia, J.; Sanchez-Sicilia, L.; Montero, A.: Magnesium excretion in idiopathic hypercalciuria. Nephron *40:* 446–450 (1985).

8 Coe, F.L.; Favus, M.J.: Hypercalciuria states. Mineral Electrolyte Metab. *5:* 183–200 (1981).

M. Gonella, MD, Servizio di Nefrologia e Dialisi, Ente Ospedaliero,
I-15033 Casale Monferrato (Italy)

Contr. Nephrol., vol. 58, pp. 115–117 (Karger, Basel 1987)

Magnesium Excretion in Recurrent Calcium Urolithiasis

Evaluation of 46 Hypercalciuric Patients

P. Piana, G. Casetta, C. Giona, M. Petrillo, A. Tizzani

Università degli Studi di Torino, Facoltà di Medicina e Chirurgia, Istituto di Nefro-Urologia, Cattedra di Urologia (Director: Prof. S. Rocca Rossetti), Torino, Italia

Recent studies about clinical and experimental aspects of urolithiasis reported very contrasting results regarding the importance and possible role of magnesium urinary excretion in affecting the formation and growth of oxalocalcic stones. Our previous experience on in vitro crystallization kinetics showed an inhibitory effect of Mg on monohydrated Ca oxalate crystallization at concentrations of 10^{-3} and 10^{-6} mol. We tried therefore to check the importance of Mg excretion related to Ca excretion in a clinical study and to verify the effective value of Ca_u/Mg_u ratio in 46 hypercalciuric patients and 24 non-stone-forming controls.

Materials and Methods

All patients underwent a complete metabolic evaluation to investigate possible predisposing factors. Briefly we evaluated, first on standard diet, the urinary and serum contents of Na, K, Ca, Cl, Mg, P and uric acid; the renal clearances, 24-hour oxaluria, serum parathyroid hormone (PTH), proteins, albumin, alkaline phosphatase were checked as well, together with Brand's test for cystinuria, urine analysis and culture. Urinary salts and renal clearance evaluation were repeated after 4 days at 400 mg/day Ca dietary intake; on the same day Nordin's test was performed. After 4 days at 1 g/day Ca dietary intake the whole set of determinations was repeated. All lithiasic patients had passed spontaneously or had undergone urological surgery for more than 1 oxalocalcic stone. The controls did not show any previous episode of urolithiasis. The results were statistically analyzed by Student's t-test.

Table I. Results on different dietary Ca intakes. Means (± SD) are shown

Results on standard diet			
Controls	Ca	183 mg/24 h	(49.85)
	Mg	70 mg/24 h	(14.18)
	Ca_u/Mg_u	2.63	(0.66)
Absorbtive hypercalciuria	Ca	363	(72.39)
	Mg	99	(31.15)
	Ca_u/Mg_u	3.97	(1.01)
Renal hypercalciuria	Ca	491	(57.91)
	Mg	113	(0.66)
	Ca_u/Mg_u	4.24	(0.19)
Results on 400 mg Ca diet			
Controls	Ca	134	(40.95)
	Mg	63	(16.97)
	Ca_u/Mg_u	2.15	(0.67)
Absorbtive hypercalciuria	Ca	242	(85.53)
	Mg	86	(21.30)
	Ca_u/Mg_u	2.69	(0.48)
Renal hypercalciuria	Ca	385	(89.73)
	Mg	98	(20.38)
	Ca_u/Mg_u	3.95	(0.20)
Results on 1 g Ca diet			
Controls	Ca	180	(50.63)
	Mg	71	(18.46)
	Ca_u/Mg_u	2.55	(0.67)
Absorptive hypercalciuria	Ca	349	(95.60)
	Mg	87	(30.71)
	Ca_u/Mg_u	4.24	(1.05)
Renal hypercalciuria	Ca	426	(89.87)
	Mg	110	(11.33)
	Ca_u/Mg_u	4.01	(0.34)

Results

The results of urinary Ca and Mg excretion, together with the Ca_u/Mg_u ratio at different diets are shown in table I. Patients with absorptive and renal hypercalciuria had on standard diet a significantly higher Mg urinary excretion ($p < 0.001$) in relation to the controls. Ca_u/Mg_u ratio was very different from the controls ($p < 0.001$). Serum Mg did not vary significantly among the groups. During low Ca diet, urinary Ca excretion decreased, especially in absorptive patients; urinary Mg excretion diminished as well. Ca_u/Mg_u ratio remained abnormal in renal hypercalciuria and fell in the normal range in absorptive hypercalciuria. After 1 g Ca diet Ca excretion varied as expected; magnesiuria was constant in controls and again elevated in hypercalciuric patients. Ca_u/Mg_u ratio was always statistically different as compared to controls, whilst similar among the patient groups.

Discussion

The evaluation of Ca_u/Mg_u ratio may be used as a clinical guide when treatment of calcium oxalate lithiasis is performed with Mg oxide. In patients with absorptive hypercalciuria, Mg excretion is higher than in controls on standard diet but this does not counterbalance the striking rise of Ca excretion. During low Ca diet the Ca_u/Mg_u ratio falls in the normal range; treatment with Mg oxide is therefore not useful, since the low Ca intake seems to suffice. In renal hypercalciuria thiazide therapy usually succeeds in normalizing Ca excretion. Treatment with Mg oxide has not therefore a definite indication since there is no evidence of Mg depletion with thiazide therapy.

On the other hand, patients treated with Mg oxide should be carefully controlled. Some side effects could occur, such as hypercalciuria due to tubular competition between Ca and Mg, as well as a reduction of inhibitory activity of citrates, due to formation of Mg-citrate complexes.

Prof. Alessandro Tizzani, MD, st. Ponte Isabella a San Vito 131, I–10133 Torino (Italy)

Contr. Nephrol., vol. 58, pp. 118–121 (Karger, Basel 1987)

Is Urinary Prostaglandin E_2 Excretion Correlated to Urinary Excretion of Calcium, Sodium and Potassium?

R. Pfab[a], *M. Hegemann*[a], *M. Weitbrecht*[a], *I. Böttger*[b], *S. Nigam*[c]

Departments of [a]Urology and [b]Nuclear Medicine,
Technical University of Munich, Munich, FRG;
[c]Prostaglandin Research Unit, Free University of Berlin, Berlin

Hypercalciuria is well recognized as an important factor in the cause of idiopathic calcium stone disease. It is now well established that renal prostaglandins (PG) influence intrarenal hemodynamics and tubular electrolyte excretion [1, 3].

PG seem to influence calcium and sodium reabsorption producing either hypercalciuria and natriuresis or sodium retention and hypocalciuria. Buck et al. [2] treated 43 hypercalciuric patients with a PG inhibitor for periods ranging from 2 to 4 weeks, and all patients showed a significant fall in urinary calcium excretion to within the normal range. Contrary to these results are the measurements of Rocco et al. [5]: they administered indomethacin, ketoprofen and aspirin to normal volunteers. These non-steroidal anti-inflammatory drugs decreased urinary sodium excretion but had no effect on creatinine clearance or urinary calcium excretion. For further investigation of this hypothesis we measured the urinary PGE_2, calcium, sodium and potassium excretion in patients with recurrent calcium urolithiasis.

Material and Methods

Patient Data. 18 unselected patients with recurrent, sterile, metabolically active stone formation, 11 males and 7 females; average age 42 years.

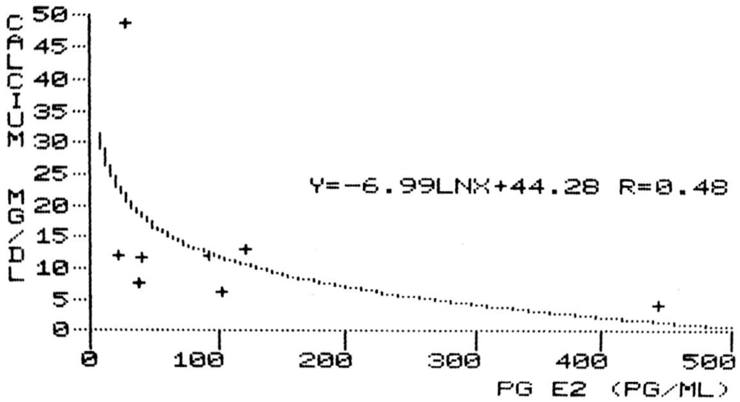

Fig. 1. Correlation between urinary PGE_2 excretion and urinary calcium concentration using the Nigam assay.

Study Protocol. Stone formers participated in an outpatient study. None of the patients took medication which could affect the metabolism of calcium. Pretest urine was sterile. All patients were maintained on the customary outpatient diet until 8 p.m. the night before testing. From then on they fasted until the beginning of the test procedures the following morning. 24-hour urine was collected from all patients while consuming random diet.

Analyses. Urinary calcium, sodium and potassium concentration was examined by a Technicon SMA 12 autoanalyzer and by flame photometry.

Urinary PGE_2 concentration was determined by two different methods: (1) By a method published by Nigam et al. [4]: PGE_2 was extracted from acidified urine, separated by chromatography on silica gel columns and by high pressure liquid chromatography and was then measured by radioimmunoassay. (2) By NEN PGE_2 (^{125}I) Ria Kit: The urine sample was acidified to pH 4.0 and extracted twice with an equal volume of chloroform. The extract was then assayed without further chromatographic separation.

Results

Our results (fig. 1, 2) showed only poor correlation between urinary PGE_2 excretion and urinary calcium concentration (Nigam et al. [4]: $r = 0.48$; NEN: $r = 0.16$). Further on, our results indicated that irrespectively of the method there was no significant correlation between urinary PGE_2 excretion and urinary sodium concentration (Nigam: $r = 0.44$; NEN: $r = 0.11$).

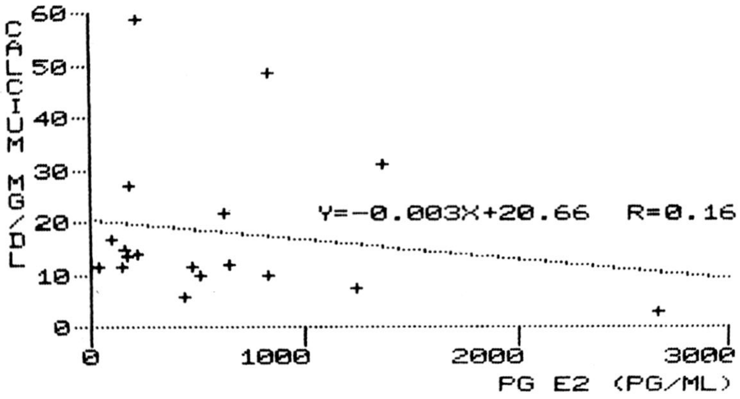

Fig. 2. Correlation between urinary PGE_2 excretion and urinary calcium concentration using the NEN assay.

A high significant correlation ($p < 0.01$) between urinary PGE_2 excretion and urinary potassium concentration was measured, when the method described by Nigam was applied ($r = 0.90$). However, if we used the NEN Ria Kit, there was no significant correlation between urinary PGE_2 excretion and urinary potassium concentration ($r = 0.02$).

Discussion

In contrast to Buck et al. [2], who investigated the influence of renal PG on urinary calcium excretion by inhibition of the PG synthetase, we tried to measure the real concentration of PGE_2 in the 24-hour urine of recurrent calcium stone formers.

Our data did not show any apparent correlation between urinary PGE_2 concentration and urinary sodium or calcium concentration.

These results can be due to two possibilities: For whatever reason the results of our assays do not represent the real PGE_2 urinary concentrations; or PG are only of secondary importance in the modulation of urinary calcium and sodium excretion. No ready explanation can be given for the significant correlation between urinary PGE_2 concentration and urinary potassium excretion in the Nigam assay [4].

References

1 Bello, I.; Ruilope, L.; Alcaraz, F.; Garcia-Robles, R.; Tresguerres, J. F.; Alcazar, J. M.; Barrientos, A.; Sancho, J.; Rodicio, J. L.: Pathogenesis of hypertension in renal lithiasis. Mineral Electrolyte Metab. *6:* 302–307 (1981).

2 Buck, A. C.; Lote, C. J.; Sampson, W. F.: The influence of renal prostaglandins on urinary calcium excretion in idiopathic urolithiasis. J. Urol. *129:* 421–426 (1983).

3 Favre, L.; Williams, G.; Favre, H.; Paunier, L.; Vallotton, M. B.: Relationship of renal prostaglandins to distal transport of sodium chloride in normokalemic and hypokalemic man. Mineral Electrolyte Metab. *11:* 186–191 (1985).

4 Nigam, S.; Becker, R.; Rosendahl, U.; Hammerstein, J.; Benedetto, C.; Barbero, M.; Slater, T. F.: The concentrations of 6-keto-PGF 1-alpha and TXB 2 in plasma samples from patients with benign and malignant tumours of the breast. Prostaglandins *29:* 513–527 (1985).

5 Rocco, V. K.; Sakhaee, K.; Pak, C. Y. C.; Brater, D. C.: Lack of effect of prostaglandin inhibition on calcium excretion in normal volunteers. J. Urol. *133:* 1093–1094 (1985).

Rudolf Pfab, MD, Department of Urology, Technical University of Munich,
Ismaningerstrasse 22, D–8000 München 80 (FRG)

Contr. Nephrol., vol. 58, pp. 122–126 (Karger, Basel 1987)

Tubular Dysfunction in Nephrolithiasis: A Consequence of the Stone

Ph. Jaeger[a], *L. Portmann*[a], *J. M. Ginalski*[b], *P. Burckhardt*[a, 1]

Departments of [a]Internal Medicine and [b]Radiology, University Hospital, Lausanne, Switzerland

It has been known for almost 30 years that some patients with nephrolithiasis present renal tubular leaks of lithogenic substances such as calcium or phosphate [1, 2]. Meanwhile, evidence has been obtained that various other signs of tubular dysfunction can be encountered in renal stone formers [3–9]. Therefore, a concept has emerged that a primary leak of lithogenic substances, as part of a generalized renal tubular dysfunction, might be the first step of a cascade leading to renal stone disease. Recently, however, we challenged this hypothesis and raised the question whether the stone itself might be responsible for this apparent tubulopathy [10].

Patients and Methods

Two hundred and fourteen renal stone formers were included in this study. Based on an ambulatory protocol detailed elsewhere [10], the following 9 diagnoses were made: primary hyperparathyroidism (8 patients), medullary sponge kidneys (21 patients), hyperuricemia with or without concomitant hyperuricosuria (10 patients), cystinuria (2 patients) and struvite stone disease (6 patients); the remaining 167 patients were idiopathic stone formers with either normocalciuria (66 cases) or hypercalciuria (101 cases), the latter being classified into the absorptive (25 patients), dietary (69 patients) or renal (7 patients) subtype.

To evaluate the renal tubular function of these patients, the following parameters have been measured in fasting condition: theoretical renal threshold for phosphate (TmP/GFR)

[1] The authors wish to thank Miss A. F. Jacquet who performed the acid-base analyses, Mrs E. Temler who measured insulin and Miss M. C. Evraere who typed the manuscript. This study was supported in part by the Swiss National Science Foundation, Grant No. 3.923.0.83.

[11], excretion of lysozyme and of γ-glutamyl-transferase (γ-GT), fractional excretion of glucose, insulin, K and Mg; tubular acidification processes were studied by measurements of fasting urinary pH before and after a 3-day load in NH_4Cl (3 to 6 g/24 h) and by determination of fractional excretion of HCO_3 after a 3-day load of alkali (15.7 g/day of Ca gluconate and lactate and 2.4 g/day of Ca carbonate).

Results

One-third of the patients tested presented a low TmP/GFR, 17% a leak of lysozyme or of γ-GT, 8% a leak of glucose or of insulin, 3% a leak of Mg and 7% a leak of K. In 28% of the patients tested, fasting urinary pH was found on two occasions above 5.85; a NH_4Cl loading test was performed in most of them which led fasting urine pH to below 5.4 in all patients but one who had overt distal renal tubular acidosis (RTA). 13% of the patients tested had HCO_3 leak after alkali loading, leading to the diagnosis of incomplete proximal RTA (incomplete because of normal blood acid-base status). There was a relatively even distribution of these various tubular defects amongst the 9 categories of patients tested, with the following exceptions: a particularly high prevalence of lysozymuria in patients with struvite stone disease and in those with renal hypercalciuria, an anticipated strong incidence of low TmP/GFR in primary hyperparathyroidism, an absence of high urinary pH in patients with hyperuricemia, a marked prevalence of high urinary pH in patients with primary hyperparathyroidism and in those with struvite calculi, the latter presenting also frequent K and/or Mg leaks. Details are given in table I.

To study the cause of the tubular dysfunction the following parameters have been taken into account in two subsets of patients, i.e. 15 patients with at least 3 tubular defects and 17 patients without any tubular defect: age, sex, family history of nephrolithiasis, history of previous nephrotomies, number of stones ever formed or formed during the last 2 years, and presence of stones within the pyelocaliceal system at the time of the work-up. As apparent from table II, no significant difference between both subpopulations could be detected with respect to the first 6 parameters. On the other hand, as shown in figure 1, the number of stones present within the pyelocaliceal system at the time of the work-up was significantly larger amongst patients with tubular defects than in the control group; in particular the prevalence of cases with large stones in place was particularly high (33%) in patients with 'leaky' tubules, whereas no such case was found in the control group.

Table I. Number of patients with tubular dysfunction (number of patients tested)

	TmP/GFR < 0.8 mmol/l	Lysozyme > 17 kU/g creatinine	γ-GT > 21 U/g creatinine	FE glucose $> 525 \times 10^{-6}$	FE insulin $> 55 \times 10^{-4}$	FE Mg $> 4.5 \times 10^{-2}$	FE K $> 25 \times 10^{-2}$	pHu > 5.85	FE HCO_3 $> 15{,}000 \times 10^{-6}$
Primary hyperparathyroidism	5 (8)	1 (7)	0 (7)	0 (6)	2 (6)	0 (5)	0 (7)	6 (7)	0 (1)
Medullary sponge kidneys	6 (18)	5 (18)	1 (12)	1 (3)	0 (4)	0 (7)	0 (6)	6 (18)	1 (10)
Hyperuricemia	3 (10)	3 (10)	2 (4)	1 (2)	0 (2)	0 (3)	1 (4)	0 (10)	1 (3)
Cystinuria	1 (2)	0 (2)	0 (1)	0 (1)	0 (1)	0 (1)	0 (1)	2 (2)	1 (1)
Struvite stone disease	1 (4)	6 (6)	2 (6)	1 (3)	2 (3)	2 (3)	2 (4)	6 (6)	0 (0)
Idiopathic stone formers with normocalciuria	17 (64)	5 (63)	5 (36)	2 (24)	3 (24)	0 (26)	1 (26)	9 (66)	2 (33)
Absorptive idiopathic hypercalciuria	7 (25)	4 (24)	4 (18)	1 (14)	0 (14)	0 (16)	1 (17)	7 (24)	2 (18)
Dietary idiopathic hypercalciuria	19 (64)	7 (64)	6 (32)	1 (30)	1 (29)	1 (28)	1 (28)	21 (64)	8 (31)
Renal idiopathic hypercalciuria	2 (7)	4 (6)	1 (4)	0 (2)	0 (2)	0 (3)	1 (3)	3 (7)	0 (5)

Table II. Characteristics of patients with multiple tubular defects and without defects

	Multiple tubular defects (n = 15)	No tubular defects (n = 17)	p
Sex	6 M / 9 F	11 M / 6 F	n.s.
Age, years	49.0 ± 3.4	41.7 ± 2.4	n.s.
Occurrence of stones in family	3+ / 15	8+ / 17	n.s.
Occurrence of previous nephrotomy	4+ / 15	4+ / 17	n.s.
Number of stones formed (total)	5.97 ± 2.47	5.18 ± 1.14	n.s.
Number of stones formed (last 2 years)	1.47 ± 0.19	2.12 ± 0.38	n.s.

$\overline{X} \pm$ SEM. Adapted from reference 10 with permission from the publisher.

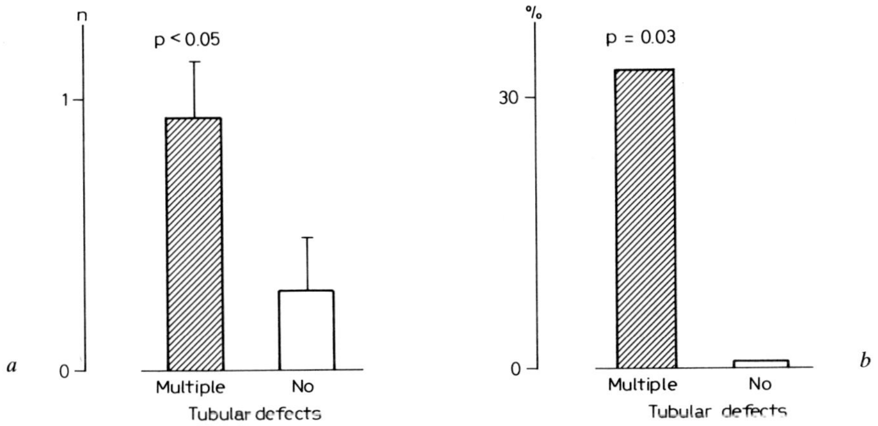

Fig. 1. Mean number of stones (*a*) and prevalence of large stones (*b*) in the pyelocaliceal systems at the time of analyses in patients with multiple tubular defects (hatched bars) and in those without such defects (open bars).

Discussion

The present study confirms that signs of tubular dysfunction can be encountered in renal stone formers, and that these leaks are not limited to lithogenic substances. On the contrary, this study shows that the defects may involve various transport systems located not only in the proximal tubule, but also in more distal nephron segments, and that the defects occur with a relatively even prevalence amongst the various categories of patients.

With respect to the pathogenic role of the renal tubular dysfunction, the data do not support the hypothesis that the defect comes first and the stone second: in particular no genetic trend could be detected. Conversely, a marked prevalence of tubulopathies was noted amongst stone formers who had stones, and in particular large stones, in place within the pyelocaliceal system at the moment when the tubular defects were diagnosed. This observation is interpreted as to show that the tubulopathy associated with nephrolithiasis is the consequence rather than the cause of the stone.

References

1 Albright, F.; Henneman, P.; Benedict, P. H.; Forbes, A. P.: Idiopathic hypercalciuria. A preliminary report. Proc. R. Soc. Med. *46:* 1077–1081 (1953).

2 Bordier, P.; Ryckewart, A.; Gueris, J.; Rasmussen, H.: On the pathogenesis of so-called idiopathic hypercalciuria. Am. J. Med. *63:* 398–409 (1977).

3 Ching, K. N.; Karam, J. H.; Choy, F. B.; Kolb, F. O.; Grodsky, G. M.; Forsham, P. H.: Hyperinsulinuria in patients with renal calculi. Clinica chim. Acta *40:* 383–389 (1972).

4 D'Angelo, A.; Pagano, F.; Ossi, E.; Lupo, A.; Messa, P.; Tessitore, N.; Maschio, G.: Renal tubular defects in recurring bilateral nephrolithiasis. Clin. Nephrol. *6:* 352–360 (1976).

5 Sutton, R. A. L.; Walker, V. R.: Responses to hydrochlorothiazide and acetazolamide in patients with calcium stones. New Engl. J. Med. *302:* 709–713 (1980).

6 Backman, U.; Danielson, B. G.; Johansson, G.; Ljunghall, S.; Wikström, B.: Incidence and clinical importance of renal tubular defects in recurrent renal stone formers. Nephron *25:* 96–101 (1980).

7 Fellström, B.; Backman, U.; Danielson, B. G.; Johansson, G.; Ljunghall, S.; Wikström, B.: Urinary excretion of urate in renal calcium stone disease and in renal tubular acidification disturbances. J. Urol. *127:* 589–592 (1982).

8 Baggio, B.; Gambaro, G.; Ossi, E.; Favaro, S.; Borsatti, A.: Increased urinary excretion of renal enzymes in idiopathic calcium oxalate nephrolithiasis. J. Urol. *129:* 1161–1162 (1983).

9 Anton, F. M.; Puig, J. G.; Gaspar, G.; Martinez, M. E.; Ramos, T.; Martinez-Pineiro, J. A.: Renal tubular acidosis in recurrent renal stone formers. Eur. Urol. *10:* 55–59 (1984).

10 Jaeger, P.; Portmann, L.; Ginalski, J. M.; Jacquet, A. F.; Temler, E.; Burckhardt, P.: Tubulopathy in nephrolithiasis: consequence rather than cause. Kidney int. *29:* 563–571 (1986).

11 Walton, R. J.; Bijvoet, O. L. M.: Nomogram for the derivation of renal threshold phosphate concentration. Lancet *ii:* 309–310 (1975).

Ph. Jaeger, MD, Department of Internal Medicine, University Hospital (CHUV),
BH 10, CH–1011 Lausanne (Switzerland)

Contr. Nephrol., vol. 58, pp. 127–136 (Karger, Basel 1987)

Concerning the Pathogenesis of Idiopathic Hypercalciuria[1]

Arthur E. Broadus, William J. Burtis, Dan A. Oren, Leonardo Sartori, Linda Gay, Alice F. Ellison, Karl L. Insogna

Department of Internal Medicine, Yale University and the West Haven Veterans Medical Center, New Haven and West Haven, Conn., USA

In this brief review, we would like to touch on three areas: (1) the frequency of 'dietary' hypercalciuria in patients screened on their 'free' or habitual diets; (2) the operational definition of what we have come to refer to as 'constitutional' hypercalciuria, and (3) the criteria for diagnosis, frequency, and details of pathogenesis of the syndrome of absorptive hypercalciuria. For brevity, we will confine ourselves largely to our own work in the area and will make no attempt to review the subject of the hypercalciurias in a comprehensive fashion.

Materials and Methods

We have recently summarized the results from the first 400 patients screened in the Renal Stone Clinic at Yale [1]. Stone analyses were available from 363 patients and, of these, 282 had garden-variety calcium stone disease (pure calcium oxalate or mixed calcium oxalate-calcium phosphate stones). In order to fully appreciate the data in the following sections, it is necessary to describe in some detail the manner in which the patients were screened for hypercalciuria and further evaluated.

Patients arrived for their first visit having collected a 24-hour urine specimen on their 'free' or habitual diet and having kept a 3-day diet diary, the last day corresponding to the day of the urine collection. A number of routine fasting measurements were performed on this morning, including the renal tubular phosphate threshold (TmP/GFR). The patients were then instructed on a 1,000-mg calcium, 1 g/kg protein, and 100-mEq sodium diet for a 3-day period, with a 24-hour urine collection being performed on the third day of this diet.

[1] Supported in part by grants (RR 125 and AM 31998) from the National Institutes of Health, by the Veterans Administration, and by the Adult General Clinical Research Center of the Yale-New Haven Hospital.

All consenting patients found to be hypercalciuric on either their 'free' diet or the defined 1,000-mg calcium diet, or both, were evaluated in more detail. The minimum such evaluation was a 24-hour urine specimen and performance of an oral calcium tolerance test on an outpatient basis after 7–10 days on a restricted calcium (400-mg) and sodium (100-mEq) diet, and the maximum such evaluation was a 5-day admission to a metabolic ward, with study on a restricted (400-mg) calcium diet, performance of the calcium tolerance test, and restudy on an unrestricted (1,000-mg) calcium diet [2–4]. Additional details concerning the further study of selected subgroups of patients are given in the text below.

As will be discussed, *both* the limits used in defining hypercalciuria *and* the dietary conditions under which patients were screened turned out to be important considerations in constructing the study populations of hypercalciuric patients described below. We chose to accept patients as hypercalciuric if they exceeded either an absolute excretion rate limit (> 300 mg/day in males and > 250 mg/day in females) or a weight-adjusted limit (> 4 mg/kg/day in either sex) on *either* the 'free' diet or the defined 1,000-mg calcium diet. The upper-normal limit of the calciuric response to the calcium tolerance test is Δ <0.20 mg calcium/dl GF [2], and the normal range for the plasma concentration of 1,25-$(OH)_2D$ is 22–66 pg/ml [3, 4].

'Dietary' Hypercalciuria

Using the criteria given above, 122 (43%) of the 282 patients with calcium stone disease were classified as hypercalciuric. As shown in table I, these 122 patients could be subclassified into four groups: (1) those patients who were hypercalciuric only on the 'free' diet (group A); (2) those patients who were hypercalciuric on both diets but who demonstrated a pronounced fall in calcium excretion (> 50 mg/day) on the 1,000-mg calcium diet relative to the 'free' diet (group B); (3) those patients with essentially the same results on both diets (group C), and (4) those patients who were hypercalciuric only on the defined 1,000-mg calcium diet (group D).

The 44 patients in groups A and B were regarded as examples of 'dietary' hypercalciuria. On average, these patients were consuming about 700 mg/day of calcium on their 'free' diets, yet when screened on an even higher calcium intake of 1,000 mg/day, they demonstrated a paradoxical fall in calcium excretion averaging nearly 100 mg/day. Clearly, some dietary factor other than calcium must have been contributing to the hypercalciuria in these patients on their habitual diets. A variety of lines of evidence indicated that by far the most important dietary factor in this regard was sodium [1]. These data included (a) significantly ($p < 0.001$) higher figures for sodium intake and sodium excretion in patients with 'dietary' hypercalciuria than in nonhypercalciuric patients or the hypercalciuric patients in groups C and D, (b) a striking parallel between the reductions in calcium

Table I. Screening results from 122 hypercalciuric patients

Diet on which hypercalciuria was detected	Calcium excretion on 'free' diet mg/day	Calcium excretion on 1,000-mg calcium diet mg/day	Number of patients	Number of patients evaluated in detail
A 'Free' diet only	334	236	27	17
B Both 'free' and 1,000-mg calcium diets but calcium excretion fell > 50 mg/day on the 1,000-mg diet	422	331	17	12
C Both 'free' and 1,000-mg calcium diets	354	365	41	34
D 1,000-mg calcium diet only	224	328	37	28

The data are given as mean values.

excretion and sodium excretion on the two diets in patients with 'dietary' hypercalciuria, and (c) a strong positive correlation ($r = 0.50$, $p < 0.001$) between sodium excretion and calcium excretion on the 'free' diet in the entire hypercalciuric population (groups A–D). In addition, multiple linear regression analysis indicated that sodium was far more strongly correlated with calcium excretion on the 'free' diet than other dietary factors which might be considered as important influences on calcium absorption and/or excretion (e.g. dietary calcium, protein, or carbohydrate).

Seventeen patients in group A were evaluated in detail, and 14 were found to be metabolically normal (mean calciuric response to the calcium tolerance $\triangle$ 0.14 mg calcium/dl GF and mean plasma 1,25-$[OH]_2D$ 51 pg/ml). In contrast, and in keeping with the findings in the other groups found to be hypercalciuric on the defined 1,000-mg calcium diet (see below), patients in group B were enriched for the syndrome of absorptive hypercalciuria. That is, 12 patients in group B were evaluated in detail, and 8 patients were classical examples of absorptive hypercalciuria (mean calciuric response to the calcium tolerance test $\triangle$ 0.28 mg calcium/dl GF and mean plasma 1,25-$(OH)_2D$ 70 pg/ml).

We conclude from these data (1) that 'dietary' hypercalciuria is common, contributing to if not causing hypercalciuria in as many as one half of patients found to be hypercalciuric on their habitual diets, (2) that the principal culprit appears to be sodium, (3) that apparent sodium-induced hypercalciuria can occur in individuals who appear to be otherwise metabolically normal or may be superimposed on other well-recognized mechanisms such as absorptive hypercalciuria, and (4) that a study population defined on a 'free' diet is likely to be quite heterogeneous with respect to mechanism, a point which probably has a great deal to do with the controversy in the literature with respect to the pathogenesis of so-called idiopathic hypercalciuria. Our findings complement those of Muldowney et al. [5] and clearly support the notion that apparent sodium-induced hypercalciuria is clinically important.

'Constitutional' Hypercalciuria

The defined 1,000-mg calcium diet employed in the outpatient studies described above is identical to that employed in our inpatient evaluation [2–4] and is designed (a) to maximize the appreciation of hypercalciuria in any patient in whom the hypercalciuria is based, wholely or in part, on gastrointestinal hyperabsorption of calcium, and (b) to minimize dietary influences other than calcium (see previous section). It has been our experience that a study population of hypercalciuric patients so defined is highly enriched for patients with true metabolic abnormalities in calcium metabolism, most particularly the syndrome of absorptive hypercalciuria. This was also the experience in the present series: of the 74 patients in groups B–D of table I evaluated in detail, 58 (78%) proved to have the syndrome of absorptive hypercalciuria. Additional details concerning this syndrome are presented in the next section.

The remaining 16 patients from groups B–D were initially regarded as unclassifiable. However, in reexamining the data from these 16 patients, a typical phenotype was observed in 10. These 10 patients were all of large size, were hypercalciuric when calcium excretion was expressed on an absolute excretion rate but not on a weight-adjusted basis, and were metabolically quite normal. We have come to use the term 'constitutional' hypercalciuria in connection with such patients. The findings in these 10 patients are contrasted in table II with those in patients of similar large size who proved to have the syndrome of absorptive hypercalciuria and also with

Table II. 'Constitutional' hypercalciuria

Patient populations	Weight kg	Calcium excretion on 1,000-mg calcium diet		Calciuric response to calcium tolerance test △ mg calcium/dl GF	Plasma $1,25\text{-}(OH)_2D$ pg/ml	Sex M/F
		absolute mg/day	weight-adjusted mg/kg/day			
Constitutional hypercalciuria	101	363	3.6	0.12	44	9/1
Patients of large size with absorptive hypercalciuria	94	411	4.4	0.25	66	11/1
Patients of small size with absorptive hypercalciuria	52	252	4.6	0.29	66	2/15

All data are given as mean values.

those in patients of small size who proved to have the syndrome of absorptive hypercalciuria (who were predominately females). The data in table II clearly indicate that weight-adjusted values for calcium excretion are the single most reliable means of expressing and interpreting the results for calcium excretion in a patient population with a greater than 2-fold range of body size and also are highly predictive of an underlying error in calcium metabolism. That is, if only patients exhibiting a calcium excretion rate ≥ than 4.0 mg/kg/day on the 1,000-mg calcium diet were accepted as hypercalciuric, then 58 of 64 patients (91%) proved to have the syndrome of absorptive hypercalciuria.

Pathogenesis and Criteria for Diagnosis of Absorptive Hypercalciuria

This section summarizes a series of studies which has led us (1) to conclude that absorptive hypercalciuria is regularly a $1,25\text{-}(OH)_2D$-mediated syndrome, (2) to question the validity of the measurement of fasting calcium excretion as a criterion for patient classification, and (3) to propose that the pathogenesis of absorptive hypercalciuria is due to a disordered regulation of 1,25-$(OH)_2D$ production, the precise nature of this defect being as yet unknown.

Our initial clinical study involved 50 patients with absorptive hypercalciuria, 25 normal subjects, and 25 non-hypercalciuric patients with stone disease [3]. The patients with absorptive hypercalciuria were required to fulfill *each* of three criteria for purposes of inclusion: (1) hypercalciuria on the 1,000-mg calcium diet, (2) an abnormal calciuric response to the calcium tolerance test, and (3) normal or suppressed parathyroid function in the fasting state [2–4].

The principal conclusions of this study were four [3]. First, elevated values for plasma 1,25-$(OH)_2D$ were observed in 80% of the patients with absorptive hypercalciuria, with high-normal values being observed in the remaining 20%. Second, a 'severe' clinical and biochemical form of the disorder could be identified simply by selecting those patients whose plasma level of 1,25-$(OH)_2D$ exceeded the normal mean by more than four standard deviations. Third, a majority of patients with absorptive hypercalciuria demonstrated an increase in fasting calcium excretion and also in fasting fractional calcium excretion (or calcium clearance), but these results were negatively correlated with fasting parathyroid function, indicating that this 'renal leak' of calcium was secondary to chronic parathyroid suppression. Fourth, when the results for TmP/GFR or the serum phosphorus concentration in the non-hypercalciurics were considered, there was no correlation or predictable relationship between these values and the plasma concentration of 1,25-$(OH)_2D$, a finding which does not support the phosphate-leak hypothesis of pathogenesis.

Interpretation as to the basis of the increase in fasting calcium excretion in patients with absorptive hypercalciuria is of some general importance, given the rather widespread use of this measurement as a key if not definitional criterion for classifying patients with idiopathic hypercalciuria. We therefore sought to confirm this observation and interpretation experimentally. This was done by creating a 'model' of absorptive hypercalciuria in normal subjects by administering a supraphysiological dose of 1,25-$(OH)_2D$ [6]. Fasting calcium excretion increased by 50% in this 'model' and was entirely the result of an increase in fasting calcium clearance, which was in turn the result of the hyperabsorption-induced suppression of parathyroid function [6]. These findings corroborate the clinical data described in the previous paragraph and suggest that, by itself, fasting calcium excretion is an entirely non-specific criterion for patient classification. A virtually identical result and interpretation has been published by Adams et al. [7].

We next sought to confirm that the increased plasma concentration of 1,25-$(OH)_2$D observed in patients with absorptive hypercalciuria was a reflection of an increased production rate of the hormone rather than an alteration in its metabolic clearance. This study was performed using the infusion equilibrium technique and revealed an identical metabolic clearance rate in normal subjects and patients with absorptive hypercalciuria [8]. The average production rate of 1,25-$(OH)_2$D in the patients with absorptive hypercalciuria was 3.4 μg/day, some 50% higher than the mean value observed in normal subjects [8].

At this point, we concluded that we had been able to construct a rather homogeneous study population and that the next level of questioning should focus on the control of 1,25-$(OH)_2$D production in patients with absorptive hypercalciuria. Our initial hypothesis in this regard was that 1,25-$(OH)_2$D production might be relatively autonomous in these patients and that a suppression test could be devised which would bring such an abnormality into stark relief. This suppression test was fashioned from our 5-day inpatient protocol by resampling patients on the morning of day six, some 72 h after the dietary calcium intake had been increased from 400 to 1,000 mg/day [4].

What we observed was quite the opposite of what was predicted by the autonomy hypothesis. The circulating concentration of 1,25-$(OH)_2$D turned out to be remarkably sensitive to an increase in calcium intake in patients with absorptive hypercalciuria (fig. 1). This sensitivity was such that, whereas there was virtually complete segregation of values for plasma 1,25-$(OH)_2$D between non-hypercalciuric patients and patients with absorptive hypercalciuria on the restricted calcium diet, there was essentially complete overlap of these values between the groups on the 1,000-mg calcium diet (fig. 2). Indeed, on the 1,000-mg calcium diet the mean value of 49 pg/ml for plasma 1,25-$(OH)_2$D in the patients with absorptive hypercalciuria was nearly identical to our normal mean of 44 pg/ml [4].

Six inpatients who had been through the short-term protocol were discharged on the 1,000-mg calcium diet and restudied at 14 days. These patients demonstrated an apparent 'escape' phenomenon, in which circulating 1,25-$(OH)_2$D rebounded toward initial values and TmP/GFR plummeted to values which were lower even than those observed initially on the restricted calcium diet [8].

Our conclusions from this study were basically two. First, it was apparent that the plasma concentration of 1,25-$(OH)_2$D in patients with absorptive hypercalciuria is highly fluid as a function of calcium intake and that

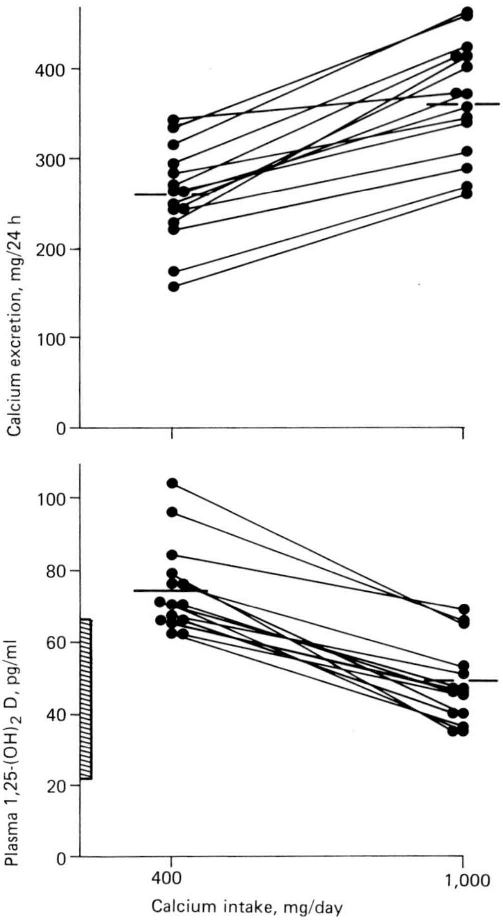

Fig. 1. Plasma 1,25-$(OH)_2D$ and 24-hour calcium excretion in 15 patients with absorptive hypercalciuria studied initially on a restricted (400-mg) calcium diet and again 72 h after being placed on an unrestricted (1,000-mg) calcium diet. The hatched area indicates the normal range for plasma 1,25-$(OH)_2D$, and the horizontal bars represent mean values.

values ranging from low-normal to some two times the normal mean could be seen in individual patients based on the conditions of study. This point is considered to be particularly relevant to the study design employed in the metabolic evaluation of hypercalciuric patients and likely explains much of the disagreement in the literature regarding the results for plasma 1,25-$(OH)_2D$ in hypercalciuric patients. Second, these data suggest disor-

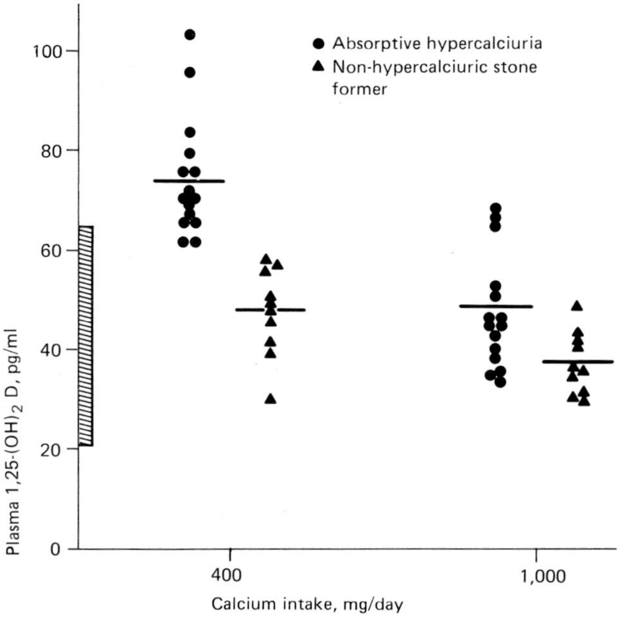

Fig. 2. Individual values for plasma 1,25-$(OH)_2D$ in 15 patients with absorptive hypercalciuria and 10 non-hypercalciuric patients with stone disease studied on both a 400- and a 1,000-mg calcium diet. The hatched area indicates the normal range, and the horizontal bars represent mean values.

dered control rather than autonomy as the basis for the increase in the production rate of 1,25-$(OH)_2D$ in patients with the syndrome of absorptive hypercalciuria.

We are presently in the midst of a systemic evaluation of the control(s) of 1,25-$(OH)_2D$ production in patients with absorptive hypercalciuria. One hypothesis under consideration is that patients with absorptive hypercalciuria might display a hypersensitivity to phosphate deprivation in terms of 1,25-$(OH)_2D$ production. What we have observed is again quite the opposite of what might have been predicted, in that patients with absorptive hypercalciuria have displayed a blunted if not entirely absent 1,25-$(OH)_2D$ response to a phosphopenic stimulus [9]. These data would appear to represent evidence for a frankly qualitative defect in the control of 1,25-$(OH)_2D$ production in patients with absorptive hypercalciuria. An alternate hypothesis, and one which is considered to be particularly attractive on intuitive grounds, is that the pathogenetic basis of absorptive hypercalciuria could relate to a proximal tubular hypersensitivity to the effects of parathyroid hormone. Such a defect could explain all of the data summarized in the preceding paragraphs. This hypothesis is under current study, employing the infusion of a slightly supraphysiological dosage of $bPTH^{1-34}$ as a stimulus. The findings to date are intriguing but too preliminary to merit inclusion in this manuscript.

References

1 Burtis, W.J.; Oren, D.A.; Insogna, K.L.; Lang, R.; Kliger, A.S.; Sartori, L.; Gay, L.F.; Ellison, A.F.; Broadus, A.E.: Metabolic evaluation of 363 consecutive patients in a renal stone clinic (submitted).

2 Broadus, A.E.; Dominguez, M.; Bartter, F.C.: Pathophysiologic studies in idiopathic hypercalciuria. J. clin. Endocr. Metab. *47:* 751–760 (1978).

3 Broadus, A.E.; Insogna, K.L.; Lang, R.; Mallette, L.E.; Oren, D.A.; Kliger, A.S.; Ellison, A.F.: A consideration of the hormonal basis and phosphate-leak hypothesis of absorptive hypercalciuria. J. clin. Endocr. Metab. *58:* 161–169 (1984).

4 Broadus, A.E.; Insogna, K.L.; Lang, R.; Ellison, A.E.; Dreyer, B.E.: Evidence for disordered control of 1,25-dihydroxyvitamin D in absorptive hypercalciuria. New Engl. J. Med. *311:* 73–80 (1984).

5 Muldowney, F.P.; Freaney, R.; Moloney, M.F.: Importance of dietary sodium in the hypercalciuric syndrome. Kidney int. *22:* 292–296 (1982).

6 Broadus, A.E.; Erickson, S.B.; Gertner, J.M.; Cooper, K.; Dobbins, J.W.: An experimental human model of 1,25-$(OH)_2D$-mediated hypercalciuria. J. clin. Endocr. Metab. *59:* 202–206 (1984).

7 Adams, N.D.; Gray, R.W.; Leman, J.; Cheung, H.S.: Effects of calcitriol administration on calcium metabolism in healthy men. Kidney int. *21:* 90–97 (1982).

8 Insogna, K.L.; Broadus, A.E.; Dreyer, B.E.; Ellison, A.F.; Gertner, J.M.: Elevated production rate for 1,25-dihydroxyvitamin D in patients with absorptive hypercalciuria. J. clin. Endocr. Metab. *61:* 490–495 (1985).

9 Insogna, K.; Lang, R.; Ellison, A.; Broadus, A.: Qualitative abnormality in 1,25-dihydroxyvitamin D response to phosphorus deprivation in patients with absorptive hypercalciuria. Clin. Res. *33:* 433A (1985).

Arthur E. Broadus, PhD, Division of Endocrinology, Fitkin I,
Department of Internal Medicine, Yale University, 333 Cedar Street,
New Haven, CT 06511 (USA)

Contr. Nephrol., vol. 58, pp. 137–142 (Karger, Basel 1987)

Increased Plasma Concentrations of Total and Free 1,25-$(OH)_2$ D_3 in Calcium Stone Formers with Idiopathic Hypercalciuria

P. Bataille[a], *R. Bouillon*[b], *A. Fournier*[a], *H. Renaud*[a], *J. Gueris*[c], *A. Idrissi*[a]

[a]CHU, Amiens, France; [b]Clinique St. Rafaël, Leuven, Belgique; and [c]Hôpital Lariboisière, Paris, France

The role of 1,25-$(OH)_2D_3$ vitamin D in the pathophysiology of hypercalciuria frequently observed in calcium stone formers remains controversial. As a matter of fact elevated plasma concentrations (P) of 1,25-$(OH)_2D$ have been reported with a widely variable frequency ranging from zero [1, 2] to 80% [3]. These discrepancies may be explained by genetic differences but this seems unlikely since absence of increased P 1,25-$(OH)_2D$ has been observed in Chicago [1] and Amsterdam [2]. More likely the discrepancies may be explained by the criteria of selection of the patients and by the dietary conditions. The latter are of primary importance since it has been shown that P 1,25-$(OH)_2D$ are highly sensitive to calcium diet [4]. Furthermore, although 1,25-$(OH)_2D$ assays have been available for more than 10 years, their reliability is not consistent and explains why data are still rare and come only from a few highly specialized laboratories. Radioimmunoassay methods recently introduced seem to have higher reproducibility and higher sensitivity than the receptor assays [5]. Finally the D-binding protein may alter the fraction of free 1,25-$(OH)_2D$, i.e. the biologically active fraction and this parameter has heretofore not been taken into account in the 1,25-$(OH)_2D$ interpretation in calcium stone formers.

Therefore, we have studied the plasma concentrations of 1,25-$(OH)_2D$ measured by radioimmunoassay simultaneously with measurement of the D-binding protein and the other usual phosphocalcic parameters in calcium stone formers after 4 days of calcium-restricted diet (CaRD), strictly classified on the basis of the calcium excretion, fasting calcium:creatinine urinary ratio and plasma concentrations of parathyroid hormone (PTH) before and after 1 g of calcium load, in comparison to a control group studied in the same conditions.

Patients and Methods

51 normocalcemic patients and 12 controls were studied as outpatients. They collected their 24-hour urine on free diet and after 4 days of CaRD (400 mg/day). After 12 h fasting, 2-hour fasting urines were collected for determination of the uCa/uCr. Before 1 g calcium load at 9 a.m., blood samples were taken and analyzed for calcium, creatinine, phosphate, protein, PTH and 1,25-$(OH)_2D_3$. PTH was again evaluated at 1 p.m.

Values of plasma calcium were corrected according protein concentration with Parfitt's formula. The renal tubular phosphate threshold ($TmPO_4$/GFR) was derived by means of a nomogram [6]. PTH C terminal determined by radioimmunoassay has a normal range between 20 and 45 pg/ml on normal calcium diet. Normal mean (± SD) for serum 1,25-$(OH)_2D$ determined by radioimmunoassay as described by one of us [5] on a free diet is 42 ± 13 pg/ml. The normal mean (± SD) for DBP measured by serial radial immunodiffusion [7] is 333 ± 58 mg/l. The free 1,25-$(OH)_2D$ index was calculated as the molar ratio of this steroid and DBP. Normal mean ± SD on free diet is 1.8 ± 4 (molar ratio $\times 10^{-5}$).

Classification of Patients

Based on our own control data previously published [8], 19 patients were normocalciuric on a free diet (NCa). After CaRD, 9 patients became normocalciuric and were considered as having dietary hypercalciuria (DH). Their fasting uCa/uCr and plasma PTH levels were in the normal range. In the remaining were found patients with absorptive hypercalciuria (AH), defined by increased calciuria on free as well as on CaRD but with normal fasting uCa/uCr and normal PTH levels, and 2 patients with renal hypercalciuria (RH), defined by increased calciuria on free as well as CaRD but with elevated fasting uCa/uCr and higher PTH levels than in controls on the same restricted diet, which normalized after calcium load.

Some patients were classified in a group of undetermined idiopathic hypercalciuria (UH). These patients were hypercalciuric on free diet as well as on a CaRD. Their fasting uCa/uCr was elevated but with fasting PTH levels in the range of controls values that excluded the diagnosis of RH according to the criteria of Pak et al. [9].

Results

Table I shows first the expected increases of uCaV on free and CaRD and the increase of fasting uCa/uCr urinary ratio according to the classification criteria. Then it shows that plasma calcium tends to be lower than in controls, in the calcium stone formers with normocalciuria, dietary hypercalciuria and absorptive hypercalciuria. Plasma phosphate and Tm PO_4/GFR are significantly lower than in control in UH and still more in AH.

Table II shows that fasting PTH is only increased in the 2 patients with RH (this increase and its normalization by calcium load are in fact definition criteria for RH), whereas it is in the lower range of normal in the other patients with idiopathic hypercalciuria and significantly lower in pa-

Table I. Basic biological data (mean ± SEM)

Calcium stone former groups	Sex ratio M/F	uCaV-free diet mmol/ 24 h	uCaV CaRD mmol/ 24 h	Fasting uCa/uCr mmol/ mmol	PCa mmol/l corrected for protein	PPO_4 mmol/l	$TmPO_4$/ GFR mmol/l
Normo-calciuria	7/12	5.1 ±0.3	2.1 ±0.2	0.13 ±0.01	2.27 ±0.06*	0.90 ±0.08	0.86 ±0.03
Dietary hyper-calciuria	6/3	10.3 ±0.7***	4.2 ±0.3	0.17 ±0.02	2.27 ±0.06*	0.93 ±0.06	0.85 ±0.03
Absorptive hypercalciuria	6/2	10.4 ±1.5***	7.5 ± 0.9***	0.15 ±0.02	2.28 ±0.08	0.82 ±0.09***	0.70 0.04***
Renal hyper-calciuria	1/1	8.3 −15.7***	6.5 −7.1***	0.45 −0.67**	2.37 −2.56	0.97 −1.19	0.75 −1.1
Undetermined hypercalciuria	9/4	10.8 ±1***	7.7 ±0.6***	0.39** ±0.03	2.37 ±0.05	0.88 ±0.06*	0.77 ±0.05**
Controls	7/5	5 ±2.2	3.7 ±1	0.17 ±0.02	2.39 ±0.09	1.05 ±0.12	0.96 ±0.04

Significance of the comparison versus controls: * $p < 0.05$; ** $p < 0.01$; *** $p < 0.001$.

tients with normocalciuria and dietary hypercalciuria. The D-binding protein levels of the patients are comparable with those of the controls. Plasma concentrations of total 1,25-$(OH)_2D$ as well as of free 1,25-$(OH)_2D$ index are significantly increased above the normal mean + 2 SD not only in the 2 patients with RH but also in 5 out of the 8 patients with AH and in 6 out of 13 patients with UH.

In the AH group PPO_4 and $TmPO_4$/GFR are negatively correlated to total P 1,25-$(OH)_2D$ ($r = -0.90$, $n = 8$, $p < 0.01$; $r = -0.86$, $n = 8$, $p < 0.01$) and to the free 1,25-$(OH)_2D$ index ($r = -0.87$, $n = 8$, $p < 0.01$; $r = -0.75$, $n = 8$, $p < 0.01$). In the UH group the free 1,25-$(OH)_2D$ index was negatively correlated to PTH ($r = -0.59$, $n = 13$, $p < 0.05$), but no correlation was found between PPO_4, PCa and free P 1,25-$(OH)_2D$. No correlation was found between PTH and fasting uCa/uCr.

Table II. Basic biological data (mean ± SEM)

Calcium stone formers groups	PTH fasting pg/ml	D-binding protein μg/ml	P 1,25-$(OH)_2D$ pg/ml	Molar ratio 1.25-$(OH)_2D$/DBP 10^{-5}
Normocalciuria	19* ±3	401 ±16	61 ±3	2.05 ±0.1
Dietary hypercalciuria	19* ±4	306 ±17	59 ±6	2.05 ±0.19
Absorptive hypercalciuria	28 ±7	357 ±17	72 ±6**	2.7 ±0.24**
Renal hypercalciuria	62 −96**	389 −317	88 −78**	3.08 −3.27**
Undetermined hypercalciuria	30 ±5	389 ±16	72 ±7**	2.47 ±0.24**
Controls	42 ±6	390 ±23	50 ±4	1.75 ±0.14

Significance of the comparison versus controls: * $p < 0.05$; ** $p < 0.01$.

Discussion and Conclusions

D-binding protein is normal in calcium stone formers and does not affect interpretation of the plasma concentration of 1,25-$(OH)_2D$.

Total and free plasma concentrations of 1,25-$(OH)_2D$ are increased in 60% of idiopathic hypercalciuria. This is observed in the 2 patients with renal hypercalciuria who presented a state of secondary hyperparathyroidism and in patients with absorptive hypercalciuric according to the criteria of Broadus et al. [3], which include absorptive and undetermined hypercalciuria in the classification of Pak et al. [9].

A decreased plasma phosphate, observed in these latter subgroups of Pak's classification, is more marked in the absorptive subgroup which therefore corresponds more precisely to the type 3 of the absorptive hypercalciuria of Pak et al. [9]. Only in this subgroup strong negative correlations between P 1,25-$(OH)_2D$ (free or total) and PPO_4 or $TmPO_4/GFR$ ($r = -0.9$, and $r = -0.86$, respectively, $p < 0.01$) were found. These correlations are compatible either with the phosphate leak hypothesis [10, 11] or with the hypothesis of a complex disorder of the proximal tubule associating phosphate leak and increased 1,25-$(OH)_2D$ synthesis [3].

The significant negative correlation found between free P 1,25-$(OH)_2D$ and PTH ($r = -0.59$, $p < 0.05$) in the undetermined hypercalciuria suggests that PTH is suppressed by a primary increase of 1,25-$(OH)_2D$ synthesis. In this subgroup it has to be pointed out that no other correlation has been found between P 1,25-$(OH)_2D$ and the other potentially stimulating factors of 25-OH vitamin D_1 α-hydroxylase, i.e. low plasma concentrations of calcium or phosphate, suggesting an independent dysregulation of 1,25-$(OH)_2D$ in this subgroup. Since different pathophysiological correlations have been found with P 1,25-$(OH)_2D$ in the 2 subgroups of idiopathic hypercalciuria (absorptive and undetermined) the distinction on the basis of fasting uCa/uCr ratio normality seems justified.

In our urolithiasis populations, renal hypercalciuria with increased but suppressive PTH secretion is a rare pathophysiological condition since it occurs in only 4% of the calcium stone formers.

References

1 Coe, F.L.; Favus, M.G.; Crockett, T.; Strauss, A.L.; Parks, J.H.; Porat, A.; Gantt, C.L.; Sherwood, L.M.: Effect of low calcium diet on urine calcium excretion, parathyroid-function and serum 1,25-$(OH)_2D_3$ levels in patients with idiopathic hypercalciuria and in normal subjects. Am. J. Med. *72:* 25–32 (1982).

2 Metelen Bos, J.C.; Jongen, M.J.M.; Wim, J.F.; Van der Vijgh, P.; Van Ginkel, J.: Vitamin D status in urinary calcium stone formation. Archs intern. Med. *145:* 681 684 (1985).

3 Broadus, A.E.; Insogna, K.L.; Lang, R.; Mallette, L.E.; Oren, D.A.; Gertner, J.M.; Kliger, M.S.; Ellison, A.: A consideration of the hormonal basis and phosphate leak hypothesis of absorptive hypercalciuria. J. clin. Endocr. Metab. *58:* 161–169 (1984).

4 Insogna, K.; Lang, R.; Kliger, A.; Ellison, A.; Broadus, A.E.: Evidence for hypersensitivity of 1,25-$(OH)_2D_3$ production in absorptive hypercalciuria. Clin. Res. *30:* 525A (1982).

5 Bouillon, R.; De Moor, P.; Baggiolini, E.G.; Uskukovic, R.: A radioimmunoassay for 1,25-dihydroxycholecalciferol. Clin. Chem. *26:* 562–567 (1980).

6 Bijvoet, O.L.M.: Kidney function in calcium and phosphate metabolism; in Avioli, Krane, Metabolic bone disease, pp. 49–410 (Academic Press, New York 1977).

7 Bouillon, R.; Van Assche, F.A.; Van Boelen, M.; Meyns, W.; De Moar, P.: Influence of the vitamin D binding protein on the serum concentration of 1,25-dihydroxy vitamin D_3. J. clin. Invest. *67:* 589–596 (1981).

8 Bataille, P.; Charransol, G.; Gregoire, I.; Fournier, A.: Effect of calcium restriction on renal excretion of oxalate and the probability of being a stone former. J. Urol. *130:* 218–281 (1983).

9 Pak, C.Y.C.; Britton, F.; Peterson, R.; Ward, D.; Northcutt, C.; Breslau, N.; McGuire, J.; Sakhae, K.; Bush, S.; Nicar, M.; Norman, D.A.; Peters, P.: Ambulatory evaluation of nephrolithiasis. Classification, clinical presentation and diagnostic criteria. Am. J. Med. *69:* 19–30 (1980).

10 Gray, B.W.; Wilz, D.R.; Caldas, A.E.; Lemann, J.: The importance of phosphate in regulating plasma 1,25-$(OH)_2$ D levels in humans: studies in healthy subjects, in calcium stone formers and in patients with primary hyperparathyroidism. J. clin. Endocr. Metab. *45:* 299–306 (1977).

11 Shen, F.H.; Baylink, D.Y.; Nelsen, B.L.; Sherrard, D.Y.; Ivey, J.L.; Haussler, M.R.: Increased serum 1,25-$(OH)_2D_3$ in idiopathic hypercalciuria. J. Lab. clin. Med. *90:* 955–961 (1977).

A. Fournier, MD, Néphrologie, Médecine Interne, Hôpital Sud,
BP 3009, F–80030 Amiens Cedex (France)

Contr. Nephrol., vol. 58, pp. 143–147 (Karger, Basel 1987)

Lack of Effects of an Increased Pool of 25-Hydroxyvitamin D_3 on Urinary Excretion of Calcium in Healthy Subjects

Tomas Berlin, Ingemar Björkhem

Departments of Urology and Clinical Chemistry, Huddinge University Hospital, Huddinge, Sweden

The role of vitamin D_3 and its metabolites in hypercalciuria is a matter of controversy. In a pilot study 5 years ago we showed that a group of normocalcemic hypercalciuric renal stone formers had significantly higher blood levels of 25-hydroxyvitamin D_3 than a group of normocalciuric stone formers [1]. 25-Hydroxyvitamin D_3 was determined by a highly specific and accurate method based on isotope dilution-mass spectrometry [2]. In a later study our finding that there is a relationship between serum levels of 25-hydroxyvitamin D_3, and hypercalciuria was confirmed [3]. The levels of 25-hydroxyvitamin D_3, 1,25-dihydroxyvitamin D, urinary excretion of calcium and some other parameters were measured on two occasions, in March and again in September the same year, in 108 normocalcemic male stone formers. In both March and September the hypercalciuric patients had significantly higher mean serum levels of 25-hydroxyvitamin D_3 than the normocalciuric ones and stone formers with intermediate excretion of calcium had 25-hydroxyvitamin D_3 levels between those of the other two groups. With respect to 1,25-dihydroxyvitamin D, however, there was no difference between the hypercalciuric and the normocalciuric patients. The correlation between urinary excretion of calcium and serum level of 25-hydroxyvitamin D_3 in the individual patient was low (0.37), and there was no correlation to 1,25-dihydroxyvitamin D or between 25-hydroxyvitamin D_3 and 1,25-dihydroxyvitamin D.

When only the patients with extremely high and extremely low urinary calcium excretion in both March and September were considered the difference with respect to 25-hydroxyvitamin D_3 levels was even greater. When the hypercalciuric patients were classified as hyperabsorbers, as calcium leakers, as phosphate leakers or assigned to a mixed group according to Jongen's procedures [4] the hyperabsorbers were found to have the highest mean serum level of 25-hydroxyvitamin D_3. When the hypercalciuric patients were classified using the calcium load test described by Pak et al. [5] the hyperabsorbers had even higher mean serum level of 25-hydroxyvitamin D_3, significantly higher than that of the hypercalciuric group as a whole. There was, however, no statistically significant difference in the mean serum level of 1,25-dihydroxyvitamin D between the hyperabsorbers and the hypercalciuric group as a whole when classified according to Jongen or Pak.

In order to study the possible importance of 25-hydroxyvitamin D_3 per se in the development of hypercalciuria, we have increased its circulating level in healthy subjects more than twofold and studied the effects of this increase on urinary calcium excretion and some other parameters [6]. The level of 25-hydroxyvitamin D_3 was increased by two means – oral vitamin D_3 and irradiation with UVB light.

Materials and Methods

These two studies were performed in the period February to April, when the serum levels of 25-hydroxyvitamin D_3 in Sweden are lowest. In one study 12 healthy male volunteers (mean age of 31 years) were given 18,000 IU vitamin D_3 by mouth three times a week for a total dose of 396,000 IU. Twelve other healthy men (mean age of 31 years) were used as a control group.

In the second study 15 healthy female volunteers (mean age of 30 years) were exposed to UVB light, illuminating the whole body three times a week for 7 weeks for a total mean dose of 6.5 J/cm^2 (range 3.9–8.5 J/cm^2). At the start of the two studies none of the subjects had been exposed to extreme sunlight or drugs containing vitamin D. All subjects were tested for the various parameters both before and after giving vitamin D_3 or exposure to UVB light. 24-Hour urine samples were collected (over 15 ml 6 *M* HCl) for each of 3 consecutive days. The excretion values given are the means of the three determinations. During the urine sampling periods the subjects were told to drink half a liter of milk products daily and to avoid cheese. Blood samples for determining serum 25-hydroxyvitamin D_3, 1,25-dihydroxyvitamin D, calcium, phosphate, creatinine, urate, ALAT, albumin and parathyroid hormone (PTH) were taken after overnight fasting on the mornings after the urine sampling periods. On the same mornings calcium load tests (1 g of calcium by mouth) were performed as described by Pak et al. [5]. 25-Hydroxyvitamin D_3 was determined by a method based on isotope dilution-mass spectrometry [2] and 1,25-dihydroxyvitamin D by radioreceptor assay [7].

Results

Subjects Given Vitamin D_3

At the start of the study there was no statistically significant difference (Student's t-test) between the test and control groups with respect to any of the parameters determined. After giving vitamin D_3, mean serum levels of 25-hydroxyvitamin D_3 were markedly increased in the test group ($p < 10^{-6}$), whereas there was only a very small increase in the control group ($p < 10^{-5}$) (table I). The difference between the test group after receiving vitamin D_3 and the control group was also highly significant ($p < 10^{-6}$). However, no statistically significant changes were found in either group with respect to serum levels of 1,25-dihydroxyvitamin D, urinary calcium excretion or any of the other parameters measured.

Subjects Exposed to UVB Light

As expected there was a marked increase in the serum level of 25-hydroxyvitamin D_3 ($p < 10^{-7}$) (table II). There was no statistically significant increase in the amount of calcium excreted in the 24-hour urine. The molar ratio of calcium to creatinine in fasting urine was, however, significantly increased after exposure to UVB irradiation ($p < 0.025$) and there was a slight decrease in mean serum level of 1,25-dihydroxyvitamin D ($p < 0.05$). No statistically significant changes were found with respect to any of the other parameters measured.

Discussion

Three different theoretical explanations may be offered for the previously observed relationship between high 25-hydroxyvitamin D_3 levels and hypercalciuria in renal stone formers: (1) High 25-hydroxyvitamin D_3 levels may be the primary cause of hypercalciuria. If so, an elevated level, whatever the cause, would be expected to result in increased absorption and urinary excretion of calcium in otherwise healthy subjects. (2) A high concentration of 25-hydroxyvitamin D_3 may be secondary to increased absorption and excretion of calcium. (3) The primary cause of the hypercalciuria may be an increased sensitivity to the action of vitamin D metabolites, both 1,25-dihydroxyvitamin D_3 and 25-hydroxyvitamin D_3, in the intestine. Subjects with a high 25-hydroxyvitamin D_3 level would then develop an even higher degree of hypercalciuria.

Table I. Biochemical parameters before and after receiving vitamin D_3 (means ± SEM)

	Test group (n = 12)		Control group (n = 12)	
	before vitamin D_3	after vitamin D_3	at the start	at the end
S-25OHD$_3$, ng/ml	15.2 ± 1.4	49.3 ± 2.0	14.8 ± 0.9	19.3 ± 1.1
S-1,25(OH)$_2$D, pg/ml	28.5 ± 2.5	26.5 ± 2.3	34.9 ± 5.6	30.9 ± 7.1
U-Ca, mmol/24 h	4.8 ± 1.0	6.2 ± 0.8	4.2 ± 0.7	4.3 ± 0.5
U-Ca/crea (fasting value)	0.14 ± 0.02	0.20 ± 0.04	0.20 ± 0.04	0.16 ± 0.03
U-Ca/crea (after Ca load)	0.38 ± 0.04	0.36 ± 0.06	0.42 ± 0.09	0.39 ± 0.07

Table II. Biochemical parameters before and after exposure to UVB irradiation (means ± SEM)

	Before exposure (n = 15)	After exposure (n = 15)
S-25OHD$_3$, ng/ml	17.3 ± 1.1	51.7 ± 2.0
S-1,25(OH)$_2$D, pg/ml	20.2 ± 1.3	16.2 ± 1.4
U-Ca, mmol/24 h	4.2 ± 0.4	5.2 ± 0.4
U-Ca/crea (fasting value)	0.11 ± 0.02	0.21 ± 0.04
U-Ca/crea (after Ca load)	0.30 ± 0.05	0.37 ± 0.04

The results obtained in the present study seem to rule out the first hypothesis. Despite a threefold increase in the level of 25-hydroxyvitamin D_3, there were only negligible effects on the urinary excretion of calcium in the healthy subjects studied. The only statistically significant finding was an increased ratio of calcium to creatinine in fasting urine of the women exposed to UVB light. Since no such effect was observed in the group of subjects given oral vitamin D_3, and since there was no significant increase in the total excretion of calcium in either of the groups, it may be concluded that an increase in 25-hydroxyvitamin D_3 up to about 50 ng/ml has little or no effect on calcium homeostasis in healthy subjects. It should be pointed out that the levels of 25-hydroxyvitamin D_3 obtained here were similar to or higher than those we have observed in hypercalciuric stone formers with urinary calcium excretion levels more than twofold that of the present subjects.

The above conclusions concerning the effect of 25-hydroxyvitamin D_3 per se are based on the assumption that the level of the most active metabolite, 1,25-dihydroxyvitamin D, was unaffected by the procedures. This was clearly the case with the subjects given oral vitamin D_3, whereas there was a slight decrease (about 20%) in the level of 1,25-dihydroxyvitamin D in the subjects who were exposed to UVB light. In any case, the small changes observed here in the levels of 1,25-dihydroxyvitamin D cannot affect the major conclusions of the study.

References

1 Berlin, T.; Björkhem, I.; Collste, L.; Holmberg, I.; Wijkström, H.: Relation between hypercalciuria and vitamin D_3-status in patients with urolithiasis. Scand. J. Urol. Nephrol. *16:* 269–273 (1982).

2 Björkhem, I.; Holmberg, I.: Mass fragmentographic assay of 25-hydroxyvitamin D_3. Meth. Enzym. *67:* 385–393 (1980).

3 Berlin, T.; Holmberg, I.; Björkhem, I.: High circulating levels of 25-hydroxyvitamin D_3 in renal stone formers with hyperabsorptive hypercalciuria. Scand. J. clin. Lab. Invest. *46:* 367–374 (1986).

4 Jongen, M.: The role of vitamin D in the pathogenesis of urinary calcium stone disease; thesis, Amsterdam (1983).

5 Pak, C.; Kaplan, R.; Bone, H.; Townsend, J.; Waters, O.: A simple test for the diagnosis of absorptive, resorptive and renal hypercalciurias. New Engl. J. Med. *292:* 497–500 (1975).

6 Berlin, T.; Emtestam, L.; Björkhem, I.: Studies on the relationship between vitamin D_3 status and urinary excretion of calcium in healthy subjects: effects of increased levels of 25-hydroxyvitamin D_3. Scand. J. clin. Lab. Invest. *46:* 723–729 (1986).

7 Reinhard, T.; Horst, R.; Orf, J.; Hollis, B.: A microassay for 1,25-dihydroxyvitamin D_3 not requiring HPLC. Application to clinical studies. J. clin. Endocr. Metab. *58:* 91–98 (1984).

Tomas Berlin, MD, Department of Urology, Huddinge University Hospital, S–14186 Huddinge (Sweden)

Contr. Nephrol., vol. 58, pp. 148–151 (Karger, Basel 1987)

Plasma Membrane Ca-ATPase in Idiopathic Hypercalciuria

G. Vezzoli[a], *A. Elli*[a], *P. Palazzi*[a], *D. Cusi*[a], *T. Cova*[a], *D. Menghetti*[a], *M. Scabini*[a], *S. Ortolani*[a], *L. Soldati*[a], *M. Surian*[b], *F. Quarto di Palo*[a], *G. Bianchi*[a]

[a]Istituto di Scienze Mediche, Scuola di Specializzazione in Nefrologia Medica, Università di Milano, Milano; and [b]Servizio di Nefrologia e Dialisi, Ospedale di Lodi, Lodi, Italia

Idiopathic hypercalciuria is a familial defect which is attributed to an increased Ca intestinal absorption or to a reduced Ca reabsorption by renal tubule [1]. The absorptive hypercalciuria may be caused both by a primitive increase of Ca transport across intestinal epithelial cells or by an altered 1,25-OHD_3 production [1].

An outward Ca pump takes part in the intestinal Ca absorption [2], it is on the basolateral membrane of the epithelial cells, its activity is stimulated by 1,25-OHD_3 and biochemical characteristics are the same found in the erythrocytes [3, 4], but the erythrocyte enzyme does not appear influenced by the hormonal levels of vitamin D [5].

Because of the erythrocyte Ca pump independence of the hormonal feedback systems which regulates Ca homeostasis, we have studied the Ca-ATPase activity in the erythrocyte membrane ghosts from hypercalciuric subjects affected by Ca kidney stone disease, to test whether a primitive defect of active Ca transport across cell membrane is present.

Patients and Methods

Fourty-one Ca kidney stone formers were studied; 21 (18 males, 3 females; age range 21–64) were hypercalciuric (urinary Ca higher than 0.1 mmol/kg body weight/24 h) [1]; 20 (15 males, 5 females; age range 18–52) were normocalciuric. No patient had erythrocyte defects in volume, enzyme or hemoglobin; their kidney function was normal, their urine sterile. None was in therapy for at least 3 months.

Fourty-four normal controls were studied too (22 males, 22 females; age range 14–59). Calciuria in 24-hour urine and plasma free Ca were measured in patients and controls after 14 days of diet containing approximately 25 mmol of Ca; in 22 patients (12 hypercalciuric, 10 normocalciuric) parathyroid hormone (PTH) mid molecule and 1,25-OHD_3 were determined in plasma. Only in patients calciuria was also determined in morning 2-hour urine specimens collected after overnight fast and 14 days of low Ca diet containing 10 mmol of Ca, and expressed as CaE (uCa/uCr × PCr; μmol/100 ml glomerular filtrate).

Eight patients (4 normocalciuric and 4 hypercalciuric) continued the low Ca intake until 90 days; 24 h calciuria, plasma free Ca, 1,25-OHD_3 and PTH were measured. Erythrocyte membrane ghosts were prepared after 25 mmol Ca diet and after 90 days of low Ca intake. Ca-ATPase activity was determined at V_{max} as previously described [6]. The activity was expressed as nmol adenosine triphosphate (ATP) split/min/mg protein. Data in the text are presented as mean value ± standard error.

Results

The erythrocyte membrane ghosts from hypercalciuric subjects have higher Ca-ATPase activity (63.1 ± 3.29) than normocalciuric subjects affected by kidney stone disease (48.6 ± 7.89, $p < 0.001$ by Student's t-test for unpaired data), or not (48.6 ± 2.03, $p < 0.001$). On the contrary the group of the normocalciuric patients presents the same Ca pump activity of the controls. In the stone formers the values of Ca-ATPase correlate positively with 24-hour Ca excretion ($r = 0.38$, $p < 0.05$). The values of fasting CaE, PTH, plasma free Ca and 1,25-OHD_3 are not different in normocalciuric and hypercalciuric patients, but the latter is inversely correlated with the activity of the Ca pump ($r = -0.43$, $p < 0.05$).

Eight patients received a low Ca diet for 90 days; after this period the Ca-ATPase activity does not change from that found after a high Ca intake (54.8 ± 6.38 vs 53.9 ± 3.7), whereas 1,25-OHD_3 plasma levels increase (48.9 ± 5.95 vs. 37.1 ± 3.66; $p < 0.05$, Student's t-test for paired data), and calciuria decreases (5 ± 0.77 vs 6.5 ± 0.92; $p < 0.05$, Student's t-test for paired data).

Discussion

The results of the present work show an increase of the Ca-ATPase activity in the erythrocyte membrane ghosts of stone formers with idiopathic hypercalciuria. The activity correlates positively with the values of Ca excretion and negatively with 1,25-OHD_3 plasma levels; it does not change after a period of low Ca intake during which 1,25-OHD_3 increases in plasma.

Idiopathic hypercalciuria is often associated with kidney stone disease. Studies both in rats and man showed a genetic transmission of the defect, but the pathogenesis is still unclear [1]. A primary increase of intestinal absorption or a renal tubular leak were proposed [1]. Recently an alteration of 1,25-OHD_3 production has been shown [7]. The interrelationships among the single factors of Ca metabolism and the feedback mechanisms make it difficult to distinguish between primary and secondary modifications in idiopathic hypercalciuria [1].

The membrane Ca-ATPase activity is expression of the Ca pump, present in different cells; its biochemical characteristics are similar in erythrocytes, kidney tubular cells and intestinal mucosa cells [2–4]. In intestinal epithelial cells the enzyme is present only on the basolateral membranes; it takes part to active Ca absorption and is positively influenced by 1,25-OHD_3 [2, 3]. In erythrocytes the Ca-ATPase is the only Ca transport system and does not appear modified by 1,25-OHD_3 [4, 5].

So it is not influenced by the hormonal feedback mechanisms which make difficult to distinguish between primary and secondary alterations in Ca metabolism. Because of this we chose the erythrocyte to test the hypothesis of an alteration in active Ca transport across cell membrane in idiopathic hypercalciuria.

The study was performed on hypercalciuric patients who normalized their Ca excretion during fasting. So the most likely cause of hypercalciuria was an intestinal hyperabsorption.

The found defect in Ca-ATPase activity may be considered as apparently not affected by dietary Ca or vitamin D. Moreover, the inverse correlation between the activity of the pump and plasma 1,25-OHD_3 suggests that the vitamin D requirement may be lower in patients with a faster intrinsic Ca transport rate across their cell membranes.

The overall pattern of changes described here is consistent with the hypothesis that a genetically determined increase in Ca pump activity in cell membrane may be cause of hypercalciuria by an acceleration of intestinal Ca absorption independent of vitamin D.

References

1 Coe, F.L.; Buchinsky, D.A.: Pathophysiology of hypercalciuria. Am. J. Physiol. *247:* F1–13 (1984).

2 Ghijsen, W. E. J. M.; Os, C. H. van: Ca-stimulated ATPase in brush border and baso-lateral membranes of rat duodenum with high affinity sites for Ca ions. Nature, Lond. *279:* 802–803 (1979).
3 Ghijsen, W. E. J. M.; Os, C. H. van: 1-Alpha-25-dihydroxy-vitamin D_3 regulates ATP-dependent calcium transport in basolateral plasma membranes of rat enterocytes. Biochim. biophys. Acta *689:* 170–172 (1982).
4 Carafoli, E.; Inesi, G.; Rosen, B.; Calcium transport across biological membranes; in Sigel, Metal ions in biological systems, vol. 17, pp. 130–140 (Dekker, New York 1984).
5 Halloran, B. P.; DeLuca, H. F.; Vincenzi, F. F.: (Ca + Mg)-ATPase and calmodulin activity of rat red blood cells: lack of dependence on vitamin D. FEBS Lett. *114:* 89–92 (1980).
6 Vezzoli, G.; Elli, A.; Tripodi, G.; Bianchi, G.; Carafoli, E.: Calcium ATPase in erythrocytes of spontaneously hypertensive rats of the Milan strain. J. Hypertens. *3:* 645–648 (1985).
7 Broadus, A. E.; Insogna, K. L.; Lang, R.; Ellison, A. F.; Dreyer, B. E.: Evidence for disordered control of 1,25-dihydroxyvitamin D production in absorptive hypercalciuria. New Engl. J. Med. *311:* 73–80 (1984).

Prof. Giuseppe Bianchi, MD, Istituto di Scienze Mediche, Pad. Granelli,
Policlinico di Milano, via F. Sforza 35, I–20122 Milano (Italy)

Contr. Nephrol., vol. 58, pp. 152–155 (Karger, Basel 1987)

Hyperphosphaturia Associated with Hypercalciuria in Renal Calcium Stone Patients

Bruno Copercini, Franco Pecchini, Cosimo Romano

Division of Nephrology, Hospital, Cremona, Italy

Idiopathic hypercalciuria (IH) is commonly acknowledged as a pathogenetic basis for primary calcium nephrolithiasis as well as urine inhibitor deficiency and increased oxaluria. Lau et al. [1] have put in IH, a distinction of practical utility between 'diet-dependent' (DDH) and 'diet-independent' (or fast, FH) and have shown in the same instances a tubular leak of phosphate not due to parathormone (PTH).

Jaeger et al. [2] have recently pointed out renal phosphate wasting in most cases of nephrolithiasis. Other authors have reported that phosphate depletion is generally involved in IH, also if defined hypophosphatemia is rare. The aim of this investigation was to contribute to the study of the possible interrelations between phosphate metabolism and IH.

Patients and Methods

Forty-two consecutive adult patients, with 'idiopathic' calcium renal stones have been rectrospectively studied; their renal function was normal. 800 mg calcium was taken daily. Daily urine contents of calcium, phosphate and creatinine (routine methods), oxalate (colorimetric) [3], citrate (enzymatic from Boehringer Mannheim) and glycosaminoglycans (GAG) (spectrophotometric) [4] were determined. By means of the urine calcium/creatinine ratio, during normal calcium diet, 30 subjects with IH and 12 with normocalciuria (NC) were subdivided. Again based on urine calcium/creatinine, during a low calcium (400 mg/day) diet, and by means of Pak's [5] test, IH patients were classified thus: 21 as DDH and 9 as FH. DDH, FH and NC subgroups were statistically (Student's t-test) compared regarding phosphatemia (pPO_4), urine excretion ratio between PO_4 and creatinine (UPO_4/UCr), renal phosphate threshold ($TmPO_4/GFR$) as estimated with the Walton-Bijvoet [6] nomogram, urine oxalate (UOx), urine citrate (UCit), urine GAG (UGAG).

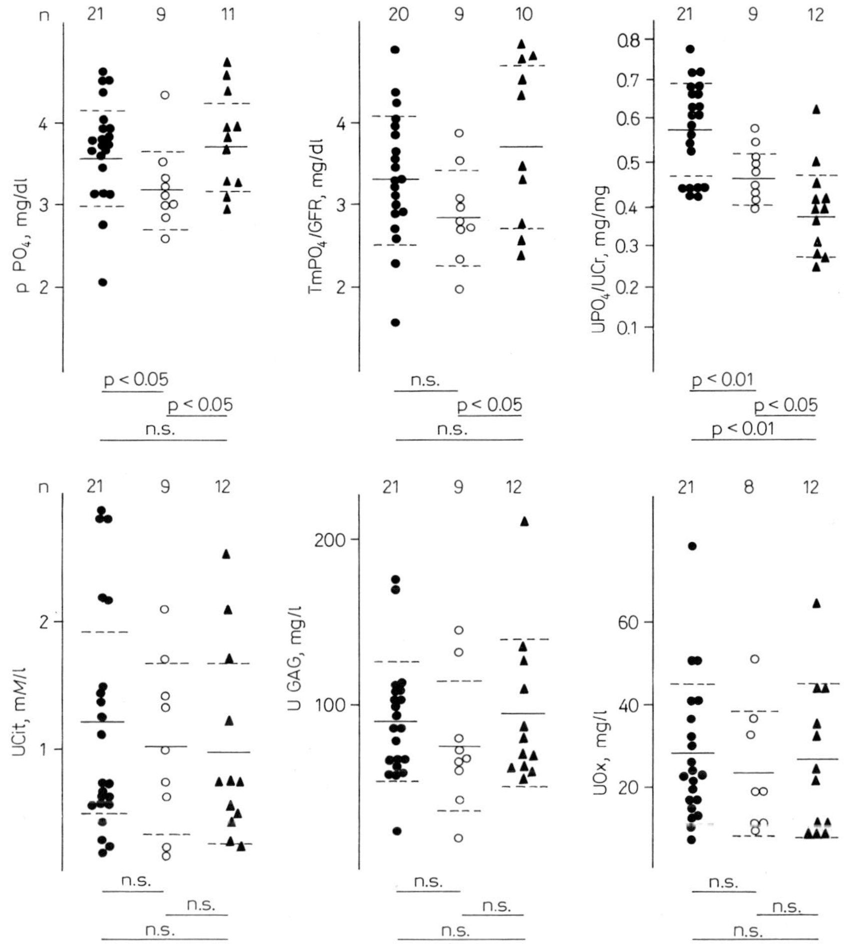

Fig. 1. Data distribution: pPO_4, $TmPO_4/GFR$, UPO_4/UCr, UCit, U GAG, UOx. Subgroups: DDH (●), FH (○), NC (▲). Number of patients on the top. Horizontal bars show mean values ± SD. Statistical comparisons at the bottom.

Results

As shown in figure 1, phosphatemia in FH is significantly lower than both DDH ($p < 0.05$) and NC ($p < 0.05$). On the contrary, there is no significant difference between DDH and NC. $TmPO_4/GFR$ of FH is also lower ($p < 0.05$) than that of NC but not than that of DDH; there is no difference between DDH and NC. The urine phosphate/creatinine ratio of patients with DDH is far greater ($p < 0.01$) than that of FH and also even greater than that of NC. However, a difference exists between FH and NC phosphate excretion too ($p < 0.05$). As regards the other considered parameters, no significant differences among subgroups are found.

Discussion

Our data confirm a connection between IH and hyperphosphaturia and show a different urine phosphate excretion in DDH subjects as compared to FH. Bordier et al. [7] pointed out a primitive phosphate depletion in 'renal' IH patients and Broadus et al. [8] demonstrated that hypophosphatemia may occur in absorptive hypercalciuria. If we consider that urine phosphate is high in our DDH patients, and gradually decreases in FH and even more in NC, we can hypothesize a deregulated renal synthesis of $1,25\text{-}(OH)_2D_3$, an overproduction of vitamin D which could promote calcium and phosphate intestinal hyperabsorption in DDH.

In the presence of FH, hypercalciuria could be induced by an increase in $25\text{-}(OH)D_3\text{-}\alpha$-hydroxylase due to tubular phosphate leak and secondary hypophosphatemia.

Sutton et al. [9] have found a defect in electrolyte tubular reabsorption that was more serious in fasting than in absorptive hypercalciuria. The DDH and FH profiles that we have drawn allow a practical therapeutic approach by exogenous phosphate restoration.

References

1 Lau, Y.K.; Wasserstein, A.; Westby, G.R.; Bosanac, P.; Grabie, M.; Mitnick, P.; Slatopolsky, E.; Goldfarb, S.; Argus, Z.S.: Proximal tubular defects in idiopathic hypercalciuria: resistance to phosphate administration. Mineral Electrolyte Metab. *7:* 237–249 (1982).

2 Jaeger, P.; Portmann, L.; Burckhardt, P.: Dysfonction tubulaire dans la lithiase rénale: cause ou consequence? Schweiz. med. Wschr. *115:* 160–162 (1985).

3 Hodgkinson, A.; Williams, A.: An improved colorimetric procedure for urine oxalate. Clinica chim. Acta *36:* 127–132 (1972).

4 Gold, E.W.: A simple spectrophotometric method for estimating glycosaminoglycan concentrations. Biochemistry, N.Y. *99:* 183–188 (1979).

5 Pak, C.Y.C.; Kaplan, R.; Bone, H.; Townsend, J.; Waters, O.: A simple test for the diagnosis of absorptive, resorptive and renal hypercalciurias. New Engl. J. Med. *292:* 497–500 (1975).

6 Walton, R. J.; Bijvoet, O. L. M.: Nomogram for determination of renal threshold phosphate concentration. Lancet *ii:* 309–310 (1975).
7 Bordier, P.; Ryckewart, A.; Gueris, J.: On the pathogenesis of so-called idiopathic hypercalciuria. Am. J. Med. *63:* 398–409 (1977).
8 Broadus, A. E.; Dominguez, M.; Bartter, F. C.: Pathophysiological studies in idiopathic hypercalciuria: use of an oral calcium tolerance test to characterize distinctive hypercalciuric subgroups. J. clin. Endocr. Metab. *47:* 751–760 (1978).
9 Sutton, R. A. L.; Walker, V. R.: Responses to hydrochlorothiazide and acetazolamide in patients with calcium stones. New Engl. J. Med. *302:* 709–713 (1980).

B. Copercini, MD, Division of Nephrology, Hospital,
Concordia Avenue, I–26100 Cremona (Italy)

Contr. Nephrol., vol. 58, pp. 156–159 (Karger, Basel 1987)

Erythrocyte Membrane Protein Phosphorylation in Urolithiasis

Bruno Baggio, Giulio Clari, Giovanni Marzaro, Giovanni Gambaro, Arturo Borsatti, Vittorio Moret

Institute of Internal Medicine and Institute of Biological Chemistry, University of Padova, Padova, Italy

We have recently shown that transmembrane oxalate flux in red blood cells (RBC) of 'idiopathic' calcium oxalate (CaOx) stone formers is faster than in healthy controls [1, 2]. We have also presented evidence that disulfonic stilbenes, which are known inhibitors of RBC anion exchanger band 3 protein [3], are capable of effacing this anomaly [4], thus pointing to band 3 protein as responsible for the faster transmembrane oxalate movement. In this study we have attempted to find out some biochemical anomalies in band 3 protein from renal stone formers.

Material and Methods

In this study RBC ghosts obtained from healthy controls and 'idiopathic' CaOx renal stone formers showing a faster than normal oxalate self-exchange were used. Ghosts were prepared according to Beutler et al. [5] and Dodge et al. [6]. The phosphorylation step was carried on according to Fairbanks et al. [7] and Waxman [8]. Protein kinase activity was assayed on exogenous β-casein in the absence and presence of Triton X-100 5% according to Hosey and Tao [9] and Clari et al. [10]. ATPase activity was determined by detecting the (^{32}P)-orthophosphate released from (γ-^{32}P)ATP as described elsewhere [11, 12].

Results

Figure 1 shows an example of the electrophoretic patterns and the corresponding autoradiograms of ^{32}P-labeled membrane proteins from ghosts of a control (A) and of a CaOx nephrolithiasis patient (B). No

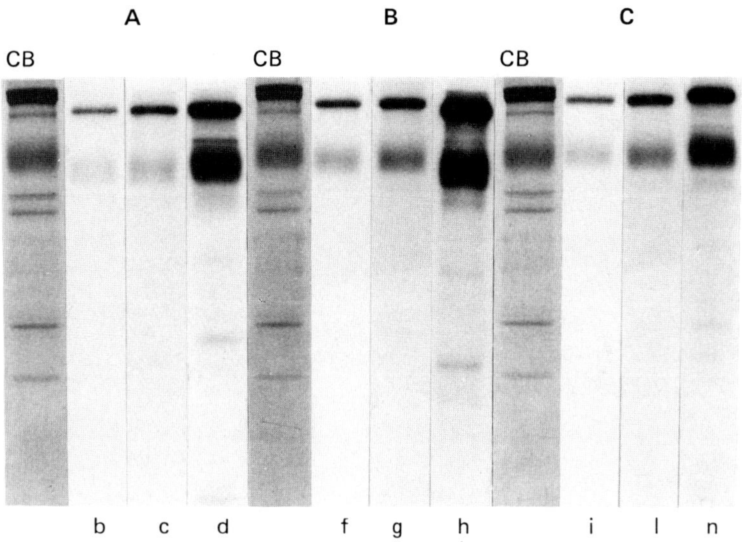

Fig. 1. Electrophoretic pattern and corresponding autoradiograms from control (A) and stone formers (B, C) (see text for further explanation).

alteration of membrane proteins was revealed by comparing Coomassie blue(CB)-stained gels of controls and nephrolithiasic patients. The time course profiles of membrane protein labeling show at 1 min (lane f), 2 min (lane g) and 10 min (lane h) of incubation time a higher ^{32}P-labeling of bands 2 and 3 from ghosts of the patient than the control (lanes b–d). ATPase activity showed an inconstant pattern since it was in the normal range in some patients and increased in others. In these last patients (an example is shown in fig. 1C) the ^{32}P-labeling of bands 2 and 3 was higher than in controls at short times (lanes i, l vs b, c), but at more prolonged incubation time (10 min) it was decreased to levels (lane n) below those in controls (lane d) and in patients with normal ATPase activity (lane h). Figure 2 exhibits an example of protein kinase activity of ghosts from a patient (lanes b, d) compared to that of a control (lanes a, c). It is quite clear that this activity is higher in the stone former both before (lane b) and after (lane d) treatment with Triton.

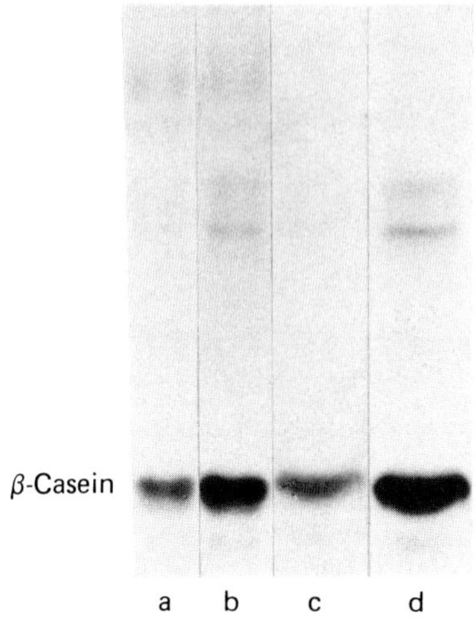

Fig. 2. Examples of protein kinase activity of ghosts from stone formers (b, d) and controls (a, c) (see text).

Discussion

The most striking data shown by this study is the abnormally high phosphorylation kinetic of both bands 2 and 3 demonstrated by stone-forming patients. This faster phosphorylation might be explained by assuming that in both bands 2 and 3 proteins have undergone a chemical or a conformational alteration of their structure, or an alteration in their topological arrangement in the membrane structure, so that new additional sites become available for phosphorylation. We have no data to rule it out, however, a primary structural defect present in two different proteins seems unfeasible. It is more likely that one or more specific kinase(s) devoted to band 3 phosphorylation has (have) an increased activity in stone formers than in controls. This might be in keeping with the higher than normal phosphokinase activity against β-casein shown by stone formers which is still present when the membrane structure organization is destroyed and ATPase activity inhibited by treatment with 5% Triton.

Since we demonstrated that the abnormal oxalate self-exchange in stone formers is normalized by inhibitors of band 3 protein, like stilbenes [4], and since we have preliminary data showing an inhibitory effect of stilbenes on band 3 protein phosphorylation, we suggest the possible existence of a link between the abnormal phosphorylation of the anion exchanger and the faster oxalate self-exchange in RBC from stone formers. Future studies will be necessary to substantiate this hypothesis.

References

1 Baggio, B.; Gambaro, G.; Marchini, F.; Cicerello, E.; Borsatti, A.: Raised transmembrane oxalate flux in red blood cells in idiopathic calcium oxalate nephrolithiasis. Lancet *ii:* 12–13 (1984).

2 Baggio, B.; Gambaro, G.; Marchini, F.; Cicerello, E.; Tenconi, R.; Clementi, M.; Borsatti, A.: An inheritable anomaly in red-cell oxalate transport in 'primary' calcium nephrolithiasis correctable with diuretics. New Engl. J. Med. *314:* 599–604 (1986).

3 Rothstein, A.; Cabantchik, Z. I.; Knauf, P.: Mechanism of anion transport in red blood cells. The role of membrane proteins. Fed. Proc. *35:* 3–10 (1976).

4 Baggio, B.; Gambaro, G.; Borsatti, A.; Clari, G.; Moret, V.: Relation between band 3 red blood cell protein and transmembrane oxalate flux in stone formers. Lancet *ii:* 223–224 (1984).

5 Beutler, E.; West, C.; Blume, K. K.: The removal of leucocytes and platelets from whole blood. J. Lab. clin. Med. *88:* 328–333 (1976).

6 Dodge, J. T.; Mitchell, C.; Hanahan, D. J.: The preparation and chemical characteristics of hemoglobin-free ghosts of human erythrocytes. Arch. Biochem. Biophys. *100:* 119–130 (1963).

7 Fairbanks, G.; Steck, T. L.; Wallack, D. F. H.: Electrophoretic analysis of the major polypeptides of the human erythrocyte membrane. Biochemistry N. Y. *10:* 2606–2616 (1971).

8 Waxman, L.: The phosphorylation of the major proteins of the human erythrocyte membrane. Archs Biochem. Biophys. *196:* 300–314 (1979).

9 Hosey, M. M.; Tao, M.: Proteinkinases of rabbit and human erythrocyte membranes. Biochim. biophys. Acta *482:* 348–357 (1977).

10 Clari, G.; Michielin, E.; Moret, V.: Interrelationships between proteinkinases and spectrin phosphorylation in human erythrocytes. Biochim. biophys. Acta *640:* 240–251 (1981).

11 Martin, J. B.; Doty, D. M.: Determination of inorganic phosphate. Modification of isobutyl alcohol procedure. Analyt. Chem. *21:* 965–957 (1981).

12 Lindberg, O.; Ernster, L.: Determination of inorganic phosphate; in Glick, Methods of biochemical analysis, vol. III, p. 2 (Interscience, New York 1956).

Bruno Baggio, MD, Istituto di Medicina Interna, Policlinico Universitario,
via Giustiniani 2, I–35128 Padova (Italy)

Contr. Nephrol., vol. 58, pp. 160–163 (Karger, Basel 1987)

Limited Role of Endogenous Glycolate as Oxalate Precursor in Xylitol-Infused Patients

A. Bär[a], *D. Löhlein*[b]

[a]Xyrofin Ltd., Basel, Switzerland, and [b]Medizinische Hochschule Hannover, Departement für Abdominal- und Transplantations-Chirurgie, Hannover, FRG

Xylitol is a known intermediate of the glucuronate pentose phosphate shunt. Its metabolism includes dehydrogenation to *D*-xylulose, phosphorylation to *D*-xylulose-5-phosphate, and subsequent transformation to fructose-6-phosphate via the pentose phosphate pathway.

In parenteral nutrition, xylitol is used as an alternative energy source to glucose. No insulin is required for its initial metabolism and its application was found to be associated with reduced gluconeogenesis and improved fatty acid oxidation [1]. However, the occurrence of a few cases of renocerebral oxalosis in xylitol-infused patients led, in the early 1970s, to the suspicion that xylitol might partly be converted to oxalate. Today, the existence of a minor catabolic pathway from xylitol to oxalate is well documented by several in vitro and in vivo studies [2–4]. On the other hand, the clinical relevance of this pathway is still controversial.

In the present study, we investigated the effect of total parenteral nutrition (TPN) with glucose and xylitol on the plasma oxalate levels and on the urinary excretion of glycolate and oxalate in order to assess whether the infusion of xylitol is associated with an increased risk of tissue oxalosis.

Materials and Methods

Eleven patients, who required major surgical treatment, were enrolled in the study. Six patients received glucose (3 g/kg/day), amino acids (1.5 g/kg/day), and lipids (100 g/day) in a volume of 2,500–3,000 ml/day for a duration of 4 days, at least (glucose group). Five patients received an identical regimen in which, however, xylitol (3 g/kg/day) was substituted for glucose (xylitol group). Prior to surgical treatment and TPN, a 24-hour urine sample and a blood

Table I. Plasma oxalate concentration and urinary glycolate and oxalate excretion in surgical patients infused with glucose and xylitol (means ± SD)

Treatment	Preop. day	Postoperative day				
		1st	2nd	3rd	4th	5th
Plasma oxalate, mg/l						
Glucose	1.633 ±0.378	0.764 ± 0.228	0.695 ± 0.196	0.689 ± 0.136	0.739 ± 0.139	0.704 ± 0.144
Xylitol	1.156 ±0.402	0.675 ± 0.202	0.675 ± 0.176	0.644 ± 0.114	0.809 ± 0.385	0.675 ± 0.179
Urine glycolate, mg/24 h						
Glucose	35.5 ± 14.2	51.7 ± 20.3	56.5 ± 37.8	59.9 ± 42.6	55.3 ± 35.4	44.0 ± 28.3
Xylitol	47.4 ± 15.9	1,107.2 ± 664.7	3,920.8 ±2,265.2	3,089.6 ±1,832.1	3,192.3 ±2,276.0	746.8 ± 454.9
Urine oxalate, mg/24 h						
Glucose	30.5 ± 8.6	40.3 ± 17.6	50.5 ± 9.8	50.2 ± 14.3	47.6 ± 14.6	43.7 ± 12.0
Xylitol	32.5 ± 9.6	57.0 ± 19.3	92.6 ± 49.0	93.3 ± 50.2	100.7 ± 46.2	61.1 ± 7.7

sample was obtained from each patient. Postoperatively and during TPN, urine and blood were collected from each patient in regular intervals.

The plasma samples were analysed for oxalate, the urine samples for glycolate and oxalate. Glycolate was determined with an enzymatic method as described elsewhere [5]. For the analysis of oxalate, a modified high performance liquid chromatographic (HPLC) method was applied which combines the advantages of previously established procedures for sample pretreatment [6] and oxalate derivatisation [7].

Results

In all patients, a decrease of the plasma oxalate levels was observed in response to TPN. Differences between the xylitol and the glucose group were not seen (table I).

Analysis of the urine samples revealed a markedly increased glycolate excretion in the xylitol-infused patients (table I). Between the second and the fourth postoperative day, the 24-hour glycolate excretion averaged 0.057 g in the glucose group and 3.401 g in the xylitol group. During the same period, the urinary oxalate excretion was only slightly higher in the xylitol-treated patients (glucose group: 49.4 mg/day; xylitol group: 95.5 mg/day) (table I).

On the fifth postoperative day, the patients started to consume liquids and the infusion regimen was accordingly discontinued stepwise. Consequently, urinary glycolate and oxalate excretion decreased again in the patients of the xylitol group.

Discussion

The present data demonstrate that the infusion of xylitol at a maximum recommended dose results in a marked increase in urinary glycolate excretion. Although glycolate is a metabolic precursor of oxalate, this effect is associated with only a small increase in the urinary oxalate excretion and with no change in the plasma oxalate levels. From the data it may be calculated that only about 0.02% of the infused xylitol was converted to oxalate. These observations which parallel those of others [8, 9] indicate that the oxidation of endogenously formed glycolate to oxalate is limited by regulatory mechanisms such as inhibition of glycolate oxidase by oxalate.

In conclusion, oxalate production from xylitol occurs in vivo. However, if xylitol is infused at recommended dose levels, the increase in plasma oxalate concentration does not reach risk levels for tissue oxalosis. An increased risk may exist, however, in patients with impaired renal function.

References

1 Georgieff, M.; Moldawer, L.L.; Bistrian, B.R.; Blackburn, G.L.: Review: xylitol, an energy source for intravenous nutrition after trauma. J. parent. enteral Nutr. *9:* 119–209 (1985).

2 Conyers, R.A.J.; Rofe, A.M.; Bais, R.; James, H.M.; Edwards, J.B.; Thomas, D.W.; Edwards, R.G.: The metabolic production of oxalate from xylitol. Int. J. Vitam. Nutr. Res. *28:* suppl., pp. 9–28 (1985).

3 Bär, A.; Oesterhelt, G.: Conversion of [U-^{13}C]xylitol and D-[U-^{13}C]glucose into urinary [1,2-^{13}C]glycolate and [1,2-^{13}C]oxalate in man. Int. J. Vitam. Nutr. Res. *28:* suppl., pp. 119–133 (1985).

4 Conyers, R. A. J.; Huber, T. W.; Thomas, D. W.; Rofe, A. M.; Bais, R.; Edwards, R. G.: A one-compartment model for calcium oxalate tissue deposition during xylitol infusions in humans. Int. J. Vitam. Nutr. Res. *28:* suppl., pp. 47–57 (1985).

5 Bais, R.; Nairn, J. M.; Potezny, N.; Rofe, A. M.; Conyers, R. A. J.; Bär, A.: Urinary glycolate measured by use of (S)-2-hydroxy-acid oxidase. Clin. Chem. *31:* 710–713 (1985).

6 Bär, A.: Effect of high oral doses of xylitol versus sucrose on urinary risk factors of urolithiasis in man. Int. J. Vitam. Nutr. Res. *28:* suppl., pp. 91–118 (1985).

7 Hughes, H.; Hagen, L. H.; Sutton, R. A. L.: Determination of urinary oxalate by high-performance liquid chromatography. Analyt. Biochem. *119:* 1–3 (1982).

8 Hauschildt, S.; Chalmers, R. A.; Lawson, A. M.; Schultis, K.; Watts, R. W. E.: Metabolic investigations after xylitol infusion in human subjects. Am. J. clin. Nutr. *29:* 258–273 (1976).

9 Ogawa, Y.: Studies on oxalate in urolithiasis. III. Effect of xylitol infusion on plasma and urinary oxalate. Jap. J. Urol. *72:* 1553–1558 (1981).

A. Bär, PhD, Bioresco Ltd., Clarastrasse 12, CH–4058 Basel (Switzerland)

Contr. Nephrol., vol. 58, pp. 164-171 (Karger, Basel 1987)

The Problem of Idiopathic Stone Formers Presenting with No Metabolic Disorders

Pathogenesis and Management

Charles Y. C. Pak

Section on Mineral Metabolism, Southwestern Medical School of the University of Texas Health Science Center at Dallas, Dallas, Tex., USA

Since 1976, we have employed a diagnostic protocol for nephrolithiasis with a classification scheme which is based on the principal underlying physiological abnormalities. Using this protocol [1], we reported in 1980 that 89.2% of patients present with 'metabolic' disturbance(s), since they could be classified into one of the following categories: absorptive hypercalciuria types I–III, renal hypercalciuria, primary hyperparathyroidism, hyperuricosuric calcium nephrolithiasis, enteric hyperoxaluria, uric acid lithiasis, infection lithiasis, renal tubular acidosis and unclassified hypercalciuria. The omission of cystinuria was not an oversight, but probably reflected absence of referral from practicing physicians because of our professed lack of expertise in the condition. The denotation of the term 'metabolic' to the classification was probably strictly inappropriate, since environmental influences could have caused or contributed to the physiological disturbances disclosed.

Thus, 10.8% of patients were believed to have 'no metabolic abnormality' in our initial report. Since then, our diagnostic protocol has been refined by the routine inclusion of urinary citrate analysis [2]. Among patients previously categorized as suffering from no metabolic abnormality, 48% had hypocitraturia. Moreover, some patients presented with a picture resembling gouty diathesis [3], with a persistent passage of unusually acid urine and calcium oxalate nephrolithiasis, sometimes accompanied by hyperuricemia and gout. In the remaining patients, comprising approximately 4% of all patients, no physiological disturbance was found, although a low urine volume reflective of environmental influence was often disclosed.

It is therefore apparent that the entity of no metabolic abnormality is comprised of at least three disorders. In this presentation, we shall consider the biochemical picture, clinical presentation and management of hypocitraturic calcium oxalate nephrolithiasis, gouty diathesis and no physiological disturbance.

It is clear that the first two conditions may coexist with other well-established conditions, e.g. hypocitraturia with various forms of hypercalciurias [2] and gouty diathesis with uric acid lithiasis [3]. They will be discussed in their 'sole' presentation, as well as in combined or full presentation with other disorders.

Hypocitraturic Calcium Oxalate Nephrolithiasis

Causes of Hypocitraturia

There are numerous reports showing that urinary citrate is low in patients with nephrolithiasis, varying from 19 to 63%. In the study at Dallas, hypocitraturia occurred alone in approximately 5% of patients and coexisted with other abnormalities in 50% of patients [2]. Hypocitraturia resulted from renal tubular acidosis [4], acquired metabolic acidosis of chronic diarrheal states [5], thiazide-induced hypokalemia [6, 7], or from unknown causes ('idiopathic'). Idiopathic hypocitraturia [8] included those who presented with hypocitraturia as the sole abnormality (48% of no metabolic abnormality or 5.2% of all patients). It also comprised hypocitraturia occurring with hypercalciuria or hyperuricosuria. In some situations, hypocitraturia may be partly dietary/environmental in origin (e.g. consumption of a high acid ash diet, an exaggerated sodium intake or strenuous physical exercise).

Pathophysiological Significance of Hypocitraturia in Calcium Stone Formation

Citrate is a well-known 'inhibitor' of the crystallization of calcium salts. First, citrate lowers ionic calcium concentration by complexing calcium, and thereby reduces the saturation of calcium oxalate and calcium phosphate [9]. Second, citrate directly inhibits the spontaneous nucleation of calcium oxalate and brushite ($CaHPO_4$ $2H_2O$). In artificial solution, addition of citrate significantly increased the formation products and permissible increments for both calcium salts [10].

In the setting of hypocitraturia, calcium stone formation (both calcium oxalate and calcium phosphate) would be expected to be enhanced be cause of the reduction in the protective action of citrate previously enumerated. Urinary saturation of calcium oxalate and calcium phosphate would be increased because of reduced citrate complexation of calcium. Crystallization process of both calcium salts would be facilitated because of the loss of the direct inhibitor activity of citrate.

Management with Potassium Citrate

Physiological Action. In patients with idiopathic hypocitraturia (occurring alone or in conjunction with absorptive hypercalciuria or hyperuricosuria) [8], potassium citrate (30–80 mEq/day in 2–4 divided doses) caused a sustained and significant rise in urinary pH and citrate throughout treatment. During treatment, mean urinary pH was kept at 6.5–7, and mean urinary citrate was maintained between 470 and 620 mg/day (within normal limits).

It has been suggested that potassium citrate may be less effective than potassium chloride in correcting the thiazide-induced hypokalemia, because of the poor reabsorbability of citrate from the renal tubules. However, in 13 patients with calcium oxalate nephrolithiasis taking thiazide who were randomized into potassium citrate and potassium chloride supplementation at equivalent dosages [6], potassium citrate was equally effective as potassium chloride in correcting thiazide-induced hypokalemia. Moreover, the addition of potassium citrate to thiazide therapy raised urinary pH and citrate [6, 7]. The citraturic response to potassium citrate was equally manifest as in idiopathic hypocitraturic calcium oxalate nephrolithiasis.

However, potassium citrate was less effective in raising urinary citrate and pH in patients with calcium nephrolithiasis due to chronic diarrheal states (such as enteric hyperoxaluria) and in those with moderate-severe distal renal tubular acidosis [5].

Physicochemical Action. In patients with idiopathic hypocitraturic calcium oxalate nephrolithiasis, potassium citrate therapy significantly reduced urinary saturation of calcium oxalate from values exceeding normal values to levels encountered in normal subjects without stones [8]. The urinary inhibitor activity against calcium oxalate crystallization, as measured by the permissible increment in oxalate [10], rose during treatment [8]. Before potassium citrate treatment, the permissible increment in oxalate of 36.7 ± 22.1 mg/l was significantly lower than that encountered in normal control subjects of 62.4 ± 25.3 mg/l ($p < 0.001$ by Student's t-test).

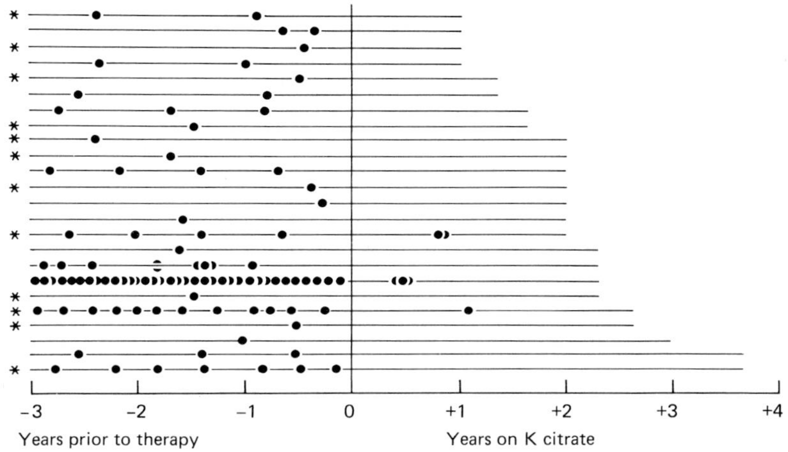

Fig. 1. Effect of potassium citrate therapy on new stone formation in idiopathic hypocitraturic calcium nephrolithiasis. Each circle represents new stone formation. Each line represents one patient. An asterisk before the line indicates presence of preexisting stone(s).

Throughout potassium citrate therapy, the permissible increment in oxalate increased significantly to the range encountered in normal subjects without stones (52.5 ± 78.1 mg/l). Thus, more soluble oxalate was needed to be added to whole urine to elicit spontaneous precipitation of calcium oxalate after treatment with potassium citrate. Similar effects of potassium citrate were encountered in patients with thiazide-induced hypocitraturia and calcium stones [7].

Clinical Response. During potassium citrate treatment [8], 89.2% of patients with idiopathic hypocitraturic calcium nephrolithiasis were in remission, all patients experienced reduced stone formation rate, and group mean stone formation rate declined by 86.7%. The results in those receiving potassium citrate alone are shown in figure 1.

Potassium citrate therapy is also effective in incomplete distal renal tubular acidosis [4] and thiazide-induced hypocitraturia [7].

Nine patients with incomplete distal renal tubular acidosis received potassium citrate (60–80 mEq/day). Six patients did not form further stones. Three patients continued to pass stones. For this analysis, these stones passed were considered to be newly formed, although they most likely represented passage of preexisting stones. Using this assumption, remission rate was 66.7%, stone formation rate declined individually in all 9 patients, and group mean stone formation rate declined by 91.2% upon institution of potassium citrate therapy.

Thirteen patients with hypercalciuric calcium oxalate nephrolithiasis (11 with absorptive and 2 with renal hypercalciuria) continued to form calcium stones (principally calcium oxalate) when treated with thiazide (5.12 ± 10.87 stones/patient/year). Because they had hypocitraturia (250 ± 86 vs 643 ± 236 mg/day in normal subjects), potassium citrate (10–20 mEq three times/day) was added to the ongoing thiazide treatment. During combined treatment with potassium citrate and thiazide, 10 patients stopped forming new stones and all 13 had a reduced stone formation rate.

Gouty Diathesis

We have previously utilized the term 'gouty diathesis' [3] to describe the overall clinical entity of uric acid lithiasis (one of the conditions in previous classification) [1]. The invariant feature was the persistent passage of unusually acid urine (pH < 5.5) in which uric acid is sparingly soluble. Some patients had gouty arthritis or hyperuricemia. Stone analysis disclosed uric acid alone or in combination with calcium oxalate and/or calcium phosphate.

In some patients previously diagnosed as having no metabolic abnormality, we have found the above features of gouty diathesis except for the lack of uric acid on stone analysis. The stone analysis has disclosed only the presence of calcium oxalate and/or calcium phosphate. No obvious cause has been detected for the unusually low urinary pH, such as excessive intestinal alkali loss or a consumption of an animal protein-rich diet. It was presumed that urate-induced crystallization of calcium salts accounted for calcium nephrolithiasis [11].

This entity presenting with calcium oxalate nephrolithiasis probably has the same underlying pathophysiologic mechanism as the uric acid lithiasis. Thus, the two entities will be discussed together.

Pathogenesis

Unusually acid urinary environment (pH less than 5.5) may be associated with uric acid lithiasis because of the predominance of undissociated uric acid, the dissociation constant of uric acid being 5.47. Once uric acid crystallization occurs, calcium stones could form from the urate-induced crystallization of calcium salts [11, 12].

Management with Potassium Citrate

In general, the maintenance of urinary pH between 6 and 7 is desirable for the control of uric acid lithiasis and calcium oxalate nephrolithiasis. At such a pH range, the concentration of undissociated uric acid is expected to be low because most of the uric acid would be dissociated. At such pH, there would be an enhanced inhibitor activity of citrate and pyrophosphate because more of them would be in active ionic forms. Moreover, ionized calcium concentration decreases as the pH rises, because of enhanced dissociation of phosphate and citrate and calcium complexation by these anions, thus reducing the saturation of calcium oxalate.

Effect of Potassium Citrate on the Crystallization of Uric Acid. Potassium citrate treatment significantly increased urinary pH from the low mean value of 5.30 to above 6.19, but less than 7. Owing to the resulting enhanced dissociation of uric acid, the amount of undissociated uric acid significantly decreased to the range encountered in normal subjects without stones (< 150 mg/day). Thus, potassium citrate therapy significantly increased the solubility of uric acid.

Clinical Response. During potassium citrate therapy, new stone formation rate declined from 1.25 ± 1.71 to 0.01 ± 0.04 stones/year ($p < 0.001$ by χ^2-test) [3]. Remission was experienced in 94.4% of patients, and the group stone formation rate declined by 99.2%. Figure 2 shows the clinical response of patients receiving potassium citrate alone.

No Physiological Disturbance

In approximately 4% of patients, no obvious physiological disturbance could be found. Thus, they did not have hypercalciuria, hyperuricosuria, hyperoxaluria, hypocitraturia, urinary tract infection, cystinuria, or extremes of urinary pH. It is possible that they may suffer from physiological disturbances not yet disclosed.

There is some evidence for a strong environmental factor in the pathogenesis of stone formation in this entity. Many patients have low

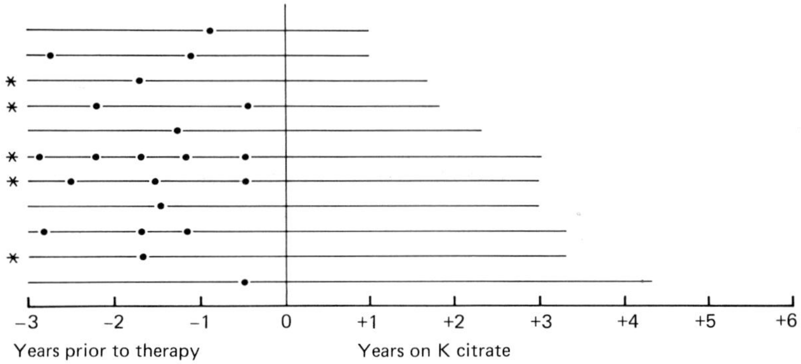

Fig. 2. Effect of potassium citrate treatment on new stone formation in gouty diathesis. Each circle represents new stone formation. Each line indicates study in a separate patient. An asterisk denotes patients with preexisting stone(s) when treatment with potassium citrate was begun.

urine output (< 1 liter/day) due to disdain for drinking fluids and excessive sweat loss. The stone disease is generally mild-moderate with an average stone formation rate of less than 1/year. Dramatic improvement in stone disease typically follows after adequate fluid intake.

References

1 Pak, C.Y.C.; Britton, F.; Peterson, R.; Ward, D.; Northcutt, C.; Breslau, N.A.; McGuire, J.; Sakhaee, K.; Bush, S.; Nicar, M.; Norman, D.; Peters, P.: Ambulatory evaluation of nephrolithiasis: classification, clinical presentation and diagnostic criteria. Am. J. Med. *69:* 19–30 (1980).

2 Nicar, M.J.; Skurla, C.; Sakhaee, K.; Pak, C.Y.C.: Low urinary citrate excretion in nephrolithiasis. Urology *21:* 8–14 (1983).

3 Pak, C.Y.C.; Sakhaee, K.; Fuller, C.: Successful management of uric acid nephrolithiasis with potassium citrate. Kidney int. (accepted).

4 Preminger, G.M.; Sakhaee, K.; Skurla, C.; Pak, C.Y.C.: Prevention of recurrent calcium stone formation with potassium citrate therapy in patients with distal renal tubular acidosis. J. Urol. *134:* 20–23 (1985).

5 Pak, C.Y.C.; Fuller, C.; Sakhaee, K.; Preminger, G.; Britton, F.: Longterm treatment of calcium nephrolithiasis with potassium citrate. J. Urol. *134:* 11–19 (1985).

6 Nicar, M.J.; Peterson, R.; Pak, C.Y.C.: Use of potassium citrate as potassium supplement during thiazide therapy of calcium nephrolithiasis. J. Urol. *131:* 430–433 (1984).

7 Pak, C.Y.C.; Peterson, R.; Sakhaee, K.; Fuller, C.; Preminger, G.; Reisch, J.: Correction of hypocitraturia and prevention of stone formation by combined thiazide and

potassium citrate therapy in thiazide-unresponsive hypercalciuric nephrolithiasis. Am. J. Med. *79:* 284–288 (1985).
8 Pak, C. Y. C.; Fuller, C.: Idiopathic hypocitraturic calcium oxalate nephrolithiasis successfully treated with potassium citrate. Ann. intern. Med. *104:* 33–37 (1986).
9 Pak, C. Y. C.; Nicar, M. J.; Northcutt, C.: The definition of the mechanism of hypercalciuria *is* necessary for the treatment of recurrent stone formers; in Berlyne, Contr. Nephrol., vol. 33, pp. 136–151 (Karger, Basel 1982).
10 Nicar, M. J.; Hill, K.; Pak, C. Y. C.: A simple technique for the assessment of the propensity for the crystallization of calcium oxalate and brushite in urine from the increment in oxalate or calcium necessary to elicit precipitation. Metabolism *32:* 906–910 (1983).
11 Pak, C. Y. C.; Holt, K.; Zerwekh, J. E.: Attenuation by monosodium urate of the inhibitory effect of glycosaminoglycans on calcium oxalate nucleation. Investve Urol. *17:* 138–140 (1979).
12 Zerwekh, J. E.; Holt, K.; Pak, C. Y. C.: Natural urinary macromolecular inhibitors: attenuation of inhibitory activity by urate salts. Kidney int. *23:* 838–841 (1983).

Charles Y. C. Pak, MD, Section on Mineral Metabolism, Southwestern Medical School of the University of Texas Health Science Center at Dallas, 5323 Harry Hines Blvd., Dallas, TX 75235 (USA)

Contr. Nephrol., vol. 58, pp. 172–175 (Karger, Basel 1987)

Medical Treatment of Idiopathic Calcium Nephrolithiasis

Maurizio Surian[a], *Fabio Malberti*[a], *Giacomo Colussi*[b], *M. Elisabetta De Ferrari*[b], *Giuseppe Rombolà*[b], *Elisabetta Benazzi*[b], *Luigi Minetti*[b]

[a]Renal Units, Ospedale Maggiore, Lodi, and [b]Ospedale di Niguarda, Milano, Italy

The efficacy of thiazides [1] or allopurinol [2] in the therapy of idiopathic calcium stones has been recently questioned either in randomized or non-randomized clinical trials. A positive effect on the prevention of stone recurrences has been shown to depend on dietary advice and close clinical supervision per se ('stone clinic effect') [3].

The aim of our study is to critically evaluate the effects on clinical activity of stone disease of thiazide and allopurinol therapy in comparison with non-pharmacological treatment.

Materials and Methods

We have retrospectively evaluated 116 idiopathic calcium stone formers (CSF) selected among 984 stone formers on file at our departments since 1976. Selection criteria were: the formation of at least 2 stones of which one in the last year, at least one year follow-up on treatment, absence of systemic diseases as well as urological abnormalities or urinary tract infection; patients with mononephrectomy and chronic renal failure (GFR < 80 ml/min) were excluded. The patients were allocated in 3 therapeutic regimens: 42 patients were treated with hydrochlorothiazide (50–100 mg/day) plus amiloride (5–10 mg/day; group T); 29 patients were treated with allopurinol (300 mg/day; group A) and 45 patients were kept without drugs (control group C). The patients with active stone disease (more than 3 stone events in the last 3 years or more than 2 stones in the last year), recent surgery, recurrences during non-pharmacological therapy were generally treated with drugs; CSF with hypercalciuria or hypertension were preferably treated with T, while A was preferably prescribed to hyperuricosuric CSF. CSF with low clinical activity, low compliance or drug side effects were allocated in the control group. A general advice to increase fluid intake (> 2 liter/day), to avoid calcium, oxalate and salt excesses was given to every CSF; a reduction of caloric intake was recommended to overweight patients. The stone recurrences were evaluated as passage of new stones or gravel or as radiological evidence of new stone or growth of a preexisting one. The clinical activity of stone disease was evaluated as individual stone formation rate (number of stones/year) or as group stone formation rate (number of stones/patient/year, in which patient/year is the product of mean duration of follow-up by the number of patients). Clinical, radiological and biochemical parameters were obtained before treatment and every 6 months during the follow-up.

Results

The groups did not differ for incidence of hypercalciuria (C = 60%, T = 69%, A = 59%), hyperoxaluria (C = 22%, T = 26%, A = 24%), while hyperuricosuria was 22% in C, 43% in T and 55% in A. The 3 groups were similar for basal urine volume (C = 2,024 ± 930, T = 2,252 ± 913; A = 2,063 ± 899 ml/day), calcium (C = 294 ± 138; T = 333 ± 137; A = 306 ± 160 mg/day), and oxalate (C = 46.3 ± 17.5; T = 43.8 ± 24.8; A = 48.8 ± 17.3 mg/day) excretion; basal uric acid excretion in C was 571 ± 191 mg/day, 643 ± 213 in T and 686 ± 128 in A ($p < 0.02$ vs C). At the end of the follow-up urine volume was similar in all groups and significantly increased ($p < 0.01$) in comparison with basal values (C = 2,470 ± 725; T = 2,641 ± 1,019; A = 2,436 ± 1020 ml/day). In comparison with basal values a significant decrease of calciuria in T (234 ± 106 mg/day, $p < 0.001$) and of uricosuria in A (477 ± 218 mg/day, $p < 0.005$) was observed. Oxaluria did not change during the study in any group. No difference for any of the metabolic parameters considered was observed among the groups at the end of the follow-up. In every group, recurrent patients did not differ from non-recurrent patients for calcium, oxalate and uric acid excretion, while only in C urine volume was lower in recurrent (1,612 ± 827 ml/day) than in non-recurrent patients (2,237 ± 882, $p<0.05$). The 3 groups were homogeneous for pre- and post-treatment follow-up (table I); stone activity (as shown by number of stones/patient-year) was lower in C than in T and A. After treatment, the number of stones/year and/or number of stones/patient-year significantly fell in all the groups; however, the effects in T and A were not greater than in C. Fifty-six hypercalciuric CSF (27 in C and 29 in T group) were evaluated apart: before treatment, the number of stones/year was 1.03 ± 1.07 in C and 1.12 ± 1.2 in T; during a follow-up of 56 patients/year in C and 64 in T, the number of stones/year fell to 0.3 ± 0.52 in C (vs pretreatment: $p < 0.002$) and 0.43 ± 0.63 in T (vs pretreatment: $p < 0.01$) without significant differences between the 2 groups.

Table I. Clinical activity of stone disease before and during therapy

	Controls (n = 45)	Thiazide (n = 42)	Allopurinol (n = 29)	p <
Pre-treatment				
Patients/year	453	383	322	n.s.
Stones	209	256	251	n.s.
Stones/year	0.83 ± 0.93	1.1 ± 1.2	1.2 ± 1.5	n.s.
Stones/patient-year	0.46	0.67*	0.78***	0.02 vs C
Post-treatment				
Patients/year	93.1	97.2	49.5	n.s.
Stones	25	39	23	n.s.
Stones/year	0.33 ± 0.52**	0.34 ± 0.56***	0.79 ± 1.45	n.s.
Stones/patient-year	0.27	0.40*	0.46**	n.s.

Versus pre-treatment: * $p < 0.05$; ** $p < 0.02$; *** $p < 0.001$.

Discussion

Our study shows that thiazide and allopurinol therapy of idiopathic calcium stone disease is not more effective than conservative treatment alone, though significantly reducing stone activity in comparison with the pretreatment period. This is in keeping with the suggestion [1] that the effects of pharmacological treatment in calcium nephrolithiasis may be, when compared to pretreatment period, at least partly obscured by spontaneous remission and co-intervention. Also our study may be biased by selection criteria since patients in treatment groups had a more active disease; however, even considering a subgroup of CSF with similar metabolic pattern (i.e. hypercalciuria) and stone activity, pharmacological therapy with thiazide was not more effective than diet and fluids in reducing stone formation rate. Similar results are reported by others in non-randomized [4] and randomized [1, 2, 5] studies. A few studies would indeed suggest a positive effect of thiazide over conservative treatment [6, 7]. Even if this was the case, dietary advice, increased fluid intake and close clinical supervision (the so-called 'stone clinic effect') would seem to be highly effective in most patients [1, 3, 7]. We think its efficacy is to be evaluated in every patient before drugs be prescribed.

References

1 Churchill, D.; Taylor, W.: Thiazides for patients with recurrent calcium stones: still an open question. J. Urol. *133:* 749–751 (1985).

2 Smith, M.J.V.: Placebo versus allopurinol for renal calculi. J. Urol. *117:* 690–692 (1977).

3 Hosking, D.H.; Erickson, S.B.; Van Den Berg, C.J.; Wilson, D.M.; Smith, L.H.: The stone clinic effect in patients with idiopathic calcium urolithiasis. J. Urol. *130:* 1115–1118 (1983).

4 Marangella, M.; Tricerri, A.; Sonego, S.; Ronzani, M.; Fruttero, B.; Daniele, P.G.; Bruno, M.; Linari, F.: Critical evaluation of various forms of therapy for idiopathic calcium stone disease. Proc. Eur. Dial. Transpl. Ass. *20:* 434–437 (1983).

5 Trinchieri, A.; Mandressi, A.; Zanetti, G.P.; Favini, P.; Ruoppolo, M.; Quadraccia, A.; Luongo, P.; Rocco, F.: Allopurinol versus placebo for calcium renal stones treatment: a double-blind evaluation during two years of follow-up. Mineral Metab. Res. Italy *4:* 13–17 (1983).

6 Laerum, E.; Larsen, S.: Thiazide prophylaxis of urolithiasis: a double-blind study in general practice. Acta med. scand. *215:* 383–389 (1984).

7 Backman, U.: Agents other than thiazide diuretics in the treatment of calcium oxalate nephrolithiasis; in Robinson, Dennis, Ferris, Glassock, Kokko, Tisher, Nephrology, pp. 1011–1024 (Springer, Berlin 1984).

Maurizio Surian, MD, Servizio di Dialisi, Ospedale Maggiore, I–20075 Lodi (Italy)

Contr. Nephrol., vol. 58, pp. 176–180 (Karger, Basel 1987)

Do Indomethacin, Thiazide, Pyridoxine or Allopurinol Prevent Calcium Oxalate Stones?

J. M. Reis-Santos, P. Guimarães, R. Correia, A. M. Ferreira[1]

Department of Urology, Curry Cabral Hospital, Faculty of Medical Science, Lisbon, Portugal

Apart from dietetic methods, several drugs have been pointed out as having a preventive effect on the recurrence of calcium oxalate stones. The therapeutic results do not always concur and it is difficult to evaluate epidemiological data due to the number and variety of parameters outside the study. Also we know that there is no one ideal experimental model for studying calcium oxalate urinary stones, some are too acute and others too chronic and difficult to reproduce [1–5]. We have used a modified version of the model described by Okada et al. [6] and have tried to compare the protective effect of various drugs on urolithiasis, produced by ethylene glycol (EG) plus a synthetic form of vitamin D, in a rat model.

Material and Methods

Male Wistar rats, weighing between 200 and 300 g, were divided into six groups. All had free access to water with 0.5% EG, with the exception of group I (control) which was given plain water. After the third week the quantity of EG added to the water was increased to 0.8%. 0.25 μg 1α-(OH)D_3 (vitamin D) was given orally once a day, four times a week, to all rats except those in group I. Group II (placebo) was given a placebo, group III 4 mg/kg

[1] We wish to thank Prof. Adolfo Coelho and Dr. Fernanda Carvalho for their assistance in the histological study; Dr. J. M. Santos-Coelho for doing the CT scans; the directors of the 'Instituto Gulbenkian de Ciências', in Oeiras, for all the facilities put at our disposal, and especially Mr. J. Romão for his help, and Miss Aida Pinto for secretarial assistance.

body weight/day indomethacin, group IV 3.2 mg/kg body weight/day hydrochlorothiazide, group V 8.0 mg pyridoxine HCl/100 g body weight/day and group VI 10 mg/kg body weight/day allopurinol. Blood serum calcium, phosphate, creatinine and blood urea nitrogen (BUN) were measured at the beginning and at the end of the study. 24-hour urine collections were obtained the day before and every day during the last 3 days of the sixth week of the study, to determine calcium, phosphate, oxalate, creatinine and urea values. After 6 weeks the rats were anaesthetised and the urinary apparatus was exposed and photographed to determine the degree of hydronephrosis. The urinary apparatus was removed in block and fixed. Soft X-ray films and computerised tomography (CT) were taken to determine the number of stones. The kidneys were prepared for histological examination by staining with haematoxilin-eosin and von Kossa. The von Kossa stain allowed us to determine metastatic calcification areas. Stones found in the ureters were removed and analysed by infrared spectroscopy. Results are presented as the mean ± SD, and the statistical significance of differences was assessed by Student's t-test. Values of less than $p < 0.05$ were considered significant.

Results

Table I shows serum calcium, phosphate, BUN, creatinine and urinary excretions of calcium, phosphate, oxalate, creatinine and urea in the rats after the 6-week study period.

Calcium urinary excretion increased in all groups (table I) with one exception of those protected by indomethacin and thiazide ($p < 0.01$). The allopurinol group had the highest calcium oxalate and the lowest phosphate excretion values.

Table II shows the number of dilated ureters compared with the other parameters tested, and also the number of stones counted by contact radiography. The analysis of these calculi reveals calcium oxalate monohydrate.

The urinary apparatus was examined using CT. The histologic examination revealed total absence, or insignificant patches, of metastatic calcification in any of the kidneys. The number of tubular crystals and the degree of crystal aggregation was greater in rats treated with allopurinol than in those of group II (placebo).

Rats treated with indomethacin and thiazide rarely presented dilated tubules and where crystals did exist they were few and were not aggregated (table II). Lesions in the renal structure of these two groups were rarely found.

There was a good correlation between X-ray films, CT data and the number of aggregated, intratubular crystals found by histological examination.

Table I. Serum calcium, phosphate, creatinine and BUN; urinary excretion of calcium, phosphate, oxalate, creatinine and urea in the various groups of rats after 6 weeks of study

	Group I (control I)	Group II (placebo)	Group III (indomethacin)	Group IV (thiazide)	Group V (pyridoxine)	Group VI (allopurinol)
Blood						
Calcium mg/100 ml	9.57 ± 0.78 (10)	11.46 ± 3.76 (10)	10.26 ± 1.74 (8)	11.57 ± 3.43 (8)	8.4 ± 3.43 (8)	11.12 ± 1.14 (8)
Phosphate mg/100 ml	7.87 ± 0.72 (10)	8.13 ± 1.85 (10)	9.32 ± 1.30 (8)	6.33 ± 2.37 (8)*	7.30 ± 1.35 (8)	8.05 ± 0.97 (8)
BUN mg/100 ml	48.9 ± 6.26 (10)*	54.05 ± 5.84 (10)	46.13 ± 10.10 (8)*	53.22 ± 10.48 (8)	50.28 ± 10.70 (8)	55.92 ± 10.87 (8)
Creatinine mg/100 ml	1.23 ± 0.41 (10)*	0.97 ± 0.15 (10)	1.07 ± 0.21 (8)	1.07 ± 0.25 (8)	1.32 ± 0.07 (8)*	1.13 ± 0.21 (8)*
Urine						
Calcium mg/100 ml	4.08 ± 1.90 (10)***	16.63 ± 4.85 (10)	5.83 ± 1.40 (8)***	9.25 ± 5.34 (8)***	14.3 ± 11.17 (8)	17.83 ± 14.17 (8)
Phosphate mg/100 ml	98.1 ± 103.9 (10)***	104.73 ± 90.9 (10)	80.2 ± 88.3 (8)	55.6 ± 111.2 (8)	3.73 ± 3.50 (8)***	3.36 ± 4.64 (8)***
Oxalate mg/day	2.23 ± 0.32 (10)***	5.12 ± 0.49 (10)	4.87 ± 0.87 (8)	5.01 ± 3.02 (8)	2.29 ± 1.12 (8)***	5.63 ± 1.16 (8)
Creatinine mg/100 ml	138.6 ± 96.3 (10)	202.6 ± 103.6 (10)	122.16 ± 57.7 (8)*	200.4 ± 113.2 (8)	114.33 ± 58.22 (8)	116 ± 124.35 (8)
Urea mg/100 ml	4.48 ± 3.08 (10)**	2.06 ± 1.78 (10)	3.88 ± 2.1 (8)*	1.67 ± 3.35 (8)	3.5 ± 0.96 (8)	2.01 ± 1.98 (8)

Values are expressed as the mean ± SD. Figures in parentheses indicate numbers of rats. The urine values represent the average of the last 3 days.
Significantly different from group II (placebo): * $p < 0.05$; ** $p < 0.025$; *** $p < 0.01$.

Discussion

The rat model studied confirmed some of the data obtained in humans with the therapeutic use of thiazides, prostaglandin synthetase inhibitors and pyridoxine. As this model for testing the efficiency of these and other drugs [unpublished material] has proved easy to reproduce, we recommend it for future investigation. Less toxicity and a higher percentage of

Table II. Relationship between number of stones, dilated tubules, intratubular crystals, crystal aggregation and dilated ureters found in the different groups

	Control	Placebo	Indomethacin	Dichlotride	Pyridoxine	Allopurinol
Rats	10	10	8	8	8	8
Stones	0	49	10	8	28	55
Dilated tubules	0	+++	+	+	++	++++
Intratubular crystals	0	+++++	+	+	++	++++
Crystal aggregation	0	++++	0	0	++	++++
Dilated ureters	0	12	2	0	6	16

stones at the end of the sixth week was shown by us by beginning the experimental model with a lower dose of EG and increasing it after the third week [unpublished data].

Hydronephrosis, resulting from obstruction of the ureter by calculi, was also responsible for some alterations in renal function. The failure of allopurinol to control hyperoxaluria and hypercalciuria may explain the results obtained in this group. The results obtained with pyridoxine were perhaps better because, although it did not control the calciuria, it lowered the oxaluria to similar values to those of the control group. Allopurinol has been held as a prophylactic for calcium oxalate urolithiasis in humans but, as we have not been able to demonstrate any preventive usefulness of this drug in our rat model, it suggests that further investigation is required.

References

1 Vermeulen, C.W.; Lyon, E.S.: Mechanisms of genesis and growth of calculi. Am. J. Med. *45:* 684 (1968).

2 Jordan, W.R.; Finlayson, B.; Luxenberg, M.: Kinetics of early time calcium oxalate nephrolithiasis. Investve Urol. *15:* 465 (1978).

3 Werness, P. G.; Knoz, F. G.; Smith, L. H.: Low phosphate diet in rats: a model for calcium oxalate urolithiasis; in Smith, Robertson, Finlayson, Urolithiasis research, p. 731 (Plenum Press, New York 1981).
4 Tanret, P.; Thomas, J.; Cottenot, F.: Evolution des dépôts oxaliques et lipidiques au cours de la lithiase rénale expérimentale par l'éthylèneglycol et l'acide oxalique. Soc. Biol. *155:* 1025 (1961).
5 Lyon, E. S.; Borden, T. A.; Vermeulen, C. W.: Experimental oxalate lithiasis produced with ethylene glycol. Investve Urol. *15:* 465 (1978).
6 Okada, Y.; Kawamura, J.; Kuo, Y. J.; Yoshida, O.: Experimental model for calcium oxalate urolithiasis; in Ryall, Brockis, Marshall, Finlayson, Urinary stone, pp. 378–383 (Churchill-Livingstone, Edinburgh 1984).

José Manuel Reis-Santos, MD, Universidade Nova de Lisbon,
Faculty of Medical Science, Department of Urology, Curry Cabral Hospital,
P–1000 Lisbon (Portugal)

Contr. Nephrol., vol. 58, pp. 181–183 (Karger, Basel 1987)

Are Calcium Antagonists Potential Antilithiasic Drugs?

Giovanni Gambaro, Elisa Cicerello, Francesco Marchini, Carlo Paleari, Arturo Borsatti, Bruno Baggio [1]

Institute of Internal Medicine, Postgraduate School of Nephrology, University of Padova, Padova, Italy

Recently reported data indicated that the calcium antagonist, nifedipine, reduces urinary calcium and oxalate excretion in patients, with idiopathic calcium oxalate (CaOx) nephrolithiasis [1]. This report describes the effect of another calcium antagonist, flunarizine, on some lithogenic risk factors.

Materials and Methods

This study was performed on 10 patients (5 males and 5 females, aged from 30 to 45 years) with recurrent idiopathic CaOx nephrolithiasis, selected as previously described [2]. 10 mg/day of flunarizine was administered for 14 days. Patients followed a standard Italian diet and were not taking any other drug. At the beginning and at the end of the study, urinary excretion of oxalate (enzymatic method using the Sigma kit), calcium, phosphate, urate and citrate were evaluated as previously reported [2], as well as erythrocytic oxalate self-exchange [3, 4]. Statistical analysis was performed by Student's t-test for paired data, and the 'r' coefficient of linear correlation.

Results

The results, summarized in table I, show that flunarizine reduced both oxalate excretion and erythrocyte self-exchange of oxalate significantly. These decreases were correlated with their respective basal values

[1] We are grateful to Zambeletti SpA, Milan, for the generous gift of the drug.

Table I. Biochemical results of flunarizine treatment

	Before flunarizine	After flunarizine	t	p <
Oxalate, mg/day	52.02 ± 18.39	36.82 ± 12.32	2.51	0.05
Calcium, mg/day	328.30 ± 157.13	292.00 ± 112.58	1.18	n.s.
Phosphate, mg/day	1,111.70 ± 312.96	1,243.80 ± 497.63	0.78	n.s.
Citrate, mg/day	582.43 ± 366.53	503.29 ± 359.45	1.38	n.s.
Uric acid, mg/day	544.80 ± 136.57	591.30 ± 216.02	0.80	n.s.
Volume, ml/day	1,567.00 ± 322.98	1,410.00 ± 366.52	2.03	n.s.
RBC oxalate self-exchange, $K \times 10^{-2}$ min^{-1}	3.05 ± 0.93	1.14 ± 1.06	4.81	0.001

($p < 0.01$ for oxalate and $p < 0.001$ for erythrocyte self-exchange). No effect on urinary excretion of phosphate, urate, citrate and calcium was observed.

Discussion

The results of this study show that flunarizine is effective in reducing urinary oxalate excretion, and the effect is proportional to the basal oxalate excretion levels. Unlike nifedipine [1], no significant effect on urinary calcium excretion was observed. This dissimilar effect on calcium levels may perhaps be explained by the different composition of the patient groups treated with the two calcium antagonists, with specific reference to the different frequency of hypercalciuria. In fact, in the present study, only 4 of the 10 patients were hypercalciuric, compared to 7 of 12 patients in the nifedipine study, which demonstrated that the calcium reduction was correlated with basal calcium levels. Like nifedipine, flunarizine does not determine modifications in the other urinary parameters of lithogenic risk (phosphate, citrate). The effect of flunarizine at the cellular level on oxalate self-exchange [3, 4] may provide a possible explanation of how flunarizine reduces oxalate levels. It is possible that it alters body handling of oxalate by modifying cellular flow of this anion at the intestinal and/or renal epithelial level.

The data reported above constitute a further suggestion that drugs exerting a calcium antagonist effect may be useful in preventing calcium nephrolithiasis recurrence, since they bring about a favorable modification in the equilibrium between lithogenic ions and inhibitory substances.

References

1 Baggio, B.; Gambaro, G.; Marchini, F.; Cicerello, E.; Borsatti, A.: Effect of nifedipine on urinary calcium and oxalate excretion in renal stone formers. Nephron *43:* 234–235 (1986).

2 Baggio, B.; Gambaro, G.; Oliva, O.; Favaro, S.; Borsatti, A.: Calcium oxalate nephrolithiasis: an easy way to detect an imbalance between promoting and inhibiting factors. Clinica chim. Acta *124:* 149–155 (1982).

3 Baggio, B.; Gambaro, G.; Marchini, F.; Cicerello, E.; Borsatti, A.: Raised transmembrane oxalate flux in red blood cells in idiopathic calcium oxalate nephrolithiasis. Lancet *ii:* 12–13 (1984).

4 Baggio, B.; Gambaro, G.; Marchini, F.; Cicerello, E.; Tenconi, R.; Clementi, M.; Borsatti, A.: An inheritable anomaly of red cell oxalate transport in 'primary' calcium nephrolithiasis correctable with diuretics. New Engl. J. Med. *314:* 599–604 (1986).

Bruno Baggio, MD, Istituto di Medicina Interna, Policlinico Universitario,
via Giustiniani 2, I–35128 Padova (Italy)

Contr. Nephrol., vol. 58, pp. 184–186 (Karger, Basel 1987)

The Effect of Fenquizone on the Urinary Inhibitors of Calcium Oxalate Urolithiasis

A. Cupisti, F. Ciardella, E. Morelli, L. Dani, S. Lupetti, S. Luchi, M. Meola, G. Barsotti

Clinica Medica I, Università degli Studi, Pisa, Italia

In a recent work we demonstrated that fenquizone (Idrolone®, Farmaceutici Maggioni, Milano, Italy), a quinazolinone diuretic, exerts a significant hypocalciuric effect in patients with recurrent calcium oxalate stone disease and hypercalciuria [1].

The aim of the present investigation was to evaluate the effect of fenquizone therapy on the urinary excretion of some inhibitors of calcium oxalate crystallization, such as citrate, glycosaminoglycans and magnesium in patients with calcium oxalate nephrolithiasis.

Patients and Methods

We studied 16 normo- or hypercalciuric patients (11 males and 5 females) aged between 24 and 52 years, with recurrent calcium oxalate urolithiasis, before and during fenquizone therapy (10 mg daily by mouth as a single dose in the morning). During the study period (2.7 ± 1.0 months) they followed a free-mixed diet with a controlled calcium content (1 g/day). The 24-hour urine output was collected during 3 consecutive days immediately before and at the end of the study period without any preservative, for the determination by methods described elsewhere of the daily excretion of calcium (uCa), oxalic acid (uOx), citrate (uCit), glycosaminoglycans (uGAG), magnesium (uMg) and urinary volume. The uCa/uCit ratio was also evaluated as an index of lithogenic activity [2].

The statistical analysis of the results was performed by using Student's t-test for paired data.

Results

During fenquizone therapy the uCit increased significantly as compared with the values observed in the control period (from 2.84 ± 1.11 to 3.60 ± 1.59 mmol/day; $p < 0.001$, table I). The uGAG showed a similar

Table I. Effects of fenquizone therapy (mean ± SD)

	uCa mg/day	uCit mmol/day	uGAG mg/day	uCa/uCit mmol/mmol
Control	288.5 ± 62.5	2.84 ± 1.11	68.1 ± 33.4	3.10 ± 1.76
Treatment	209.8 ± 56.5	3.60 ± 1.59	111.8 ± 48.8	1.69 ± 0.77
	p < 0.001	p < 0.001	p < 0.005	p < 0.001
	Urinary volume ml/day	uOx mg/day	uMg mg/day	
Control	1,994 ± 796	25.3 ± 6.8	69.8 ± 20.1	
Treatment	2,300 ± 840	24.7 ± 7.0	76.2 ± 30.8	
	p < 0.05	n.s.	n.s.	

significant increase (from 68.1 ± 33.4 to 111.8 ± 48.8 mg/day; $p < 0.005$) while the uMg was unchanged (table I). The uOx excretion did not decrease, while the uCa was significantly reduced (from 288.5 ± 62.5 to 209.8 ± 56.5 mg/day; $p < 0.001$, table I). The daily urinary volume slightly increased and, finally, the uCa/uCit ratio was significantly lowered from 3.1 ± 1.76 to 1.69 ± 0.77; $p < 0.001$ (table I).

Discussion

These results confirm the hypocalciuric effect of fenquizone in hypercalciuric as well as in normocalciuric patients with calcium oxalate stone disease. In addition, this drug shows other beneficial properties, as the increase in the urinary excretion of some inhibitors of calcium oxalate crystals growth, such as uCit and uGAG [3]. The thiazide diuretics also reduce the uCa excretion, but they do not have any hypercitraturic action. On the contrary, some authors described a decrease of uCit during thiazide therapy [4].

As a consequence of the lowering of uCa and the increase of uCit, the fenquizone treatment causes a significant reduction of the uCa/uCit ratio which must be regarded as an important index of lithogenic activity [2]. We can then conclude that fenquizone, for its properties and its good tolerance [5], may be safely used for the long-term prevention of relapses in patients with calcium oxalate stone disease.

References

1 Cupisti, A.; Morelli, E.; Lupetti, S.; Ciardella, F.; Dani, L.; Carbone, C.; Luchi, S.; Giovannetti, E.; De Giorgi, A.R.; Barsotti, G.: Fenquizone for the treatment of idiopathic hypercalciuria in patients with recurrent calcium stone disease. Curr. Ther. Res. *38:* 293–297 (1985).

2 Denis, M.C.; Aveynier, M.; Sirajeddin, M.; Vialtel, P.: Mean of discrimination between controls and stone-formers (Abstract). Mineral Electrolyte Metab. *11:* 8–9 (1985).

3 Fleish, H.: Inhibitors and promoters of stones. Kidney int. *13:* 361–375 (1978).

4 Churchill, D.N.; Taylor, D.W.: Thiazides for patients with recurrent calcium stones: still an open question. J. Urol. *133:* 749–751 (1985).

5 Glorioso, N.; Bandiera, F.; Dessì Fulgheri, P.; Madeddu, P.; Oppes, M.; Tonolo, G.C.; Rappelli, A.: Once-a-day fenquizone in the treatment of hypertensive patients with impaired glucose tolerance. Curr. Ther. Res. *35:* 483–487 (1984).

Prof. Giuliano Barsotti, MD, Clinica Medica I, Università degli Studi,
I–56100 Pisa (Italy)

Contr. Nephrol., vol. 58, pp. 187–189 (Karger, Basel 1987)

Long-Term Urinary Acidification in Phosphatic Urolithiasis

F. Pizzarelli[a], *M. Peacock*[b]

[a]Centro Fisiologia Clinica CNR, Reggio Calabria, Italy;
[b]MRC, Mineral Metabolism Unit, Leeds, England

Urinary pH critically affects the degree of saturation with respect to calcium phosphate (CaP) and struvite [1, 2]. As shown by studies in animals, phosphatic stone recurrence is favored by urine alkalinization and is inhibited by urine acidification [3, 4]. In this study we analyzed retrospectively the effect of a long-term urinary acidification in human beings.

Patients and Methods

According to the results of a standard acid load test (ALT), 24 patients with recurrent stone disease of the CaP type associated with various amounts of struvite and persistently high urinary pH were divided into two groups.

Group A: 11 patients (4 men and 7 women, age 39.2 ± 16.5 years, mean ± SD) with inability to acidify urine to a pH lower than 5.5 (5.7 ± 0.2, range 5.5–6.2). Group B: 13 patients (4 men, 9 women, age 45.3 ± 11.9 years) with urinary pH during ALT lower than 5.1. Two patients of group A showed nephrocalcinosis. Ammonium sulfate in low doses, 2–3 g/day, was taken for 4.7 ± 3.7 years (range 2–12) by group A and for 6.5 ± 5.0 years (range 2–17) by group B patients.

Chemical analysis of stones, octocalcium phosphate relative saturation (OCPrs), urinary OH-proline/creatinine (OHpr/Cr) ratio and maximal tubular reabsorption of Ca (TmCa) were assessed or calculated as previously described.

Results and Discussion

In this study 24 patients, 11 with inability to properly acidify urine during ALT, were treated with low doses of ammonium sulfate. In a follow-up of 2–17 years, the treatment appeared successful in reducing urinary pH as well as OCPrs; stone formation rate (SFR) was concomitantly reduced (table I). Although the reduction in SFR was statistically significant in both groups, the effect appeared clinically meaningful only in group B. If

Table I. 24-hour urinary pH, OCPrs and SFR before (B) and during (D) treatment

	Group A		Group B	
pH				
B	6.6 ± 0.3	*	6.4 ± 0.4	**
D	6.2 ± 0.3		5.8 ± 0.5	
OCPrs				
B	0.5 ± 0.3	*	0.4 ± 0.5	**
D	–0.1 ± 0.6		–0.5 ± 0.7	
SFR				
B	1.6 [a]		1.8	a
D	1.1 [b]		0.2	

* $p < 0.025$; ** $p < 0.001$ paired t-test.
[a] $p < 0.01$ χ^2 with Yates correction.
[b] 0.45 without the two patients with nephrocalcinosis.

the 2 patients with nephrocalcinosis, who continued to pass stones as in the pretreatment period, are left out of analysis, in group A SFR was reduced from 1.1 to 0.45 stone/patient/year, a clinically relevant result.

At the low doses employed in our study, ammonium sulfate did not induce systemic acidosis as long as the renal function remained normal. Lacking of acidosis, it comes as no surprise that urinary daily excretion of Ca and TmCa did not change with time (table II).

As far as can be judged from the fasting Ca/Cr ratio (table II), no patient presented evidence of increased bone turnover. Moreover, in the 6 patients treated for 8 years or more the fasting OHPr/Cr ratio remained unchanged: 0.012 ± 0.002 mmol/mmol before, 0.011 ± 0.004 mmol/mmol during treatment.

We can argue that the eradication of infection, by intermittent antibiotic treatment, could have affected the stone recurrence by reducing the infective component of the stone, i.e. struvite. However, analysis of stones passed before and during therapy (struvite 20 vs 21%, CaP 73 vs 66%, CaOx 7 vs 13%) showed no variation in the percentage of struvite.

In conclusion acidifying agents in low doses seem useful in patients with recurrent phosphatic urolithiasis and persistently high urinary pH. With the exception of nephrocalcinosis, some benefit can be obtained even in the presence of a mild tubular acidification defect. Our results encourage undertaking properly controlled prospective trials.

Table II. Plasma and urinary variables

	Plasma		Fasting urine		24-hours urine	
	Cr µmol/l	tCO_2 mmol/l	Ca/Cr mmol/mmol	TmCa mmol/l GF	V l/day	Ca mmol/day
Group A						
Baseline	81.4 (14.3)	24.6 (1.6)	0.37 (0.19)	1.96 (0.22)	1.7 (1.0)	5.4 (3.1)
1–2 years	79.6 (23.3)	25.1 (1.5)	0.28 (0.13)	2.01 (0.17)	1.8 (0.6)	5.0 (1.7)
3–12 years	90.5 (26.0)	25.3 (1.0)	0.28 (0.11)	2.02 (0.10)	2.2 (0.4)	5.5 (1.5)
Group B						
Baseline	98.2 (23.3)	25.8 (1.7)	0.46 (0.24)	1.83 (0.14)	1.7 (0.5)	7.0 (3.8)
1–2 years	109.8 (37.6)	24.1 (3.4)	0.36 (0.21)	1.94 (0.14)	1.7 (0.5)	6.0 (3.4)
3–17 years	101.0 (17.2)	25.3 (2.1)	0.35 (0.20)	1.98 (0.15)	1.9 (0.5)	6.7 (2.4)

SD in parentheses. Changes with time in plasma and urinary variables were not significant by paired t-test.

References

1 Robertson, W. G.; Peacock, M.; Nordin, B. E. C.: Measurement of activity products in urine from stone-formers and normal subjects; in Smith, Urolithiasis: physical aspects, pp. 79–95 (National Academy of Science, Washington 1972).

2 Griffith, D. P.: Struvite stones. Kidney int. *13:* 372–380 (1978).

3 Hoar, D. W.; Emerick, R. J.; Embry, L. B.: Ovine phosphatic urolithiasis as related to the phosphorus and calcium contents and acid-base-forming effects of all-concentrated diets. J. Anim. Sci. *29:* 647–652 (1969).

4 Crookshank, H. R.: Effect of ammonium salts on the production of ovine urinary calculi. J. Anim. Sci. *30:* 1002–1004 (1970).

Francesco Pizzarelli, MD, Centro Fisiologia Clinica CNR,
via Sbarre Inferiori 39, I–89100 Reggio Calabria (Italy)

Contr. Nephrol., vol. 58, pp. 190–192 (Karger, Basel 1987)

Primary Hyperoxaluria: Effect of Treatment with Vitamin B_6 and Shock Waves

M. Amato[a], *S. Donzelli*[a], *M. Lombardi*[a], *M. Salvadori*[a], *M. Carini*[b], *C. Selli*[b], *R. Caudarella*[c]

[a]Division of Nephrology, Careggi Hospital, [b]Institute of Urology, Florence; and [c]Institute of Medical Pathology I, Bologna, Italy

Case Report

A 19-year-old man came to our hospital in January 1985. His parents were first cousins. He had a nephrocalcinosis since the age of five. Since that time he suffered from renal colics with repeated emissions of sand or oxalate stones. Nevertheless, he had normal psycho-physical growth with perfect bone maturation. Renal function had a slow and constant decrease in time, until the patient was hospitalized in our department.

Results

Diagnosis of primary hyperoxaluria was made on the basis of the anamnestic data, the radiographic picture, the high oxalate excretion (230 mg/24 h). His three sisters and the parents underwent a renal echography, a study of the renal function, tissue typing and urinary oxalate determination. Oxaluria was normal in the parents. We found the anomalous gene in the heterozygous form in the three sisters, who were genetically identical to each other with respect to the HLA system and completely different from the brother. This means that primary hyperoxaluria may eventually be related to the HLA system, even if a study on many families would be necessary to state this (fig. 1).

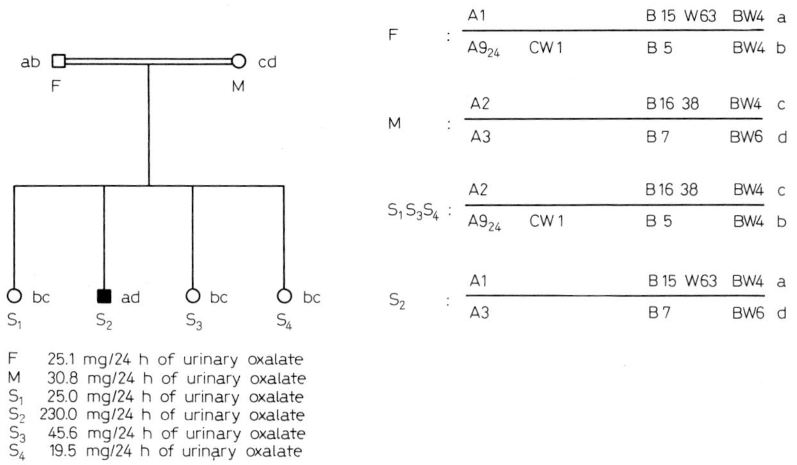

Fig. 1. Pedigree, HLA typing and urinary oxalates of the family.

Discussion

We gave the patient a high dose of vitamin B_6 (fig. 2) hoping that he would be among the few patients with primary hyperoxaluria [1] responding to this treatment [2]. In these patients a high dose of vitamin B_6 would enhance the glyoxylic acid transformation into glycine. In fact the administration of pyridoxine reduced the oxalate excretion to normal values with a slight improvement in renal function.

The patient's voluntary interruption of the treatment had dramatic results. Urinary oxalates returned to high values and the renal function suddenly decreased. This fact was also ascribed to the urinary obstruction caused by a big oxalate stone impacted in the left ureter. It was then mandatory to perform extracorporeal shock wave lithotripsy. The good results of this combined therapy are shown in figure 2.

Three main points arise from this case report: (a) According to the pedigree and the tissue typing we confirm that the primary hyperoxaluria is a hereditary, recessive illness. It is also possible that it might be linked in some way to the HLA system. (b) A vitamin B_6 treatment should always be tried from the first stages of every case of primary hyperoxaluria. (c) An extracorporeal shock wave treatment [3] seems to be mostly advisable for such patients. This is not only for acute stone episodes but also as a means of eliminating the oxalate stones in the pyelocaliceal system.

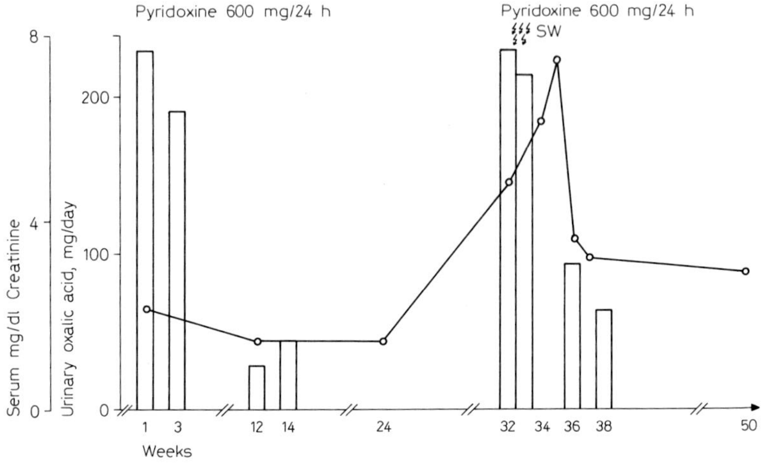

Fig. 2. Clinical course according to the therapy. SW = Shock wave.

References

1 Williams, H.E.; Smith, L.H.: Primary hyperoxaluria; in Stambury, Wyngaarden, Fredrickson, The metabolic basis of inherited disease, pp. 204–228 (McGraw-Hill, New York 1972).

2 Kasides, G.P.; Rose, A.G.: Metabolic hyperoxaluria and its response to pyridoxine; in Ryall, Brockis, Marshall, Finlayson, Urinary stone, pp. 138–147 (Churchill-Livingstone London 1984).

3 Chaussj, C.H.; Schmiedtt, E.: Shock waves treatment for stones in upper urinary tract. Urol. Clin. N. Am. *10:* 4–7 (1983).

Marcello Amato, MD, via Pisacane 11/2, I–50132 Firenze (Italy)

Contr. Nephrol., vol. 58, pp. 193–195 (Karger, Basel 1987)

Mercaptoethane Sulphonate in Cystinic Calculosis Therapy

F. Di Silverio, M. Gallucci, G. P. Ricciuti, G. Alpi, D. Fini, A. Cassanelli, C. Molinari

Università degli Studi di Roma 'La Sapienza', Patologia Urologica, Roma, Italia

Cystine is a dibasic, water-insoluble amino acid which possesses an SH-radical, which easily binds sulphydrylant drugs, thus forming a soluble complex. The main objectives of the medical treatment are: to reduce cystinuria by a low-cystine diet, to raise urine pH with alkali in order to render more soluble this amino acid and to transform cystine into a soluble compound [1–3]. Therefore mercaptoethane sulphonate (MESNA), a drug capable of forming a soluble complex with cystine, has been used in 11 patients affected by familial cystinuria.

Patients and Methods

11 patients (7 males and 4 females) affected by cystine lithiasis but stone-free at the time of the study and not receiving any drugs since 2 months, have been treated with MESNA by mouth 800 mg/day, in liquid form for 20 days. Aminoaciduria was analysed by ion-exchange chromatography, and 24-hour cystine excretion was performed before and after 20 days of therapy. Common laboratory tests were made in all patients, particularly those concerning renal and hepatic function. 15 patients treated with 1 g α-mercaptopropionylglycine for the same period were used as a control group.

Results

At least a 50% decrease of cystinuria as compared to baseline values was seen in all patients while on MESNA (fig. 1). Comparing these data to those obtained with α-mercaptopropionylglycine [1] (fig. 2) it appears that more satisfying results have been obtained with MESNA.

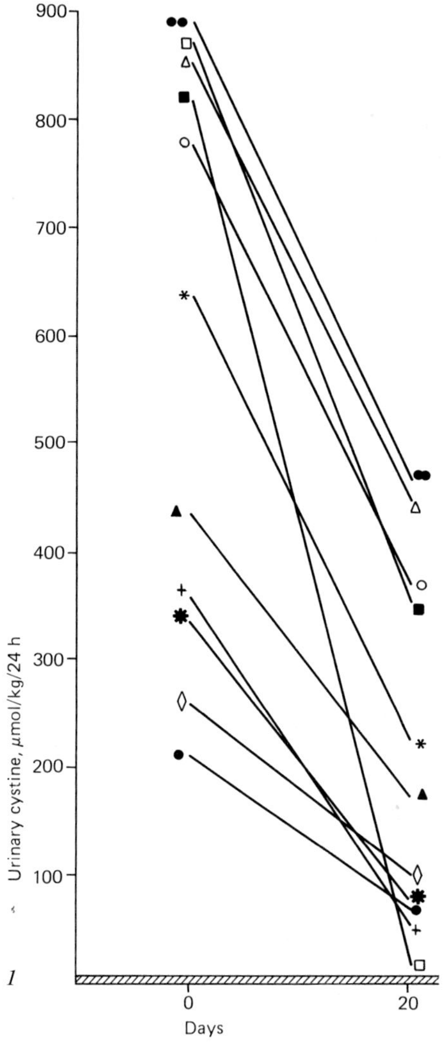

1

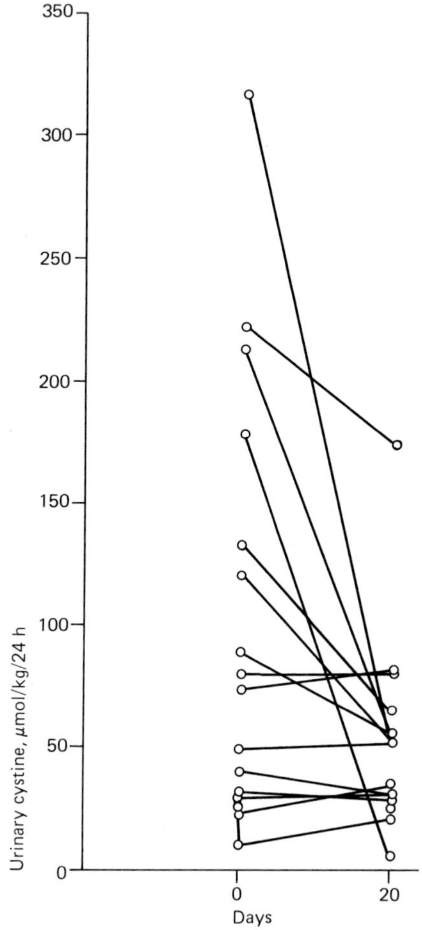

2

Fig. 1. Cystinuria 24 h before and after 20 days of treatment by MESNA 800 mg/day.

Fig. 2. Cystinuria 24 h before and after 20 days of treatment by α-mercapto-propionylglycine 1 g/day.

No noticeable side-effects have been observed. Only 1 patient had a skin rash at the end of the treatment. It is worthwhile to note that 5 of the 11 patients who had experienced side-effects with α-mercaptopropionylglycine (skin rash in 2 cases, nephrotic syndrome in 1, gastric burning in one, ageusia – reduced sensitivity to taste – in 1) entered the present study. In 7 out of 11 patients cystine crystalluria disappeared after the treatment.

Discussion

The importance of cystine lithiasis prevention justifies the efforts of research in this field. By treatment with MESNA, highly satisfying results have been obtained in controlling cystinuria. Comparing results obtained in the control group using α-mercaptopropionylglycine, a more remarkable decrease of cystinuria has been demonstrated in patients treated with MESNA. It is important to note that such a decrease ranges between 50 and 90% even in patients with very high values of cystinuria.

The absence of side-effects, at least in short-term treatment, suggests the possibility of increasing the dosage of the drug. This body of observations suggests that MESNA is a useful tool in medical therapy in this type of lithiasis.

References

1 Miano, L.; Gallucci, M.; Petta, S.: Results of medical treatment of cystine lithiasis. Eur. Urol. *5:* 229 (1979).

2 Miano, L.; Antonozzi, I.; Gallucci, M.; Morano, S.; Petta, S.: Clinical features and management of cystine nephrolithiasis. Adv. Nephrol. *375* (1981).

3 Brock, N.; Pohl, J.; Stekar, J.: Studies on the urotoxicity of oxazaphosphorine cytostatics and its prevention. I. Experimental studies on the urotoxicity of alkylating compounds. Eur. J. Cancer *17:* 595 (1981).

Michele Gallucci, MD, via Asmara 72, I–00199 Roma (Italy)

Contr. Nephrol., vol. 58, pp. 196–200 (Karger, Basel 1987)

Urease Inhibition in the Treatment of Infected Renal Stones: Propionohydroxamic Acid

A. Martelli, P. Buli, V. Cortecchia, S. Spatafora, F. Fiore, E. Tiozzi

Department of Urology, University of Bologna, Bologna, Italy

On the basis of previous experiences with inhibitors of bacteric urease, like acetohydroxamic acid, in 1981 we started the clinical study of a new hydroxamate, propionohydroxamic acid (PHA), in patients with struvite and carbonate apatite renal stones due to urea-splitting germs. As the carboxylic group is the active radical in urease inhibition, PHA with its two COOH radicals [1] was considered to be more suitable from a pharmacological point of view in the process of enzymatic inhibition than other compounds. Further toxicological studies demonstrated the good tolerance of the drug in the absence of teratogenous and mutagenic effects in test animals [2].

As for the choice of the most suitable dose, we started from the consideration that the therapeutic dose of the hydroxamates with a single radical already in use had been established at 750–500 mg/day. Hence, at the beginning of our clinical research with PHA, a dose of 375–250 mg/day was used [3].

Further pharmacokinetic studies on the drug proved that PHA has a half-life of about 15 h. Therefore, considering the accumulation fraction, the daily PHA dose was cut down to 120–60 mg/day [4]. Thus, as foreseen, effective urease inhibition together with a nearly total absence of side effects was obtained.

Patients and Methods

93 patients, between 18 and 80 years of age, underwent a therapy with PHA. 80 patients with positive urine culture due to urea-splitting germs after the complete removal of renal stones were included in the protocol together with 10 patients with residual stones and 3 patients with small clinically silent stones but with *Proteus mirabilis* urinary infection and high values of urinary ammonia and pH.

Pregnant or supposedly pregnant women, patients with serious alterations of blood hemostasis, of heart and of hepatic function and finally subjects with plasma creatinine values above 3 mg/100 ml were excluded from our research.

31 patients were administered PHA in daily doses of 375 mg (group A), 17 were treated with variable doses between 350 and 250 mg/day, 35 were first given 120 mg/day and then 60 mg/day (group B) and, finally, 10 whose kidneys were stone-free, growth of no highly urea-splitting bacteria (Pseudomonas, *Ureaplasma urealyticum*), with urinary NH_3 and pH values just above the standard, underwent a new protocol with very low dosage: 60 mg/day followed by 30 mg/day (group C).

All patients were initially treated with antibiotic therapy for 3–5 days at full dosage, according to the degree of renal failure.

Therapeutic association of PHA and antibiotic was continued until complete urine sterilization, supported by several negative urine cultures and the finding of normal urinary ammonia and pH values. In the case of in situ stones the treatment was continued ad libitum.

In the follow-up, ammonia, pH, urine culture, and various physical and laboratory parameters were evaluated, following the protocol we have previously described [4]. Plain film of abdomen was performed at the beginning of the treatment and then every 3 months. In situ stones were studied following the method described by Griffith et al. [5] for the measurement of the size of stones using a planimeter in the evaluation of their growth.

Statistic analysis of data using Student's t-test was applied evaluating the variations of urinary ammonia and pH in the patients of groups A and B, comparing the basal values to the ones of the 10th day. The same analysis was not applied to the data from group C, because of the low number of patients that can be found in this study at the moment.

Results

Urinary Alkalinity and Ammonia

Urinary pH and NH_3 have been reduced in a statistically significant way ($p < 0.001$) both in the patients of groups A and B. Figures 1 and 2 compare the changes of these parameters in subjects treated with doses of 375 and 120–60 mg/day: both curves show their fast decrease and a nearly similar pattern.

The effects of PHA at a very low dosage are visualized in figure 3: in spite of the not very high basal values no other satisfactory decreases were obtained in 4 patients. For the remaining 6, the effect, which was still valid, was not so fast as for groups A and B.

Radiographic Changes

The measurement of the size of in situ stones, carried out at least 6 months from the beginning of treatment, showed unchanged size in 77% of cases (10 patients) and an increase in the remaining 23%.

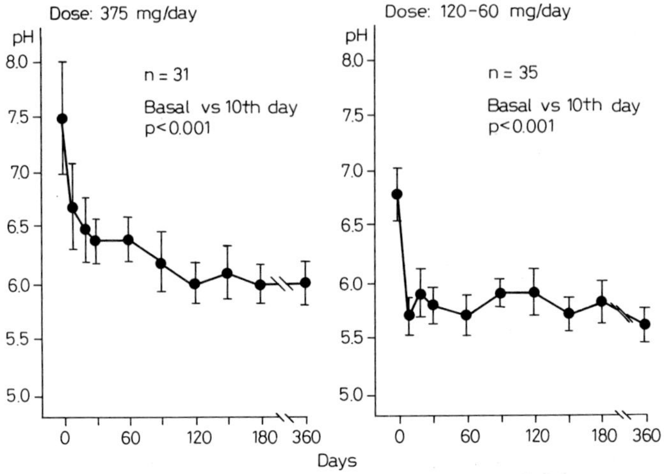

1

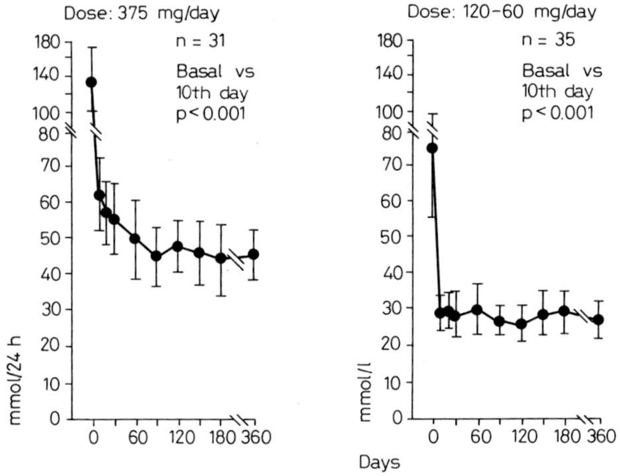

2

Fig. 1. Urinary pH changes during PHA treatment (MV ± SD): 375 vs 120–60 mg/day.
Fig. 2. Urinary NH_3 changes during PHA treatment (MV ± SD): 375 vs 120–60 mg/day.

We have never obtained stone dissolution, as reported by other authors [5].

Seventy stone-free patients, with a follow-up of at least 6 months, also underwent repeated plain films of abdomen to evaluate the presence of recurrence. The latter, from the data in literature, proves to have an incidence of 17% within 3 years [6] and 30% within 6 years [7] in patients who underwent an antibiotic therapy only. Only 3 patients (4.3%) showed

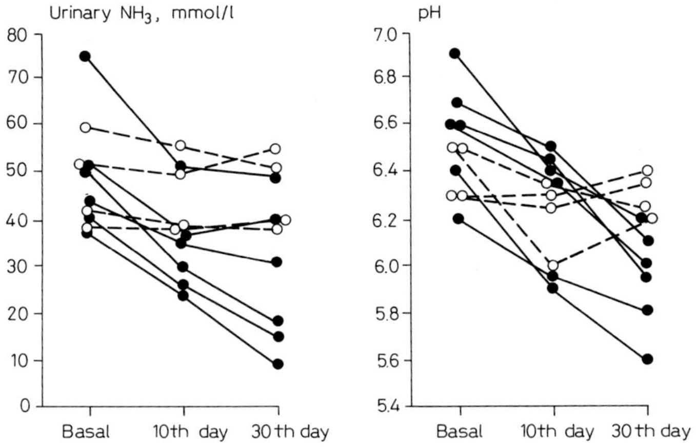

Fig. 3. Urinary NH_3 and pH changes during PHA treatment with 60–30 mg/day in 10 patients. --- = Unsatisfactory results.

recurrence, 1 belonging to group A, 1 to group B and 1 treated with 250 mg/day.

Side Effects

With the dose of 375 mg/day a low incidence of side effects was found [7]. Reduction of the dosage to 120–60 mg/day led to further diminution as can be observed in table I.

Only 1 subject in group B had to give up the therapy owing to the onset of hepatic dysfunction, which he already had at the beginning of treatment. No parameters, physical or laboratory, evaluated in the follow-up, showed any significant variation apart from the WBC decrease, probably due to improved control of infections in patients treated with PHA.

Discussion

The results obtained in the 93 patients treated with PHA have confirmed the true efficacy of the drug in the prevention of renal stone secondary to urinary infection due to urea-splitting germs. It must be pointed out that the 120–60 mg/day dose is sufficient to have good enzymatic inhibition avoiding at the same time most of the specific side effects reported by other authors with the use of hydroxamic compounds [7].

Table I. Side effects: 375–250 vs 120–30 mg/day

Side effects	375–250 mg/day 48 patients (%)	120–30 mg/day 45 patients (%)
Gastrointestinal upset	3 (6.2)	–
Hepatic dysfunction	–	1[1] (2.2)
Temporary hair loss	3 (6.2)	2 (4.4)
Temporary headache	2 (4.1)	–
Antabuse effect	3 (6.2)	2 (4.4)
Mild anemia	5 (10.4)	–
No side effects	32 (66.7)	40 (88.9)
Discontinued treatment	5 (10.4)	1[1] (2.2)

[1] Patients with pretreatment chronic liver disease.

Further reduction of posology will be possible on the basis of the results of the studies about pharmacokinetics of PHA and particularly of its accumulation fractions. About the latter, it must be pointed out that propionamide, the metabolite of the drug, is not toxic differently from the metabolites of the other hydroxamic compounds.

References

1 Von Kreibig, T.; Preussman, R.; Schmidt, W.: Chemische Konstitution und teratogene Wirkung bei der Ratte. Arzneimittel-Forsch. *18:* 645–657 (1968).

2 Wang, C. Y.; Lanfong, H. L.: Mutagenicity and antibacterial activity of hydroxamic acids. Antimicrob. Agents Chemother. *4:* 753–758 (1977).

3 Martelli, A.; Buli, P.; Brunocilla, E.: Propionohydroxamic acid in infected renal stones. A preliminary clinical report. J. Urol. *128:* 1130–1132 (1982).

4 Martelli, A.; Buli, P.; Spatafora, S.: Clinical experience with low dosage of propionohydroxamic acid (PHA) in infected renal stones. Urology *28:* 373–375 (1986).

5 Griffith, D. P.; Moskowitz, P. A.; Carlton, E. C., Jr.: Adjunctive chemotherapy of infection-induced staghorn calculi. J. Urol. *121:* 711–715 (1979).

6 Griffith, D. P.; Gibson, J. R.; Clinton, C. W.; Musher, D. M.: Acetohydroxamic acid: clinical studies of an urease inhibitor in patients with staghorn renal calculi. J. Urol. *119:* 9–15 (1978).

7 Griffith, D. P.; Martelli, A.: Round table discussion on secondary lithiasis; in Urolithiasis and related clinical research, pp. 415–421 (Plenum Press, New York 1984).

Prof. A. Martelli, MD, Department of Urology, University of Bologna,
via Massarenti 9, I-40138 Bologna (Italy)

Contr. Nephrol., vol. 58, pp. 201–206 (Karger, Basel 1987)

Propionhydroxamic Acid in the Management of Struvite Urinary Stones

P. Puppo, F. Germinale, P. Bottino, G. Ricciotti, L. Giuliani

Department of Urology, University of Genova, Genova, Italy

Infection and urinary stones are strictly related diseases. The bacterial species which play a fundamental role in the formation of infective stones (*Proteus* overall) produce the enzyme urease, which increases urinary alkalinity and the concentration of bicarbonate and ammonia ions by splitting urea and supersaturating urine with respect to struvite.

For several years a new class of drugs, i.e. the urease inhibitors, has been used in the treatment and prevention of infection-induced stones. The urease-inhibiting activity of hydroxamic acid was noted since 1962 and several works have demonstrated, between 1973 [3] and 1980 [4], that this drug can prevent stone formation and pyelonephritic changes induced by *Proteus* infection. In 1978, Smith [7] with hydroxyurea (HU) and Griffith [5] with acetohydroxamic acid (AHA) reported the first clinical applications of urease inhibitors in stone patients. In the same year we began our experience with HU [1], which 2 years later was replaced by the less toxic but not easily available AHA [2]. For the past 2 years we have adopted propionhydroxamic acid (PHA) in our protocol owing to its minor toxicity. Herein we review and compare these experiences and try to assess the usefulness of hydroxamates in consideration of the development of non-invasive techniques for stone management, such as extracorporeal shock waves and percutaneous lithotripsy.

Patients and Methods

Since 1978 we have treated with urease inhibitors 66 patients with chronic urea-splitting urinary infection. The bacterial species involved were *Proteus mirabilis* in 10 cases, *Proteus rettgeri* in 24 cases, *Proteus morganii* in 9 cases, *Proteus vulgaris* in 5 cases, *Pseudomonas*

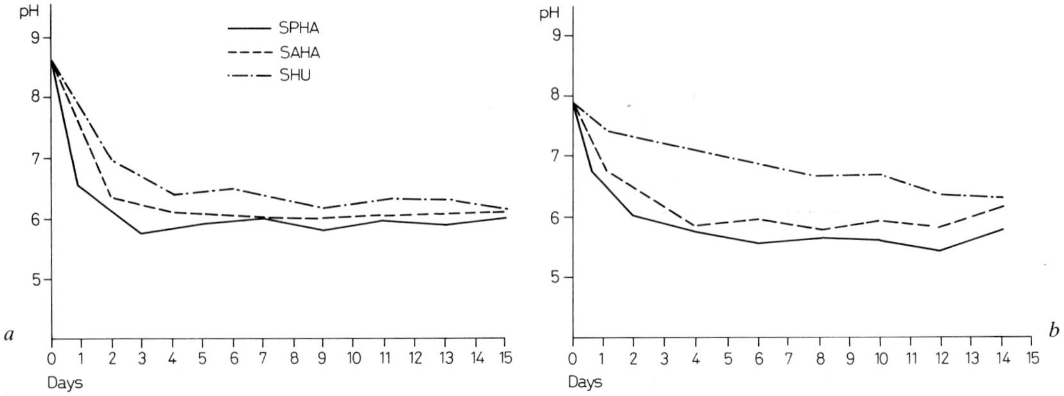

Fig. 1. Urine acidification. *a* In the presence of stones. *b* With risk of stone.

aeruginosa in 8 cases, *Serratia marcescens* in 6 cases, *Klebsiella* in 2 cases and *Providencia* in 1 case. All patients were above the age of majority, and all had a serum creatinine concentration below 1.5 mg/100 ml and a hematocrit above 25%. Patients were exluded if they could not understand the protocol; if they were pregnant, nursing, or were not using contraception; or if they had a history of varicose veins, phlebitis, pulmonary embolism or liver diseases. Thirty patients had stones, 17 had a past history of struvite stones and a persistent urea-splitting infection, 16 had been recently operated on for staghorn struvite stones, and 3 had ileal ureter and suffered from chronic urinary infection.

The patients can be subdivided in groups according to the presence of stones (S) or to the risk of stone (R) and to the different drugs used (HU, AHA and PHA). The urease-inhibitors were always associated with culture-specific oral antibiotics and administered orally as follows: HU 500 mg/day, AHA 1 g/day (afterwards reduced to 500 mg/day), PHA 120 mg/day. A complete blood count, an automated serum biochemical profile and urine culture were obtained every week during treatment. An urinary output exceeding 2 liter/24 h was maintained in every patient. The patients were instructed to measure and record their urinary pH by means of test strips in a freshly voided specimen every morning before taking the drug. Weekly pH was controlled by Bench pH meter. In 15 patients urinary ammonium excretion was monitored. All patients were treated for at least 3 months, so that we will consider this period in evaluating and comparing the results.

Results

The results were evaluated in terms of urine acidification and sterilization and they are now considered separately for each group, as is represented in figures 1 and 2. As far as urine acidification in concerned, all the drugs used gave good results, leading to pH normalization within 3 days of

a

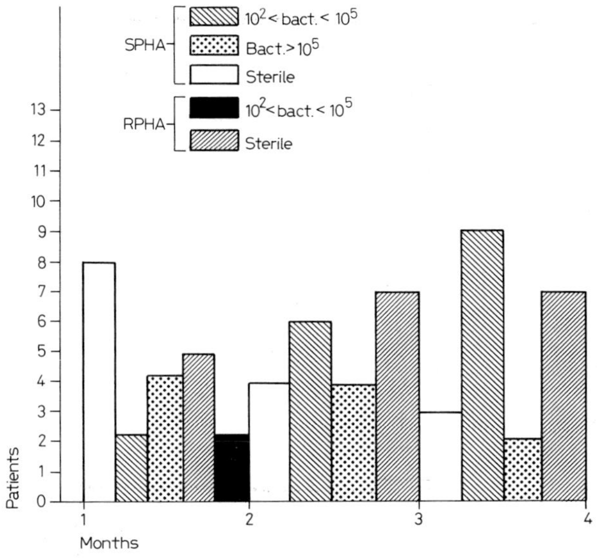

b

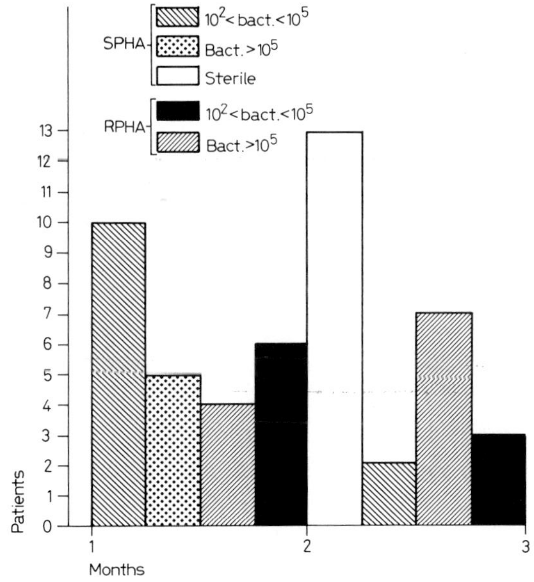

Fig. 2. Urine sterilization with *a* PHA and *b* AHA.

therapy. AHA and PHA showed a faster effect than HU, reducing urinary pH already in the second day of treatment in the majority of the cases. No significant difference was noted between the groups S and R, showing that the stone itself does not contribute to urine alkalization (fig. 1a, b). As for urine sterilization, there was a significant dramatic difference between the groups S and R. In groups SHU and SAHA no urine sterilization was achieved. In the group SPHA in 4 patients sterilization occurred (fig. 2a, b). In the group RHU, 10 out of 14 patients obtained urine sterilization in a time ranging from 1 to 8 weeks. Similarly, in the group RAHA, 13 out of 15 patients. In the group RPHA, 7 out of 7 patients showed complete recovery from urinary infections. In 15 patients of the groups SPHA and RPHA urinary ammonium decreased from a basal mean value of 262 after 10 days of therapy, to 176 after 25 days, to 155 after 40 days and to 99 after 90 days of therapy.

None of the patients with stones showed a significant increase in stone size. Conversely no dissolution or reduction in stone size could be noted. The side effects were not serious and only in 4 cases (groups SHU and RHU) compelled us to stop the therapy temporarily. In these cases white blood cells showed a considerable decrease which recovered after 15 days of interruption. The treatment was then started again with a lower dosage (250 mg/day) with no other problem.

In the other 62 cases hydroxamates provoked only a mild decrease in white blood cell count, decreasing from HU to PHA. The latter one, at the dosage of 120 mg/day, did not cause any substantial variation in white blood cell count. No other toxic effect was observed; in particular, no altered liver or renal function was revealed by routine biochemical controls.

Discussion

Treatment of struvite stones is based on a correct understanding of the etiologic factor involved. The primary objective of the treatment is to make the patient free from stones and infection and to prevent stone recurrence, while minimizing the loss of renal function. The introduction of new non-invasive techniques, such as percutaneous and extracorporeal lithotripsy, has changed the management of infected stones to that of the other stones.

The treated patients should be protected (1) from urinary obstruction by fragments and (2) from serious pyelonephritis caused by the bacteria trapped in the disrupted struvite stone. Urea-splitting organisms involved in struvite lithiasis are generally resistant to the common antibiotics and alkaline urinary pH helps bacteria to establish themselves.

Urease-inhibiting drugs can effectively acidify urine infected by urea-splitting bacteria, in the presence or absence of renal stones, a goal which is not achieved by conventional treatment. All three drugs used in our experience (HU, AHA and PHA) showed a good therapeutic activity, even if with AHA and PHA the return of urinary pH to normal values was more rapid.

The association with specific antibiotics can achieve urine sterilization in a high percentage of stone-free patients (up to 100% with PHA). In order to maintain sterile urine it is advisable to prolong the treatment for at least 1–2 months after the first negative urine culture. In patients with stones it is extremely difficult to sterilize urine also in the presence of acid pH and, furthermore, to maintain sterilization once it has been achieved. Only with PHA we have obtained some positive results. As far as stone dissolution, contrary to the positive experiences of Griffith [5] and of Martelli et al. [6] and according to those of Smith [8–9] and of Williams et al. [10], we did not observe any reduction in stone size during treatment. The effectiveness of hydroxamates depends on the concentration achieved in the urine [10]. In patients with normal renal function, the drugs are largely excreted unchanged in the urine, so that it seems that blood levels would be higher in azotemic patients given enough drug to achieve therapeutic levels in the urine. The indication for PHA treatment in struvite lithiasis should be carefully assessed on the basis of the integrated protocol of a stone center where all new techniques are available together with the surgical facilities for staghorn stones. When open surgery is planned, treatment with PHA in patients with struvite stones should be started one month before operation in order to decrease urinary alkalinitiy and, if possible, to sterilize the urine. The treatment should be suspended during the early postoperative course. In the case of percutaneous surgery the protocol should be essentially the same, while the indications are a little bit different in the case of extracorporeal lithotripsy, it being advisable to continue the therapy also during the treatment itself and in the early postoperative course. In fact the disintegration of the stone liberates the bacteria entrapped causing reinfection or overinfection of the urine already during shock wave application, as has been demonstrated by serial urine intraoperative cultures.

Whatever the technique of stone removal, once the patient is free from stone he should enter a protocol of prevention of infection (and stone) recurrence. It consists of periodic controls of urine culture and of cycles of PHA therapy if urea-splitting infection is present.

References

1 Carmignani, G.; Belgrano, E.; Puppo, P.; Cichero, A.; Giuliani, L.: Hydroxyurea in the management of chronic urea-splitting urinary infection. Br. J. Urol. *52:* 316 (1980).

2 Carmignani, G.; Belgrano, E.; Puppo, P.; Giuliani, L.: Hydroxy-Harnstoff und Acetohydrosamsäure bei der Prophylaxe und Behandlung der Patienten mit Phosphatsteinen. 32. Dt. Urol. Ges., Berlin 1980.

3 Griffith, D.P.; Musher, D.M.: Prevention of infected urinary stones by urease inhibition. Investve Urol. *11:* 228 (1973).

4 Griffith, D.P.; Musher, D.M.; Itin, C.: Urease: the primary cause of infection-induced urinary stones. Investve Urol. *13:* 346–350 (1976).

5 Griffith, D.P.: Struvite stones. Kidney int. *13:* 372–382 (1978).

6 Martelli, A.; Buli, P.; Cortecchia, V.: Acetohydroxamic acid therapy in infected renal stones. Urology *17:* 320–322 (1981).

7 Smith, M.J.V.: Hydroxyurea and infected stones. Urology *11:* 274 (1978).

8 Smith, M.J.V.: Management of infected stone disease with hydroxyurea: a five-year follow-up. Eur. Dial. Transpl. Ass. *20:* 466–468 (1983).

9 Smith, L.M.: New treatment for struvite urinary stones. New Engl. J. Med. *20:* 792–794 (1984).

10 Williams, J.J.; Rodman, J.S.; Peterson, C.M.: A randomized double-blind study of acetohydroxamic acid in struvite nephrolithiasis. New Engl. J. Med. *311:* 760–763 (1984).

P. Puppo, MD, Department of Urology, University of Genova, I–16132 Genova (Italy)

Contr. Nephrol., vol. 58, pp. 207–211 (Karger, Basel 1987)

Physicochemical Changes of Urine Environment on Propionhydroxamic Acid Therapy

M. Bruno, M. Marangella, A. Tricerri, C. Martini, F. Linari
Department of Nephrology, Mauriziano Umberto I Hospital, Turin, Italy

Although Boistelle et al. [1] have recently demonstrated that struvite crystals can form also in acidic sterile urines, i.e. that physiological urines could be sporadically supersaturated with struvite, most authors believe that struvite stones can form and grow only in the presence of urease-producing bacteria. Urease splits urea and this gives rise to an increase in urinary pH and in ammonium and in unprotonated carbonate and phosphate [2]; in the presence of calcium and magnesium, even at low concentrations, the supersaturation of urine with respect to the salts formed by the above species is easily attained. This study was designed to evaluate physicochemical changes induced by propionhydroxamic acid (PHA), a urease-inhibiting drug, on urine environment of infected stone patients.

Patients and Methods

The urine physicochemical status was periodically assessed in 18 infected stone patients on 6-month PHA therapy by measuring pH and total concentrations of ammonium, calcium, magnesium, phosphate and citrate; the saturation of urine with struvite was estimated by means of Marshall and Robertson's [3] nomograms and expressed as relative supersaturation (RS).

Patients (12 men, 6 women) were aged 44 ± 9 (mean ± SD) years (range 28–63); most of them had a history of heavy stone disease with multiple (2.6 ± 1, range 1–5) operations on urinary tract. Only 1 patient was free from calculi; 9 had unilateral and 8 bilateral calculi or residual fragments. Serum creatinine levels ranged from 0.9 to 2.1 mg/dl (mean 1.25 ± 0.30).

The drug was started at a dose of 240 mg/day and reduced within a week to 120 mg; dosage was further varied, if necessary, on the basis of the urinary assays. At the beginning PHA was associated in all the patients to a chemio-antibiotic cycle; afterwards antimicrobial treatment was not discontinued in 2 patients, while the others received intermittent cycles according to urine cultures. Results are expressed as means ± SD; statistical analysis was performed by Student's t-test and by Wilcoxon's test for paired data.

Table I. Urinary parameters (mmol/24 h) in 66 normal subjects and in 18 infected stone patients

	Normals	Patients	p <
pH	6.09 ± 0.50	7.32 ± 0.54	0.001
NH_4	25 ± 11.5	89 ± 31.4	0.001
Mg	3.5 ± 1.5	4.4 ± 3.6	n.s.
Ca	4.4 ± 1.9	4.97 ± 2.99	n.s.
P	23.9 ± 8.6	30.5 ± 11.7	0.05
Cit.	2.66 ± 1.28	1.29 ± 1.24	0.001

1

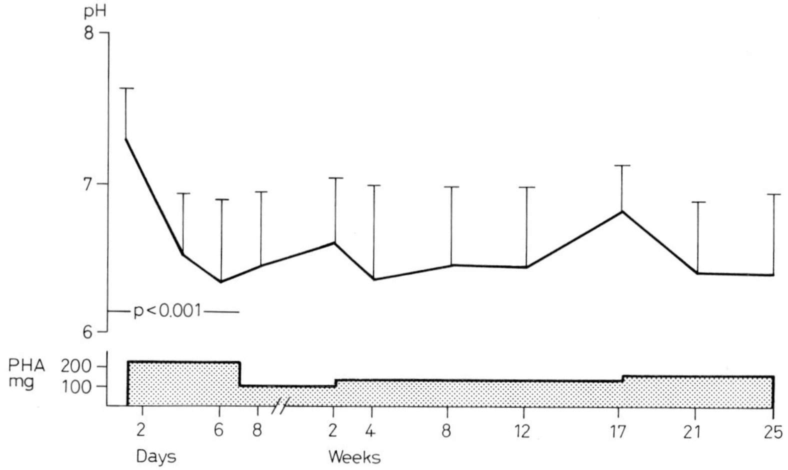

2

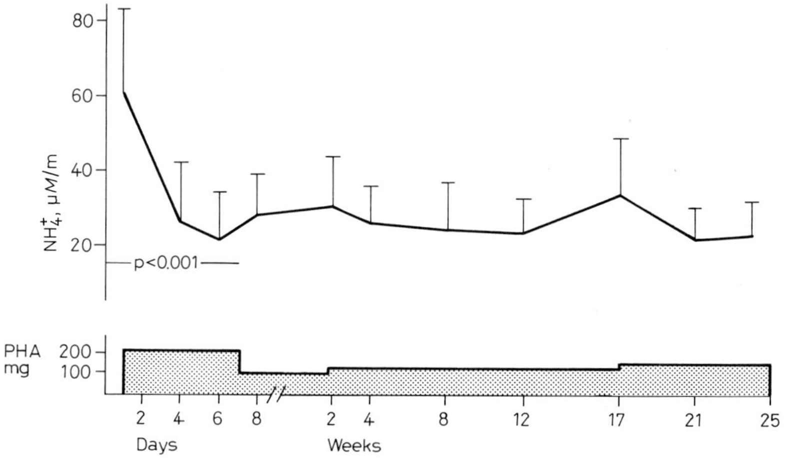

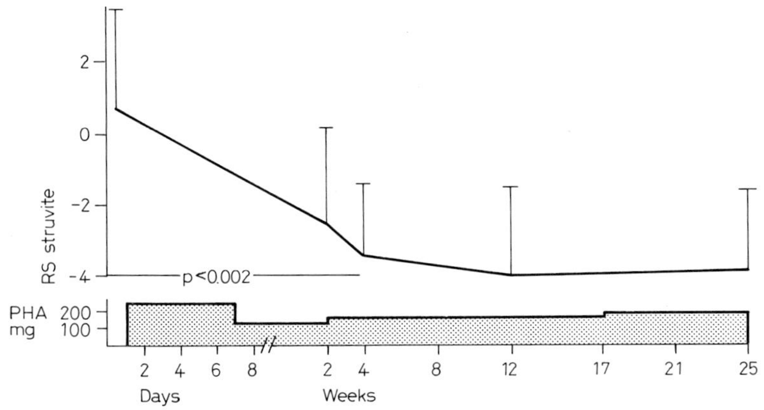

Fig. 3. Struvite RS behavior on PHA therapy.

Results

Table I compares the basal urinary parameters of the patients with those of 66 normal subjects: pH, ammonium and phosphate were significantly higher; citrate was significantly reduced. During therapy pH, ammonium and struvite RS significantly decreased in a few days (fig. 1–3); after the maintenance dose was set up, a trend toward increase in pH and ammonium was noted which required an increase in drug dosage; similar increases were observed in single patients after antibiotic was discontinued; nevertheless, urines remained undersaturated with respect to struvite in all the patients (fig. 4).

Some patients, who already had undersaturated urines at the beginning of the study, showed further reduction in struvite RS on PHA therapy. No statistically significant variation was observed in calcium, magnesium, phosphate and citrate excretions (fig. 5). Figure 6 correlates urinary pH and struvite RS under basal conditions; this good correlation persisted also during therapy.

Fig. 1. Urinary pH behavior on PHA therapy (means ± SD are shown).

Fig. 2. Urinary ammonium behavior on PHA therapy.

4
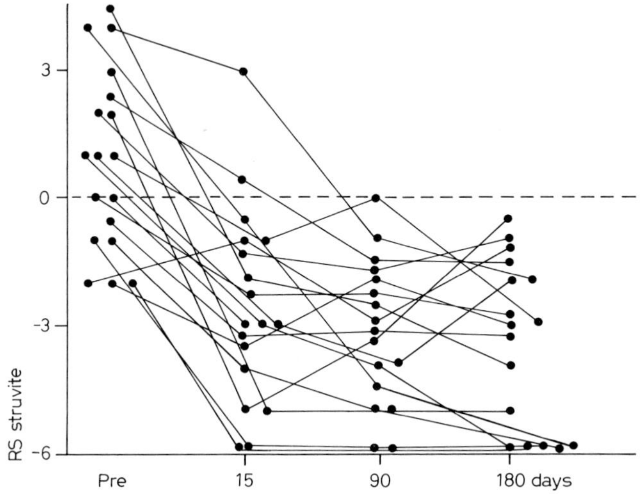

5
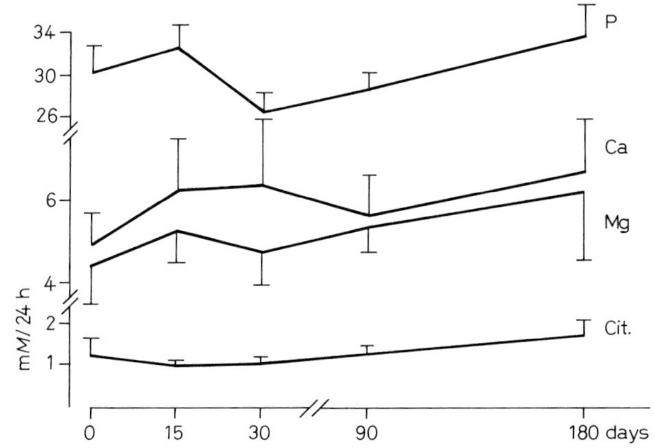

Fig. 4. Struvite RS behavior in 18 patients on PHA therapy.

Fig. 5. Calcium, magnesium, phosphate and citrate excretions on PHA therapy (means ± SEM).

Discussion and Conclusion

The increase in pH and ammonium in urines from infected stone patients ensues from urease activity; the reduction in citrate excretion may be caused either by urinary infection or by renal failure [4]; we do not know how to explain the increased phosphate in these patients.

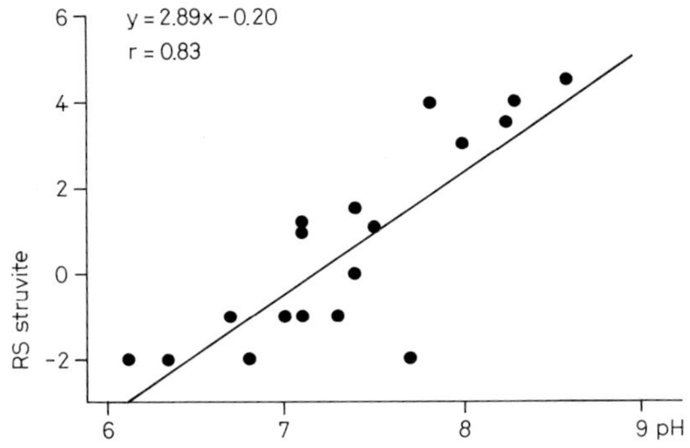

Fig. 6. Correlation between urinary pH and struvite RS in 18 infected stone patients: basal values.

The physicochemical changes in urine environment under treatment are the expected effects of the antiurease activity of PHA and/or antimicrobial activity of antibiotics: in this regard PHA and antibiotics seem to potentiate each other, but their specific role does not clearly emerge from this study. Urine pH, which well correlates with struvite RS, can be assumed as a reliable marker of the lithogenic risk.

In conclusion, PHA is effective in reducing urine RS with respect to struvite and its use, in association with antibiotics, may represent a real progress in the management of infected stone patients. The effectiveness of the above drug may be simply monitored by urinary pH determination.

References

1 Boistelle, R.; Abbona, F.; Berland, Y.; Grandvuillemin, M.; Olmer, M.: The crystallization of magnesium ammonium phosphate (struvite) in acidic sterile urine; in Schwille, 5th Int. Symp. on Urolithiasis and Related Clinical Research, Garmisch 1984. Urolithiasis and Related Clinical Research, pp. 793–796 (Plenum Press, New York 1985).

2 Griffith, D. P.: Struvite stones. Kidney int. *13:* 372–382 (1978).

3 Marshall, R. W.; Robertson, W. G.: Nomograms for the estimation of the saturation of urine with calcium oxalate, calcium phosphate, magnesium ammonium phosphate, uric acid, sodium acid urate, ammonium acid urate and cystine. Clinica chim. Acta *72:* 253–260 (1976).

4 Hodgkinson, A.: Citric acid excretion in normal adults and in patients with renal calculus. Clin. Sci. *23:* 203–212 (1962).

Michele Bruno, MD, Divisione Nefrologia e Dialisi,
Ospedale Mauriziano Umberto I, Largo Turati 62, I–10128 Torino (Italy)

Contr. Nephrol., vol. 58, pp. 212–214 (Karger, Basel 1987)

Propionohydroxamic Acid in the Treatment of Urease-Induced Calculi

Six Months Follow-Up of 19 Patients

A. Tizzani, G. Casetta, P. Piana, R. Carone, C. Giona, S. Rocca Rossetti

Università degli Studi di Torino, Facoltà di Medicina e Chirurgia,
Istituto di Nefro-Urologia, Cattedra di Urologia (Direttore: Prof. S. Rocca Rossetti), Torino, Italia

Hydroxamic acids have been proposed as inhibitors of bacterial urease in the treatment and prophylaxis of infected stone disease. Propionohydroxamic acid (PHA) proved to be a safer drug in preclinical and early clinical studies. In this work we show our experience with low-dose PHA treatment in stone-affected and stone-free patients with urinary tract infection (UTI) due to urea-splitting bacteria.

Patients and Methods

We treated 19 patients with PHA, 6 men and 13 women, aged between 20 and 68, affected by documented UTI due to urea-splitting bacteria. Twelve suffered from recurrent staghorn lithiasis and were stone-affected. 4 patients had recently undergone surgery for the same reason, the remaining had infected urine without any previous history of lithiasis. PHA was given at doses of 120 mg twice daily until normalization of urinary pH and ammonium excretion, that was usually achieved within 2 weeks. Thereafter PHA was reduced to 120 mg daily. The duration of the treatment varied between 40 and 220 days. Specific antibiotic therapy was associated in all the cases at the beginning of the treatment and later whenever urine culture turned positive again. Efficacy and tolerability of the drug were simultaneously evaluated. Urinary pH and ammonium excretion were evaluated before treatment, daily in the first 10 days, every 2 weeks until the 3rd month and monthly after then. Urine culture was repeated twice monthly until the 3rd month, then monthly. Tolerability was assessed comparing before and during therapy evaluations of haemogram, liver and kidney function, fertility and some other biological parameters. Patients were carefully interviewed monthly about the possible onset of side-effects. A complete statistical analysis of the results (Anova test) was performed concerning the first 120 days of treatment.

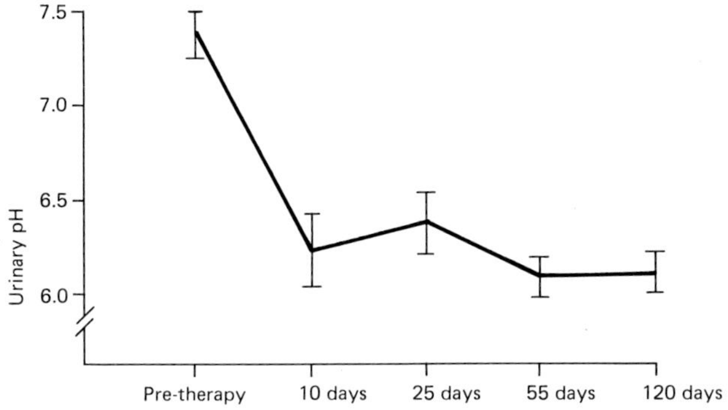

Fig. 1. Changes in mean urinary pH during PHA therapy.

Results

Fifteen patients were treated for more than 120 days, 1 patient in very poor general condition withdrew after 40 days, the remaining dropped out as not being able to attend the periodic controls. Eight patients showed mild side-effects: 4 cases of mixed neurological symptoms (dizziness, tremor, nausea, etc.), 2 cases of alcohol intolerance and 2 cases of hair loss. In 7 patients (3 stone-affected) urine sterilization was achieved, sometimes already at the first measurement, more often after one or more recurrencies or reinfections. The other 12 patients (10 stone-affected) alternated sterile urine with recurrency or reinfection periods, and urine was still infected at the end of therapy. Two patients out of these showed reinfection due to non-urea splitters. The mean urinary pH value fell promptly from 7.39 before treatment to 6.24 within 10 days of treatment and then remained quite constant until the end of the study (fig. 1). The pH reduction was highly significant ($p < 0.001$). Ammonium excretion fell from a mean pretreatment value of 189.5 to 80.5 mg/l within the first 10 days and reached the normal range after 120 days (fig. 2). This reduction is again highly significant ($p < 0.001$); moreover, a linear correlation can be drawn between ammonium excretion and time ($p < 0.02$). A significant reduction in platelet count was noted during therapy, with a minimum of 229,000/mm^3; that is, however, still in the normal range. A slight linear trend to decrease in leucocyte count was noted too, but without any pathological significance. No other evidence of pathology appeared.

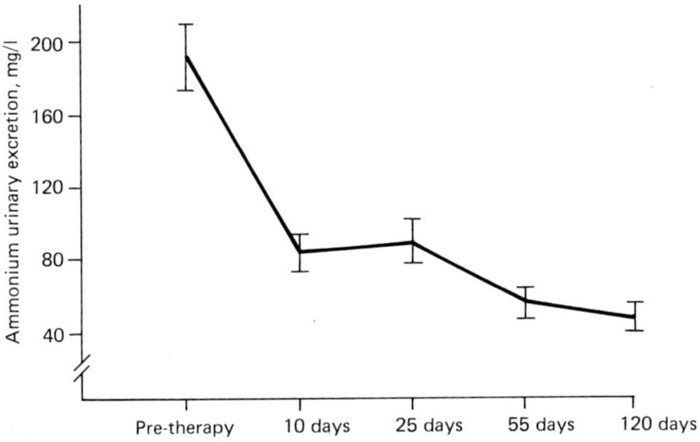

Fig. 2. Changes in ammonium excretion during PHA therapy.

Discussion

PHA confirmed its efficacy as inhibitor of bacterial urease. Normalization of urinary pH and ammonium excretion was achieved rapidly and lasted throughout the treatment with low-dose administration. Urine sterilization was not possible however, in all patients; but we could not assess a significant relation between this negative result and the stone-affecting condition. The drug showed overall a good tolerance. Side-effects have never been serious enough to advise suspension of the treatment; they resolved spontaneously or with simple additional therapy. We think that this reduction in side-effect incidence could be related to the low dose used. No patient formed new stones during treatment nor showed the growth of pre-existing ones. However, we could not achieve any reduction in stone mass.

A. Tizzani, MD, Università degli Studi di Torino, Facoltà di Medicina e Chirurgia, Istituto di Nefro-Urologia, Cattedra di Urologia, Corso Polonia 14, .
I–10126 Torino (Italy)

Contr. Nephrol., vol. 58, pp. 215–218 (Karger, Basel 1987)

Tolerance and Side Effects of Propionhydroxamic Acid

F. Di Silverio, M. Gallucci, G. Alpi, G. P. Ricciuti, D. Fini, C. Molinari
Università degli Studi di Roma 'La Sapienza', Patologia Urologica, Roma, Italy

Staghorn infected calculosis is caused by the precipitation of calcium and magnesium phosphates in an alkaline medium created by bacterial urease [1].

In order to prevent the cycle infection – alkalinization – precipitation, it is imperative to acidify the urine. Hydroxyurea has been proven as an effective acidifying drug as it can act as an inhibitor of bacterial urease. Nevertheless, it has important teratogen and mutagen effects.

In the last few years hydroxyurea derivatives have been used: these, although preserving their antiureasic properties, do not have the abovementioned side effects. The first one employed was acetohydroxamic acid with successful results, notwithstanding its high dosages [2, 3]. So propionhydroxamic acid (PHA) was introduced in therapy, which with lower dosages provides the same acidifying results [4].

Patients and Methods

We developed our experiment in open conditions and without comparison to other drugs. We studied 17 patients, 6 males and 11 females, aged from 14 to 72 years (average: 42.5), with staghorn infected renal calculosis, bilateral in 9 cases, monolateral in 7 cases, and in a surgical solitary kidney in 1 case.

All of them had pH values higher than 7 and urinary ammonium higher than normal which were assumed as indications to a treatment with urease inhibitors.

We did not consider in our series patients with pregnancy, or hematological, liver, cardiac and renal (blood creatinine level > 3 mg/100 ml) dysfunctions.

Urine pH, ammonium and cultures were periodically checked. Also liver, cardiac and renal function and patients' complaints were assessed to verify the tolerance to the drug.

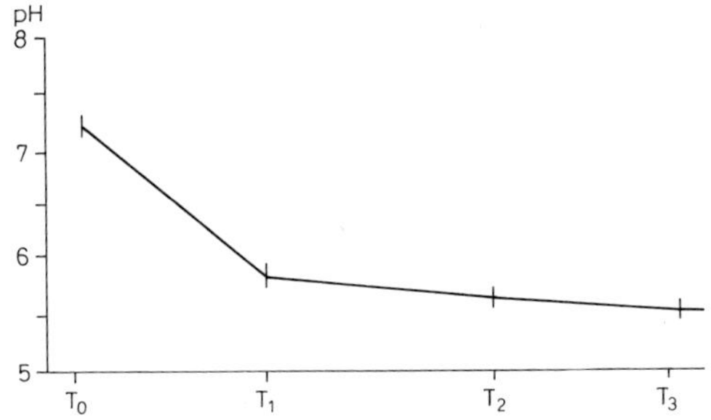

Fig. 1. Mean urinary pH variations during PHA treatment. T_0 = Start of treatment; T_1 = 10th day; T_2 = 25th day; T_3 = 55th day.

We selected four steps to calculate the medium values and to control the therapeutic effectiveness and tolerance to PHA treatment: T_0 = start of treatment, T_1 = 10th, T_2 = 25th, T_3 = 55th day of treatment.

The average values have been compared by analyzing variability (Anova) as follows: (1) T_0 vs $T_1 - T_2 - T_3$; (2) linear proceeding in $T_1 - T_2 - T_3$; (3) geometric proceeding in $T_1 - T_2 - T_3$.

The comparison had the aim to check (1) treatment effectiveness, (2) progressive effects, (3) attainment of maximum effect. The same method has been used to study other parameters. Tested patients started treatment with PHA 240 mg/day for a week, divided into two doses of 120 mg each. After that they underwent a maintenance treatment with PHA 120 mg/day, divided into two doses of 60 mg each. The treatment lasted from a minimum of 25 to a maximum of 90 days with an average treatment of 57 days. If necessary, patients also received antibiotics or chemotherapy for urinary tract infection.

Results

All patients ended their PHA treatment without any difficulty, thus showing an excellent tolerance to the drug. The analyses of the data have proved that pH and NH_4 urinary values significantly decrease due to the effectiveness of the drug (fig. 1, 2).

These results show that PHA treatment significantly affects the pH and NH_4 mean values with an early and progressive effectiveness ($p < 0.001$) which is not limited to the early phase of therapy.

We have noted a statistically significant decrease in blood leukocytes (fig. 3) progressing throughout our study, even though such a decrease is not so important from the clinical or the functional point of view; nevertheless, it is necessary to carefully measure the white blood cells. As to the

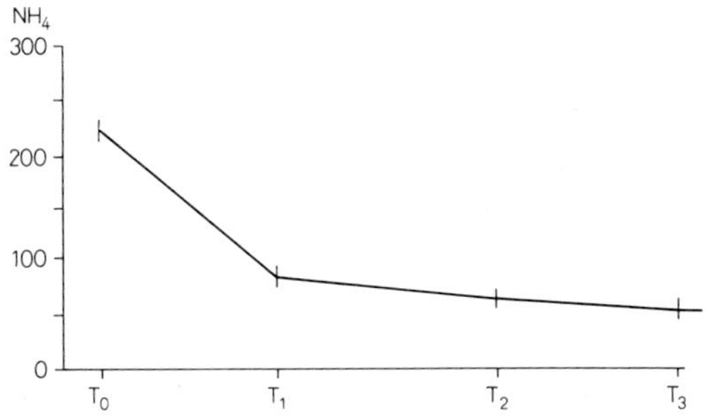

Fig. 2. Mean urinary NH_4 variations during PHA treatment (times as in figure 1).

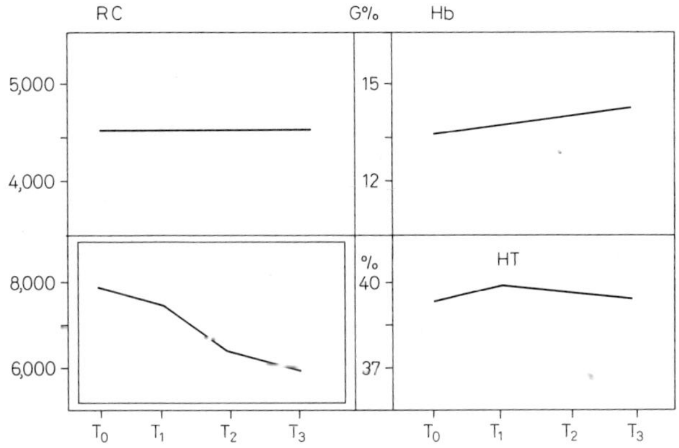

Fig. 3. Mean variations of hematological parameters during PHA treatment. T_0 = Start of treatment; T_1 = 30th day; T_2 = 60th day; T_3 = 90th day.

tolerance of the drug, we have already stated that all patients have completed the treatment without any problem.

Only 2 out of 17 cases showed gastric pyrosis during the early days of PHA treatment, which was controlled by antacid drugs, so that both patients could continue and regularly complete the treatment without modifying the PHA posology.

Another patient, aged 24, suffering from infected bilateral inferior caliceal calculosis, showed oligospermia on the 20th day of treatment. Although no previous documentation was available, this could demonstrate a cause-effect relation between the PHA treatment and the above-mentioned side effect; we decided to stop the treatment.

Conclusions

Our experiments demonstrated satisfactory anti-ureasic action of PHA up to 120 mg/day. The tolerance to these dosages seems to be good. From the clinical point of view, 2 patients showed gastric pyrosis which disappeared after a treatment with antacid drugs.

As to the hematological parameters, we observed a decrease in the number of leukocytes – not important from a clinical aspect: we must take care of this especially when dealing with long PHA treatments, and this fact must be considered in the case of higher dosages. We would like to emphasize the case of the patient showing oligospermia. We had to stop the treatment since no data previous to the PHA treatment were available. We cannot come to any conclusion about this but we suggest a careful control of this parameter, as some mutagenic effect has been reported for other derivatives of hydroxyurea [5].

References

1 Griffith, D.P.; Musher, D.M.; Itin, C.: Urease: the primary cause of infection induced urinary stones. Investve Urol. *13:* 346–350 (1976).

2 Griffith, D.P.: Struvite stones. Kidney int. *13:* 372–382 (1978).

3 Martelli, A.; Buli, P.; Cortecchia, W.: Acetohydroxamic acid therapy in infected renal stones. Urology *17:* 320–322 (1981).

4 Martelli, A.; Buli, P.; Brunocilla, E.: Propionhydroxamic acid in infected renal stones. A preliminary clinical report. J. Urol. *128:* 1130–1132 (1982).

5 Wang, C.Y.; Lanfong, H.L.: Mutagenicity and antibacterial activity of hydroxamic acids. Antimicrob. Agents Chemother. *11:* 753 (1977).

Michele Gallucci, MD, via Asmara 72, I–00199 Roma (Italy)

Contr. Nephrol., vol. 58, pp. 219–221 (Karger, Basel 1987)

Computerized in vivo Research from the Growth of Urease-Producing Bacteria in the Presence of Antibiotics Combined with Propionhydroxamic Acid

M. Rizzo[a], *P. Nicoletti*[b], *R. Bartoletti*[a], *E. Luciani*[b]

[a]Department of Urology, University of Florence;
[b]Laboratory of Bacteriology and Virology USL 10 D, Florence, Italy

Therapy as well as prophylaxis of relapses of struvite stones depend on the complete removal of the stone and on the eradication of the infection. Experimental and clinical studies have validated the program which combines antibiotics with drugs having an antiureasis action, particularly hydroxamic acids [1–3].

Previously we had carried out an in vitro study which brought out a synergism between aminoglycosidic antibiotics (particularly netilmicine, NTM) and antiureasic drugs.

In order to confirm these results from a clinical point of view, we performed an in vivo study using urine of healthy persons who had been given differentiated doses of proprionhydroxamic acid (PHA).

Materials and Methods

The growth curves were obtained using the turbidimetry method with the automatic MS 2 research apparatus as described elsewhere [4]. The culture medium was made up of a pool of urine (sterilized by filtration) from 5 healthy subjects to whom different doses of PHA had been given. The urine was placed in special holders and inoculated with 10^5 colony forming units (CFU) of a strain of *Proteus mirabilis* which had been isolated from the urine of patients affected with struvite calculosis and persistent urinary infections. Immediately after inoculation of the bacterial strain, NTM from 64 to 0.125 μg/ml was added.

Results were obtained by means of the computerized analysis of the variations of the optical density (OD) within each single holder. These data, evaluated as a function of time, permitted the elaboration of a series of curves which represented the mathematical expression of this research.

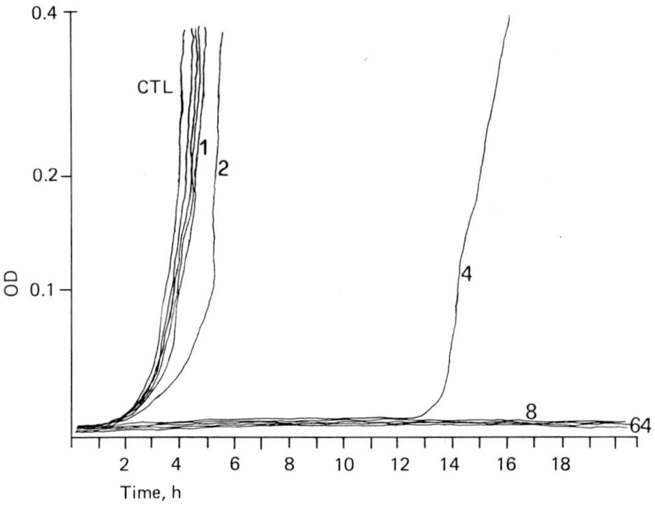

Fig. 1. Bacterial growth curves of urines from 2 subjects before PHA, added to a strain of *Proteus mirabilis* 10^5 CFU and NTM with a concentration range from 64 to 0.125 μg/ml. pH = 7.

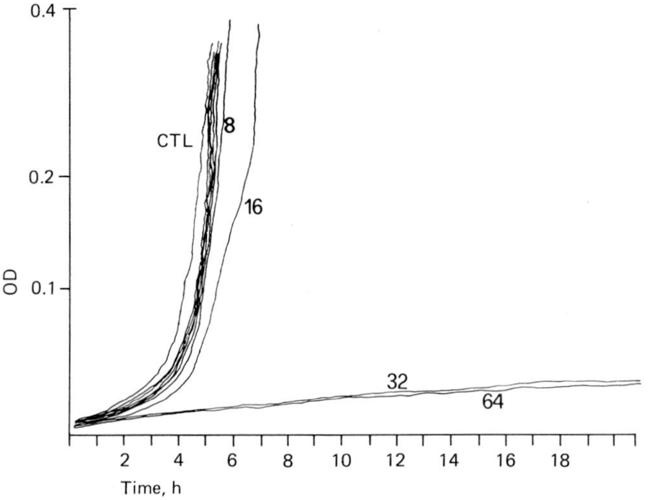

Fig. 2. Bacterial growth curves after administration of 120 mg/day PHA (same conditions as in figure 1). pH = 6.

Results

Examining the results obtained from the study of bacterial growth curves of the urine in the subjects who had received 120 mg/day PHA (fig. 1, 2), a substantial decrease in the antibacterial activity of NTM could be noted.

This result was confirmed in the urine of those given 240 mg/day PHA, where there was only partial inhibition (with regrowth after 9 h) even when a dose of 64 μg/ml of NTM added. The control graphs of the urines before and after assumption of PHA and before inoculation of *Proteus mirabilis* were superimposable.

Discussion

From our previous in vitro studies we concluded that the simultaneous administration of aminoglocosidic antibiotics and hydroxamic acids were effective in increasing the antibacterial activity [4].

The present study was designed to evaluate the true efficacy of PHA when used in combination with antibiotics. The combined activity of the two substances in the in vivo study showed an antagonistic effect which did not confirm our previous results [4]. It is likely that variations in the pH of the urine, induced by PHA, could play an important role as NTM activity seems to be decreased by an acid pH.

We conclude that sequential and not combined use of the two substances seems advisable in order to obtain satisfactory clinical results and not to further decrease renal function.

References

1 Fishbein, W. M.; Carbone, P. P.: Urease catalyses. Inhibition of the enzyme by hydroxyurea, hydroxylamine and acetohydroxamic acid. J. biol. Chem. *240:* 2407–2414 (1965).

2 Griffith, D. P.; Gibson, G. R.; Clinton, C. W.: Acetohydroxamic acid: clinical studies of urease inhibitor in patients with staghorn renal calculi. J. Urol. *119:* 9–15 (1978).

3 Martelli, A.; Buli, P.; Brunocilla, E.: Propionohydroxamic acid in infected renal stones. A preliminary clinical report. J. Urol. *128:* 1130 (1982).

4 Rizzo, M.; Nicoletti, P. L.; Bartolozzi, R.; Fattori, L.: Curve di crescita di batteri ureasi produttori in presenza di antibiotici in associazione con farmaci antiureasici. Studio con MS2 ricerca. Litiasi renale (Wichtig, Milano 1985).

Prof. Michelangelo Rizzo, MD, Clinica Urologica, Università di Firenze,
viale Pieraccini 18, I–50127 Firenze (Italy)

Contr. Nephrol., vol. 58, pp. 222–225 (Karger, Basel 1987)

Propionhydroxamic Acid for the Prophylaxis of Recurrences of Infection-Induced Renal Stones

A. Mandressi, G. Dormia, E. Montanari, A. Del Nero, A. Trinchieri, G. Zanetti, P. Tombolini, E. Pisani

Institute of Urology, University of Milan, Milan, Italy

Before and after the surgery of infection-induced renal stones it could be difficult to sterilize the urinary tract as well as to prevent recurrences. Renal stones, in fact, chronically laying in the urinary tract, produce chronic damage and some nests of infection in the renal parenchyma as well as in the mucosa. Furthermore, the infected stones harbor live bacteria and even small particles may be the source of reinfection. The infections by urea-splitting bacteria make urine supersatured with respect to struvite and carbonate apatite [1]. The most important achievement in eradicating bacteria is to lower urinary pH and ammonia to prevent stone recurrences [2]. We can reach this goal, despite of infection still present, by using antiureasic drugs [3] which unfortunately are not lacking in side effects and toxicity [4]. Recently propionhydroxamic acid (PHA) has been proposed, which seems to have greater effectiveness at lower doses than antiureasic drugs used before [8].

Patients and Methods

We treated by PHA 9 patients (6 M, 3 F; mean age 41.1 years) who had had a lot of surgical treatments for infection-induced renal stones. The treatment has been carried on for 180 days as follows: 120 mg t. i. d. for the first 15 days, 60 mg t. i. d. for the 165 days following. Urinary pH and NH_4, urine examination, urinary bacterial count, blood chemistry, arterial pressure, body weight determination and ECG were performed or measured before and after the treatment regularly. Side effects were recorded whenever they were observed.

Table I. Urinary pH

Patients	Days				
	0	10	25	40	55
V.A.	6.5	6.7	6.7	6.9	6.8
R.P.	6.6	6.6	6.3	6.2	6.1
P.M.	7	6.4	–	5.6	5.4
C.A.	6.8	6.2	6.3	5.9	5.7
M.P.	5.8	5.4	5.5	5.6	5.8
P.C.	6.7	–	6.6	6.5	5.8
D.U.	5.4	5.9	–	6	7
D.G.	6.6	7	8	7	9
M.W.	6.3	5.5	6	6.3	6.1
Mean	6.41	6.21	6.48	6.22	6.41
SD	±0.5085	±0.5743	±0.7776	±0.5093	±1.0993

Results

Out of 9 only 5 patients completed the treatment that had been scheduled in 180 days. We did not observe during the treatment any significant variation of the urinary bacterial count, which was positive in 55% of the cases before the treatment and in 66% of the cases after 55 days of treatment, nor of urinary pH and NH_4 (tables I, II), which were and remained in the normal ranges. We did not observe any significant variation of tolerability, of weight, of arterial pressure and of ECG during the treatment. Our patients dropped out the treatment because of one heavy and unique side effect: a diffuse alopecia, referred by the patients after the 55th day of treatment.

Discussion

We concluded a previous study on PHA (0.5 g/day) treatment of infection-induced renal stones writing: 'If the PHA gets a lot of side effects, then we must reduce the doses: but what would happen about efficacy?' [5]. So for the present we have employed PHA at lower doses (360 mg/day for the first 15 days and 180 mg/day for the following days of treatment) to

Table II. Urinary NH_4 concentration

Patients	Days				
	0	10	25	40	55
V.A.	21	18	23	36	41
R.P.	25	27	25	11	21
P.M.	11	26	20	19	27
C.A.	9	17	11	19	20
M.P.	14	10	15	19	20
P.C.	34	20	23	15	15
D.U.	35	42	34	30	40
D.G.	35	23	18	20	31
M.W.	15	30	27	32	29
Mean	22.11	23.66	21.77	22.33	27.11
SD	±10.576	±9.1515	±6.7966	±8.3666	±9.1028

verify the antiureasic therapy effectiveness and its tolerability. During the treatment we did not observe any variation in urinary pH nor in urinary NH_4 concentration: both parameters remained in the normal range despite the fact that infection might have persisted or recurred; then the PHA could maintain low pH and ammonia in the face of relapsing bacterial infection. We observed indeed a significant reduction of side effects; in fact, contrary to patients treated with higher doses, none out of these patients referred tremor, asthenia, nausea or headache; however, the treatment was the cause of alopecia in all the patients after 55 days. Looking at the pharmacokinetics of PHA, it has been reached a plasma peak giving a constant dose per os [6]. Moreover, looking at pharmacodynamics, we know that the PHA antiureasic effect is dose-dependent [7]. So we think that the dose we used is too low to obtain a significant beneficial result but it is necessary to avoid the heavy side effects referred by our patients.

References

1 Griffith, D.P.; Musher, D.M.; Itin, C.: Urease: the primary cause of infection induced urinary stones. Investve Urol. *13:* 346 (1976).

2 Griffith, D.P.; Musher, D.M.: Prevention of infected urinary stones by urease inhibition. Investve. Urol. *11:* 228 (1976).

3 Aroldi, A.; Mandressi, A.; Baccalin, A.; Trinchieri, A.; Zanetti, G.; Graziani, G.; Rocco, F.: Trattamento con acido acetoidrossamico (AHA) in 19 pazienti operati di calcolosi da infezione. Proc. 2nd Int. Symp. on Metabolic, Physicochemical and Therapeutical Aspects of Urolithiasis, p. 149 (Wichtig, Milano 1983).

4 Aroldi, A.; Graziani, G.; Castelnovo, C.; Colussi, G.; Surian, M.; Mandressi, A.; Mascheroni, E.; Pazardjiklian, I.; Pagano, A.; Ponticelli, C.: Acetohydroxamate in struvite stones: in vivo study. Eur. Dial. Transpl. Ass. *20:* 469 (1983).

5 Rocco, F.; Mandressi, A.; Baccalin, A.; Caimi, D.; De Cobelli, O.: Acetohydroxamic acid (AHA) versus propionhydroxamic acid (PHA) in struvite renal stones medical treatment. 6th Congr. Eur. Ass. Urology, Copenhagen, 1984, p. 2013, Abstr.

6 ZAMI 633 (propionhydroxamic acid): a new urease inhibitor (Zambeletti Research Laboratories, Milano 1984).

7 Rosenstein, I.; Hamilton-Miller, J.M.T.; Brumfitt, W.: The effect of acetohydroxamic acid on the induction of bacteria ureases. Investve Urol. *18:* 112 (1980).

8 Martelli, A.; Buli, P.; Brunocilla, E.: Propionhydroxamic acid in infected renal stones: a preliminary clinical report. J. Urol. *128:* 1130 (1982).

Alberto Mandressi, MD, Istituto di Urologia dell'Università,
via della Commenda 15, I–20122 Milano (Italy)

Contr. Nephrol., vol. 58, pp. 226–229 (Karger, Basel 1987)

The Value of Propionhydroxamic Acid in the Prevention and Therapy of Infection-Induced Stones

M. Fini, P. Romagnoli, D. Mannini, P. Maver, C. Calcopietro, D. Menniti, A. Ligabue

Divisione di Urologia I, Ospedale M. Malpighi, Bologna, Italy

This study was made to evaluate the physicochemical and bacteriological changes in urine caused by the administration of propionhydroxamic acid (PHA) for the prevention of infection-induced lithiasis.

Patients and Methods

We evaluated a group of 10 patients, 5 male and 5 female, with an average age of 36 years. Six of these patients presented monolateral or bilateral lithiasis while the other 4 were free from calculi. They all suffered from infections sustained by ureolytic germs, and all had been operated on at least once.

The study protocol included the regular measuring of urinary pH and ammonium; urinalysis, a check of the hepatic, renal and cardiac functions and blood composition were carried out approximately every 15 days. 240 mg/day of the drug was administered for the first month of treatment, and then 120 mg/day as a maintenance therapy.

Treatment lasted for 6 months. In 4 cases it was necessary to add antibiotics, for a period varying from 7 to 10 days, due to the onset of acute urinary tract infection (UTI).

Results

Following the administration of PHA, in almost all the patients we observed a progressive reduction in the pH which reached a minimum value around the 30th day (fig. 1). The same observations can be made with regard to the ammoniuria which also fell significantly ($p = 0.005$) (fig. 2). No change was observed in the bacteriological species responsible for the infection or in its load, except in one case in which, after 3 months of treatment, we observed a persistently negative urinalysis.

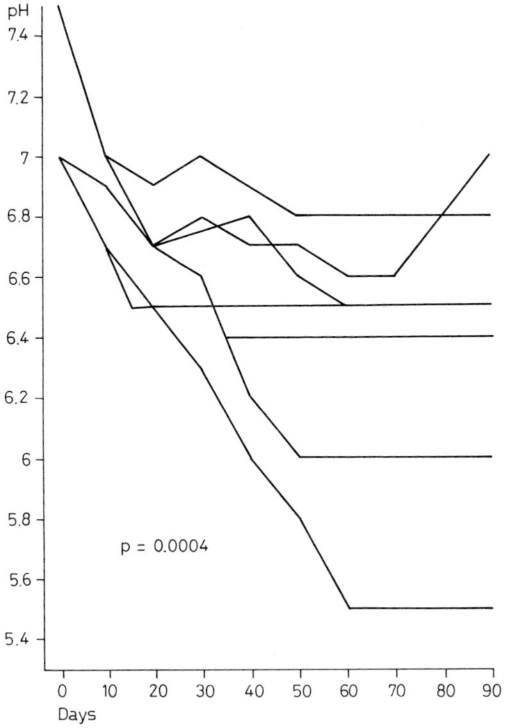

Fig. 1. Trend of urine pH before and during PHA therapy.

Renal, hepatic and cardiac functions, as well as the main blood parameters, did not change. Drug tolerance was good for the first 20 days. After 30 days all the patients showed an intolerance to alcohol, which was characterized by a significant erythema on the neck and face, accompanied by intense pruritus and, in 3 cases, by nausea. These symptoms disappeared spontaneously after 15–20 min. During the third month of treatment all the subjects studied complained of loss of hair which continued for the whole period of the study.

In 3 cases the loss of hair was so serious that the dosage had to be reduced to 60 mg. In these 3 cases it should be emphasized that although the dose was reduced by half, the pH and ammonium variations remained significant.

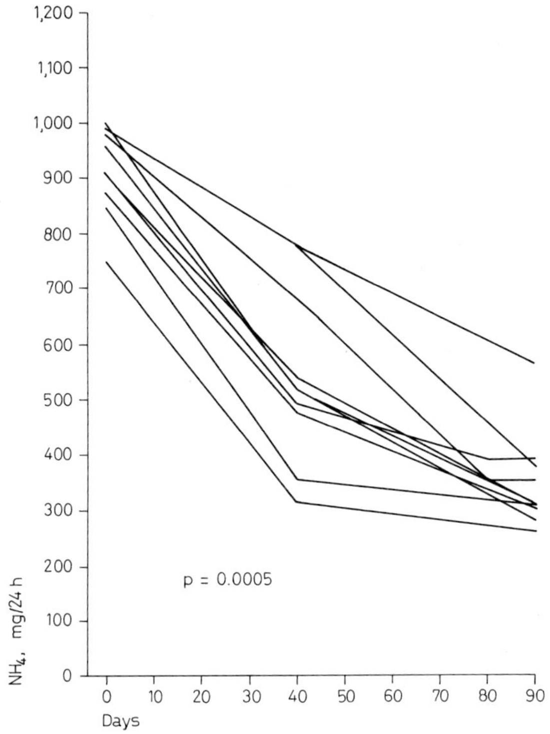

Fig. 2. Trend of ammonium excretion before and during PHA therapy.

Discussion

On the basis of our results we can confirm that PHA (like acetohydroxamic acid, AHA, already used by us [1], but with a much lower dosage) causes a modification of the physicochemical characteristics of the urine which is unfavourable to the development of recurrent lithiasis, by reducing the pH and the urinary ammonium. Naturally, these interesting biochemical modifications must be supported by equally positive clinical results. In fact, in spite of the encouraging preliminary results, it should be emphasized that our observations refer to a period of 6 months, which is too short to allow us to draw conclusions as to the prophylactic efficacy of the drug, i.e. the actual reduction in relapses, or to evaluate its real toxicity. In this respect, in agreement with previous reports [2], the drug did not alter the main blood parameters, nor those of the hepatic and renal functions.

Unfortunately, all our patients complained of a troublesome loss of hair and, in spite of constant hair re-growth at the withdrawal of PHA, this phenomenon, especially in young subjects, represented a significant cause of anxiety which made it necessary to reduce the dose in 3 cases. It is interesting to note that there was a fall in pH and ammonium even with doses lower than those normally used, and we think this warrants further studies on the subject.

References

1 Fini, M.; Ligabue, A.; Rubino, F.; Zacchini, A.; Cuzzocrea, D.: L'acido aceto idrossamico nella prevenzione della litiasi infetta. Atti della Società Italiana di Urologia 55° Congr., pp. 213–214 (1982).

2 Brunocilla, E.; Buli, P.; Martelli, A.: Trattamento con acido propionidrossamico della nefrolitiasi a stampo infetta. Urologia *5:* 809–822 (1984).

M. Fini, MD, Divisione di Urologia I, Ospedale M. Malpighi, via Palagi 9, I–40138 Bologna (Italy)

Contr. Nephrol., vol. 58, pp. 230–232 (Karger, Basel 1987)

Low-Dose Propionhydroxamic Acid Therapy in Infection-Induced Stones

Giacomo Colussi [a], *Maurizio Surian* [b], *Maria Elisabetta De Ferrari* [a], *Giuseppe Rombolà* [a], *Patrizia Rolando* [a], *Luigi Minetti* [a, 1]

Renal Units, [a]Ospedale Niguarda-Ca'Granda, Milano, and [b]Ospedale Maggiore, Lodi, Italy

Among the hydroxamic acid-derivatives so far investigated as antiureasic compounds of potential clinical benefit, propionhydroxamic acid (PHA) has been proposed as an active, low-toxicity compound. However, at dosages of 5 mg/kg body weight or more (375–500 mg/day), significant clinical symptoms and side effects have been observed. Certain pharmacokinetic properties of PHA (i.e. almost complete gastrointestinal absorption, a prolonged elimination halftime of 24.1 ± 4.2 h, a constant urine excretion during the 24 h following a single oral dose, amounting to an average excretion of 43.3% of the dose/24 h) [1] have suggested the possibility of getting therapeutic levels of the drug in urines with much lower dosages, i.e. 1 mg/kg body weight/day. We report the effects on urine physicochemical parameters of low-dose PHA therapy in 10 patients with infection-induced stones.

Cases and Protocol Study

The patients were 3 males and 7 females, aged 32–66 years, who gave informed consent to the study. All had infection stones (bilateral in 2, in a single kidney in 2, and monolateral with 2 kidneys in 6) and positive urine cultures for urease-producing bacteria at the time of the study. Glomerular filtration rate (GFR) was normal in 6, slightly reduced (75–45 ml/min) in 4. After a basal study (no therapy for at least 2 weeks), the patients underwent 3 consecu-

[1] We wish to thank Zambeletti SpA, Baranzate, for having kindly supplied PHA.

Table I. Effects on urine parameters of 3 different modes of therapy in 10 patients with infection-induced stones

	Basal	p	PHA	p	PHA+AB	p	AB
pH	6.97 ± 1.03	n.s.	6.78 ± 0.85	< 0.02	6.08 ± 0.39^{b}	< 0.02	6.38 ± 0.3
NH_4, mmol/day	52.2 ± 50.7	n.s.	68.4 ± 72.8	< 0.05	17.6 ± 9.3^{a}	n.s.	$21.3 \pm 11.5^{a, d}$
RS	-1.6 ± 3.7	n.s.	-1.6 ± 4.3	< 0.01	-6.3 ± 2.8^{c}	< 0.05	-4.7 ± 1.5^{a}

RS = Struvite relative supersaturation.
vs basal, p <: ^{a} = 0.05; ^{b} = 0.02; ^{c} = 0.001; vs PHA, p <: ^{d} = 0.05.

tive 2-week treatment regimens: PHA (120 mg/day for 2 days followed by 60 mg/day in 2 divided doses, 'PHA' study); PHA (60 mg/day) and specific antibiotic or chemotherapeutic agents ('PHA+AB' study); antibacterial therapy alone ('AB' study). At the end of each period, 24-hour urine collections (kept always at 4 °C and under mineral oil) for pH, ammonia (NH_4) and struvite relative supersaturation (RS, Marshall nomograms), a mid-stream urine culture, and fasting blood samples for hematologic, hepatic, pancreatic and renal parameters were obtained. Statistical analysis was performed by use of Student's paired t-test.

Results and Comments

As shown in table I, no significant effects on urine parameters were observed after 15 days of low-dose PHA therapy alone, suggesting insufficient inhibition of bacterial urease at these dosages; the addition of specific antibacterial therapy was indeed associated with a brisk decrease of pH, NH_4 and struvite RS, which persisted even when PHA was stopped. Some additive effects of PHA on antibacterial agent activity seem to be suggested by lower values of pH and RS during PHA+AB therapy than during AB alone: this could result from a synergistic effect of hydroxamates with antibacterial activity of antibiotics [2]. Our results suggest that, in patients with infection-induced stones, higher doses of PHA are likely to be needed in order to induce a clinically significant inhibition of bacterial urease when the drug is used alone; however, the effects of antibacterial agents might be enhanced by even small doses of PHA.

References

1 Kozma, C.; Kukovetz, W.R.; Rehm, K.D.; Johnson, K.I.: A balance, kinetic and metabolism study of radio-labelled Zami-633 in normal volunteers. IPHAR Report No. 83/929, July 1984.

2 Musher, D.M.; Saenz, C.; Griffith, D.P.: Interaction between acetohydroxamic acid and 12 antibiotics against 14 gram-negative pathogenic bacteria. Antimicrob. Agents Chemother. *5:* 106–110 (1974).

G. Colussi, MD, Renal Unit, Ospedale Niguarda-Ca'Granda,
Piazza Ospedale Maggiore 3, I–20162 Milano (Italy)

Contr. Nephrol., vol. 58, pp. 233–235 (Karger, Basel 1987)

Infectious Nephrolithiasis: Results of Treatment with Methenamine Mandelate

Alberto Jeantet[a], *Alessandra Thea*[a], *Ugo Ferrando*[b], *Maurizio Gaido*[a], *Michele Rotunno*[a], *Pier Franco Martini*[a], *Antonio Vercellone*[a]

Cattedra di Nefrologia dell'Università, Divisione di [a]Nefrologia e Dialisi, [b]Urologia, Ospedale Molinette, Torino, Italia

Infectious nephrolithiasis (struvite and carbonate apatite stones) sustained by urease-producing bacteria often resistant to usual chemico-antibiotic treatment, is difficult to manage because of the recurrence of infection, regrowth of stones and multiple surgical procedures. The aim of this study was to evaluate the results of the treatment with methenamine mandelate (MM), an acidifying bacteriostatic agent [1–3].

Patients and Methods

In a series of 466 stone-formers examined, the infrared spectrophotometric analysis of the calculus (calculi) showed the predominance of struvite in 14.6% (68/466) patients. At the start of the study 30/68 patients (male 10, female 20; mean age 40.4 ± 10.5 years; stones/patient 4.5; surgical procedures/patient 1.9; abnormalities of the urinary tract 10 = 33%; creatinine clearance 87.8 ± 18.7 ml/min) had persistent urinary tract infections due to urea-splitting bacteria resistant to the usual treatment. Fourteen patients presented renal stone(s) in situ (group A), 16 were stone-free (group B). We performed metabolic analysis on free and on standardized, differentiated as well as balanced diets, parathyroid hormone (PTH), alkaline phosphatase (APH); urothomography at the start of the study; serum pH and bicarbonate, urine pH and total bacterial count (TBC) at the start and every month; persistent urinary sterilization was defined as TBC $< 10^3$/ml for longer than 6 months. Every 6 months Cr, Ca, P, Na, K, UA; on serum and urine: oxaluria, hepatic enzymology, blood platelets, RBC, WBC; abdominal X-rays. Chemico-antibiotics were administered (i. v., per os) for 6 days plus increasing doses of MM started at day 4. Statistical analysis by Student's t-test for paired data was performed.

Table I. Results of methenamine mandelate (MM) treatment

	Before treatment	MM 4.1 ± 1.1 g/day period: 19 ± 10.5 months	
Group A			
Patients	14	14	
pH urine	7.59 ± 1.14*	5.61 ± 0.63**	
TBC	≥ 10^6/ml 14/14	≤ 10^6/ml 10/14	
Calculi		no growth 12/14	
	before treatment	MM 4.3 ± 1.1 g/day period: 12 ± 5.9 months	after treatment 8–36 months, mean 24
Group B			
Patients	16	16	12
pH urine	7.17 ± 0.54*	5.5 ± 0.43**	5.48 ± 0.55***
TBC	≥ 10^6/ml 16/16	< 10^3/ml 16/16	< 10^3/ml 12/12
Calculi	–	–	–

* vs ** p < 0.001; ** vs *** p n.s.

Results and Discussion

The metabolic analysis showed a high frequency of hypercalciuria (60%) and hyperuricosuria (43%); hyperoxaluria resulted in 13%. As a matter of fact, 15/30 patients formed calculi also of different type (CaOx and/or CaP: 11; UA: 4). Furthermore, the infrared analysis showed, in association with struvite, also CaOx in varying concentrations from 5 to 40% in 12/30 patients and ammonium urate, 33%, in 1/30 patients. Patients with metabolic disorders were treated accordingly: hypocalcic and/or hypoxalic diet for diet-dependent hypercalciuria or hyperoxaluria; hydrochlorothiazide/amiloride 50/5 mg/day for diet independent hypercalciuria; allopurinol 200/300 mg/day for hyperuricosuria; parathyroidectomy was performed in one patient. *Proteus (vulgaris, rettgerii, mirabilis, morganii)* was the most frequently detected bacteria (70%) in the two groups. Treatment with MM provided the results given in table I. In both groups urinary pH was drastically reduced to finally return to normal ranges (control group, 15 patients; pH 5.6 ± 0.5). The pH stability ensures the reduction of urinary saturation and crystallization of struvite and may account for the growth of stones (by X-ray criteria) only in 2 group A patients, while no new stones was formed by group B patients. Urine culture became negative only in 4 group A patients but in all group B patients. MM dosages were later reduced in group A patients, but discontinued in 12/16 group B patients. The latter ones were followed up after discontinuing treatment with MM and did not show modifications. Clinical and biochemical side-effects were scarce in terms of frequency, quality and quantity.

In conclusion, our results show how metabolic disturbances may predispose and aggravate infection-associated lithiasis. MM normalizes urinary pH in patients of group A and B and brings about urine sterility in stone-free subjects at the start of treatment. This study suggests the possibility of preventing the growth and the relapse of struvite renal stones with MM.

References

1 Kass, E.H.: An approach to the management of resistant urinary infectiones. Kidney int. *16:* 204–212 (1979).

2 Gleckman, R.; Alvarez, S.; Joubert, D.V.; Mattews, S.J.: Drug therapy review: methenamine mandelate and methenamine hyppurate. Am. J. Hosp. Pharm. *36:* 1509–1512 (1979).

3 Jeantet, A.; Thea, A.; Ferrando, U.; Gaido, M.; Rotunno, M.; Martini, P.F.; Vercellone, A.: Impiego del mandelato di metenamina nella litiasi da infezione: in Litiasi renale, pp. 131–136 (Wichtig, Milano 1985).

A. Jeantet, MD, Divisione di Nefrologia e Dialisi, Ospedale Molinette, Corso Polonia 14, I–10126 Torino (Italy)

Contr. Nephrol., vol. 58, pp. 236–252 (Karger, Basel 1987)

Current Status of ESWL in the Management of Renal Calculus Disease

F. Eisenberger, J. Rassweiler

Department of Urology, Katharinenhospital Stuttgart, Stuttgart, FRG

The Idea of Shock Wave Lithotripsy

The transmission of mechanical shock waves through the human body was discovered by chance in the late 1960s. A test engineer (G. Hoff) touched a target body at the very moment of impact of a high velocity projectile and felt a kind of electrical shock, though the contact point showed no damage at all [11, 14, 15].

The idea of using shock wave energy either for military purpose or for destruction of urinary calculi was born. However, there was a long way to go until the first patient was treated by the non-invasive extracorporeal shock wave lithotripsy (ESWL) (table I). The first investigations aimed at finding out whether the non-invasive disintegration of kidney stones is feasible when carried out with focussed and unfocussed shock waves, which were generated by means of light-gas guns [14]. These in vitro tests were subjected to the following items: reproducible generation of shock waves; focussing of shock wave energy; acoustic coupling to guarantee energy transfer; location of the stone; determination of optimal stone-disintegrating energy, and led to the development of the prototype of Dornier-lithotripter (table I).

Technical Principles of ESWL

Shock Wave Generation. The discharge of a high-voltage capacitor generates a spark between the two tips of an underwater electrode. The elec-

Table I. The history of the development of ESWL

1966	First observation of the transmission of mechanical shock waves through human bodies
1969	First animal experiments to study the effect of shock waves on biological tissue
1970	First in vitro destruction of urinary stones with shock waves generated by a special multistage light-gas gun
1971	Focussing of the shock waves using an ellipsoid
1974–1978	Systematic in vitro and in vivo experiments with focussed shock waves: Effect on kidney stones with different chemical composition Effect on biological tissue Development of a canine kidney stone model Development of a prototype lithotripter for animal experiments
February 7, 1980	First clinical application at the Urological Department of the University of Munich
1982	Installation of the first ESWL center at the Urological Department of the University of Munich
October 1983	Installation of the second ESWL center worldwide at Katharinenhospital, Stuttgart
Until today	More than 150 ESWL centers, more than 150,000 treatments worldwide

trode is placed at the geometric focus of a semi-elliptical reflector. The spark causes explosive evaporation of the water, which in turn produces the shock waves due to its sudden expansion. The underwater electrode guarantees reproducible constant shock wave generation. The shock wave energy (pressure) can be regulated by varying the generator voltage (15–26 kV). Every 700–1,000 shock wave releases; however, the electrode must be exchanged.

Shock waves also may be generated by use of piezoelectric elements, electromagnetic elements, impulsed laser beam, microexplosion (lead acid pellets).

Focussing. As the shock waves are generated at one focal point of the ellipsoid, all produced energy is collected again at the second focus after being reflected of the walls. Since the second focus (F2) is the point of highest shock wave energy, the patient has to be positioned in a way the stone is situated at this point. Focussing of shock wave energy substantially decreases the risk of damaging the surrounding tissue. Other principles of shock wave focussing are spheric alignment of energy sources, using an acoustic lense or pseudo-ellipsoid reflectors.

Acoustic Coupling. The acoustic resistance (impedance) of water is very close to that of most body tissue. Therefore underwater generated shock waves penetrate the body easily if the patient is put into the water. This guarantees optimal energy transfer. However, 'tubless' coupling is possible by use of a water bag but may lead to remarkable energy loss due to the different interphases (i. e. air bubbles between bag and skin).

Location of the Stone. This is achieved by use of a positioning device, which is moved under control of a two-axis X-ray system. These two X-ray converters exactly intersect in the F2 of the ellipsoid reflector. The patient who is positioned on a stretcher is moved in the three dimensions until the stone is centered on both screens. For this purpose there are three X-ray techniques with increasing radiation exposure: fluoroscopic imaging; short-time high current fluoroscopy; long-time high current fluoroscopy.

To minimize the radiation exposure of the patient, the use of high current technique should be restricted (if fluoroscopy does not provide detailed information for exact control of the degree of disintegration). Ultrasound location of the calculi principally is possible; however, there are some specific shortcomings: most ureteral stones cannot be located; determination of the degree of desintegration depends on the experience of the urologist, and is very difficult due to artifacts (reflection) superpositioning the sonographic pattern. Therefore, at the present status ultrasound location alone cannot be recommended.

Stone Disintegration

Shock waves spread through the body evenly, as the acoustic impedance of most body tissues (except lungs and bones) is close to that of water. When a shock wave reaches the stone it is partially reflected and a portion of the shock wave entering the stone is absorbed due to the abrupt change of acoustic impedance. This leads to the build up of a high-pressure gradient and subsequently to formation of tear and shear forces (consisting of tensile and comprehensible wave components), which disintegrates the stone when the limit of its comprehensive strength is exceeded. The penetrating part of the shock wave is reflected at the backfront of the stone leading to the same phenomenon. With repeated exposures the stone is finally reduced into smaller and smaller particles from the periphery to the center. Beside this mechanism further high-velocity phenomena may contribute to stone desintegration, such as cavitation.

All kinds of stones could be destroyed in vitro irrespective of their chemical composition. However, we observed a relatively big size of cystine fragments, corresponding to the fact that cystine calculi still are problematic for ESWL treatment.

In vivo Experiments

After these tests, cell cultures were examined and animals were subjected to shock waves. First trials showed that stimulation ability and the proliferative potential of human lymphocytes were not altered after repeated exposure to shock waves. Secondly it was shown that serum concentration of the hemoglobin increased slightly with the number of treatments when directly exposed to the shock waves. However, in peripheral blood there was no significant decrease of the hemoglobin level. When vital bones or bone marrow was subjected to shock waves, no damage besides minor petechial bleedings were seen, whereas bones of dead animals have been broken. After exposure of eventerated intestine and parenchymal organs of rats also no damage except minor petechial bleedings were found.

Exposure of the lungs, however, led to alveolar rupture and hemorrhage because of the different acoustic impedances between the air-filled alveoli and the parenchyma. This finally resulted in the death of all animals [5, 6]. After protection of the lungs using styrofoam, no pulmonary deterioration was observed.

First Clinical Treatment

A prototype for the treatment of humans was constructed and technically improved for clinical use. In February 1980, this method was applied on the first patient at the Urologic Clinic of the University of Munich (Head: Prof. Dr. med. E. Schmiedt) by my former coworker Christian Chaussy [3, 5] and since then more than 150,000 patients have been successfully treated worldwide [4].

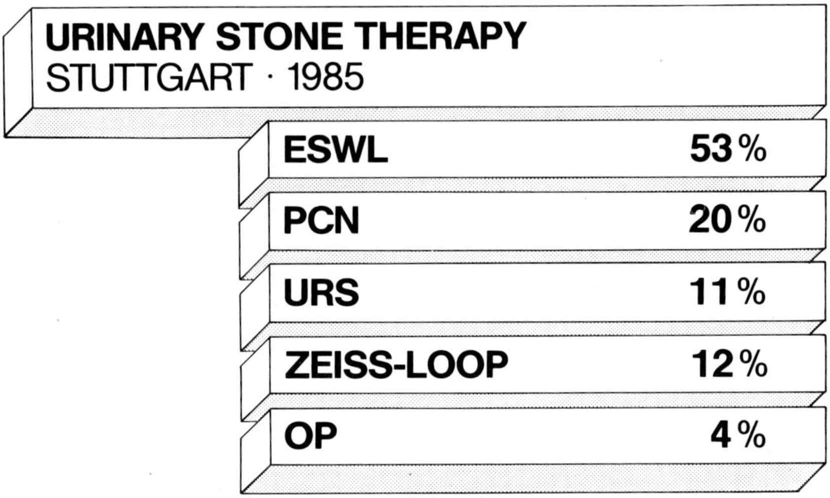

Fig. 1. Urinary stone therapy at the Urological Clinic of Katharinenhospital, Stuttgart, from October 1983 through January 1985. 3,958 treatments in 3,265 patients (2,215 ESWL, 720 PCN, 411 URS, 456 Zeiss loop, and 156 open surgery).

First Serial Lithotripter

In October 1983 the second worldwide ESWL unit was installed at our department [7, 12, 18] and since then (January 1986) more than 3,000 consecutive stone patients were treated, 2,097 of whom received ESWL treatment (fig. 1). In the FRG 22 ESWL units are operating now [4] – more than 150 lithotripters worldwide.

The first indications for the treatment of renal calculi by ESWL have been radio-opaque single pelvic or caliceal stones up to 1 cm without obstruction of the collecting system distal to the stone [3]. In the meantime, with gaining experience, indications could be extended to multiple calculi, larger stones up to partial staghorns (table II) and high ureteral concrements, i. e. above the iliac crest. Moreover, we have now first experience with successfully treated prevesical (distal ureteral) calculi. Contrast-negative stones can be treated by additional administration of contrast dye. However, localization of the fragments during shock wave exposure *still remains problematic.* We prefer for these cases percutaneous nephrolithotomy. CT density, too, did not provide any information for the

Table II. ESWL in 'easy' and 'problem' stones

	Easy stones	'Problem' stones
Complications, %		
colic	24	34
fever	5	36
Auxiliary measures, %	6	28
ureteral manipulation		
(UC, loop, ureteroscopy)	5	22
percutaneous nephrostomy	1	4
open operation	–	2
Mortality		0
Hospital days (after treatment)	4	10

ESWL treatment [22]. Presently the overall extended indications for ESWL treatment in urinary calculi can be summarized as follows: 68% of partial and complete staghorn calculi are treated by the combination PCN + ESWL. About 70% of upper ureteral calculi are treated in situ, 25% after retrograde mobilization of the stone into the renal pelvis ('push and bang'). For contrast-negative stones, we prefer percutaneous stone removal (larger calculi), percutaneous irrigation with sodium bicarbonate or alkalinization of the urine.

Contraindications are untreated bleeding disorders and gross obesity. A body weight of 130 kg represents the upper limit of the patients device. Moreover, in some patients the stone cannot be positioned into the second focus, due to enlarged subcutaneous fat at the back. Children smaller than 100 cm have to be treated surgically because they do not fit on the positioning device. However, with the use of special shaped styrofoam boards smaller children may be treated by ESWL except in case of upper caliceal calculi (increased risk of pulmonary damage).

Preoperative Preparation

Patients are prepared as before renal surgery, including mild laxatives, n.p.o. after 10 p.m. the day before and sodium-loading (1,000 ml) in the morning. Bowel preparation prevents screening difficulties because of air-filled intestine. Moreover, this avoids adverse effects on the intestine, since intestinal air represents an interphase for shock waves (risk of intestinal paralysis). In the case of urinary tract infection (UTI), antibiotics are given according to the antibiogram.

Anesthesia

We prefer the epidural catheter (90%); general anesthesia is restricted to special cases (spinal deformation, nervous patient). Furthermore, ESWL can also be performed under analgo-sedation or local cutaneous and paravertebral anesthesia. However, this cannot be recommended for general use. The advantage of the epidural anesthesia represents the fact that the catheter can be left for several days (multiple ESWL sessions, regional treatment of pain). The high-frequency jet ventilation (HFJV) technique decreases the respiratory-dependent movement of the stone and increases the efficacy of the shock wave application (about 30% less shock waves per treatment [17]). However, this kind of anesthesia is more invasive and time-consuming.

Recently we performed the majority of our cases in analgo-sedation, however, using a generator which worked on a lower level of shock wave pressure (600–800 vs 900–1200 bar). Thus, ESWL without anesthesia seems to be at the horizon.

Treatment

After location of the stone, ECG-triggered (to avoid induction of cardial arrythmia) shock wave application starts. The way of focussing and the choice of generator voltage depends on the size and localization of the stone (table III). Every 100–200 shock waves X-ray control is performed to determine the degree of disintegration and for further adjustment (fig. 2). We start at low energy (16–18 kV) to achieve fine fragmentation and to avoid scattering of the fragments, however, impacted calculi (i. e. uretereal

Table III. Recommendations for ESWL treatment

ESWL in one session	
'Crystal-like' pelvic stone (Ca-oxalate-dighydrate)	start with low energy (15–16 kV)
Impacted caliceal stone, ureteral stone	start with high energy (20–22 kV)
Multiple renal calculi	start with the smallest stone treat lower calculi first
Borderline stones/ partial staghorn calculi	start with the pelvic parts
Large, obstructive ureteric stone	focus on the upper rim of the stone
Poorly visible ureteric stone	administer contrast dye
ESWL in more sessions	
Remnants of staghorn stone following PCN	start with the stone parts in the cranial calices
ESWL monotherapy for staghorn stone	start with the pelvic and the upper caliceal parts
Maximal number of shock waves per session	
Single pelvic or caliceal stones	2,000–2,500
Multiple stones, staghorn calculi	2,500–3,000
Ureteric stones	3,000

or calyceal) need higher generator voltage (20–22 kV). The number of shock waves should not exceed 3,000 applications per kidney (mean 1,320/ treatment). The mean duration of the treatment is 40 min. Fluoroscopic time depends on the experience of the urologist (mean 11 quick pics – high current technique – and 90 s of fluorotime). The mean radiation exposure amounts to about 14 rad/patient.

Post-ESWL Management

KUB and ultrasound are performed on the 1st, 3rd and 5th days. If complete disintegration of the stone is documented and no ureteral

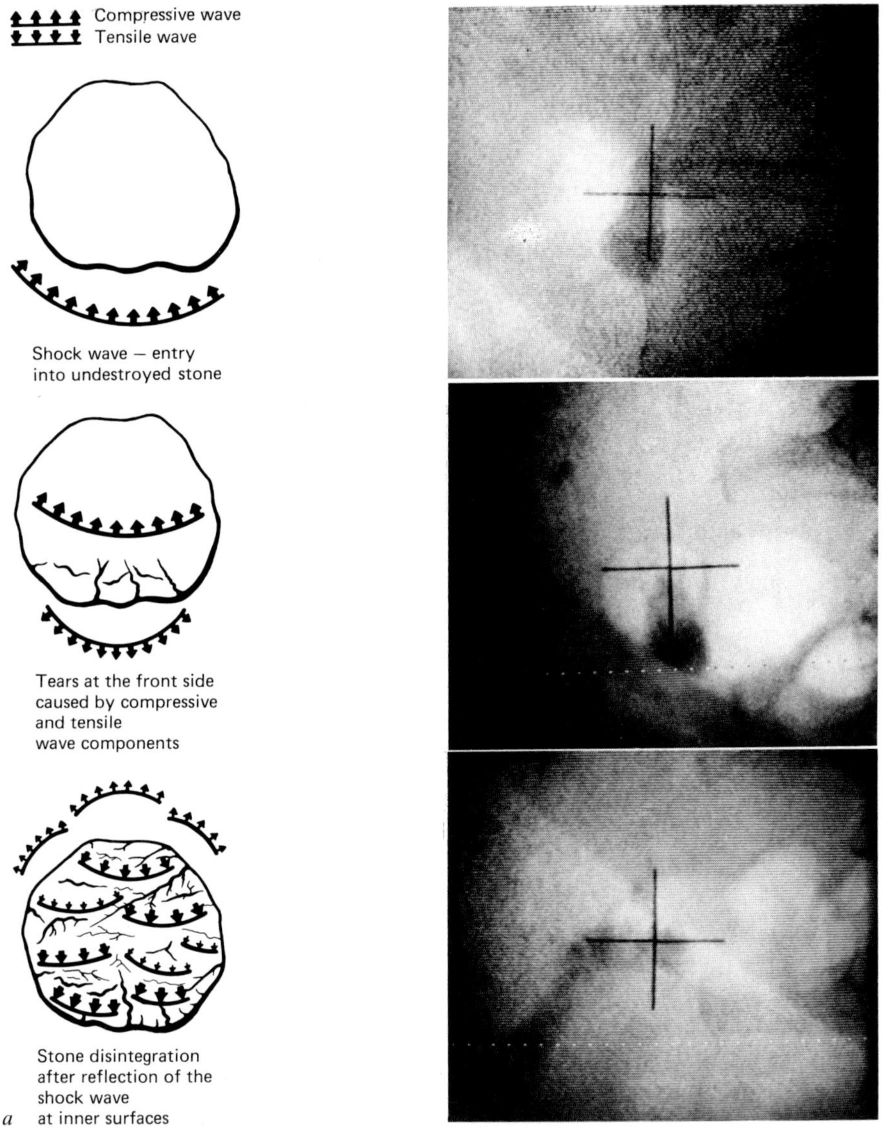

Fig. 2. a Focussing technique in the case of obstructive large ureteric (or infundibular) stones. *b* Cranial focussing of the stone at the optimal interphase between the stone and the urine (short-time high current technique, oblique monitor). *c, d* With beginning disintegration middle and lower parts are centered. *b* Short-time high current technique – 'quick pic' – after 400 shock waves, 18 kV, 'a. p.' monitor. *c* Quick pic after 900 shock waves with fragments in the lower calyceal group, 'a. p.' monitor.

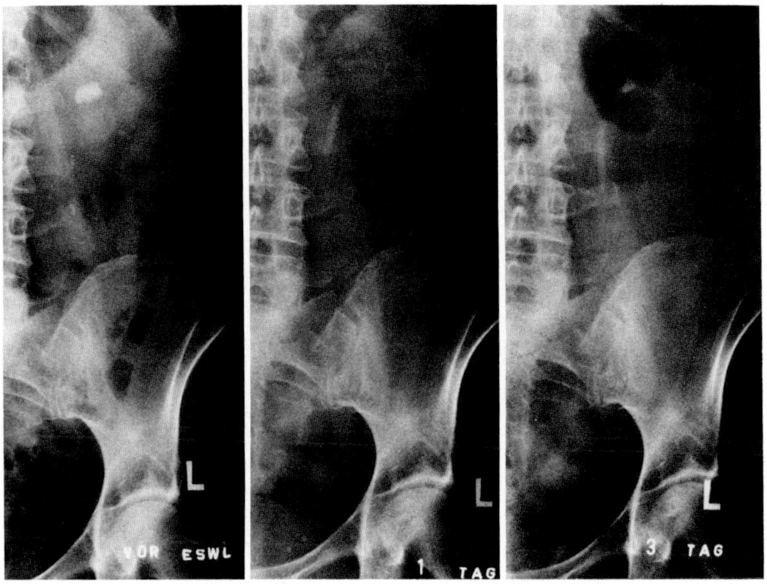

Fig. 3. Follow-up of ESWL in 'problem stones' – auxiliary measurement. KUB before and after ESWL shows complete disintegration of a large pelvic stone in the left kidney with formation of a 'steinstrasse' in the upper ureter on the first day.

obstruction or fever occurs, the patient is discharged. Ancillary measurements are indicated in the case of persistent colics or acute pyelonephritis due to ureteral obstruction ('steinstrasse') (fig. 3). We prefer in such cases the insertion of a percutaneous nephrostomy: the distended ureter is tonisized again resulting in spontaneous passage of the fragments in almost all cases. Ureteroscopy should be restricted to persistent prevesical fragments ('steinstrasse').

Complications

The rate of colic and fever during passage of stone gravel depends on the stone size (table II): 26% of all patients suffer from pain and 17% have fever above 38.8 °C. 14% of all patients have subcutaneous hematoma at the flank (particularly slim ones). Among all 2,097 treatments perirenal hematoma occurred in 5 patients which could be managed conservatively in all cases.

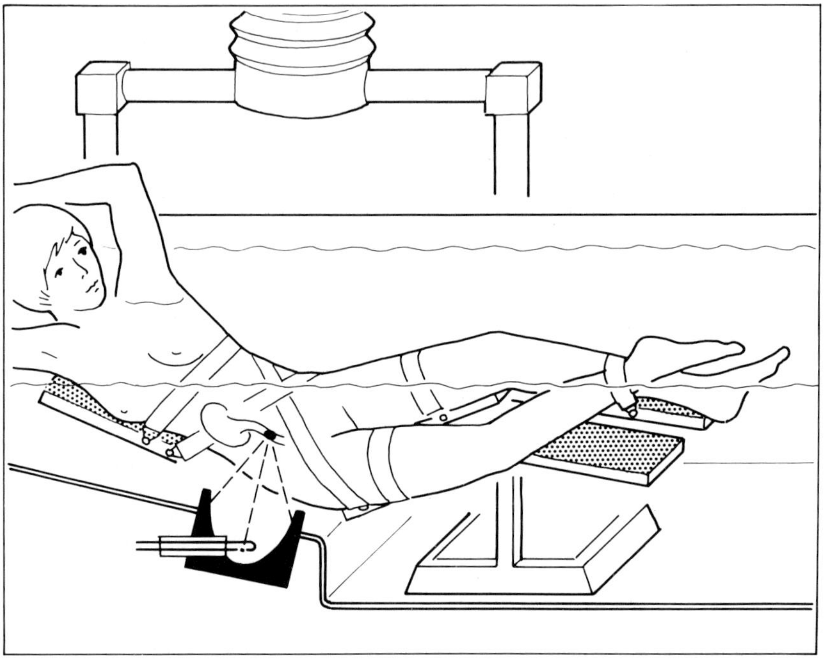

Fig. 4. In situ ESWL for upper ureteral calculi. Positioning technique. Patient is extremely rotated to the stonebearing side to avoid that the calculus is obscured by the vertebral body on the oblique monitor. Crossing of the legs stabilizes this position by fixation of the pelvis.

Upper Ureteral Stones

Using a special positioning and focussing technique (fig. 4), we could increase our success rate for in situ ESWL of upper ureteric stones to 85% (including 10% second session). Therefore, retrograde mobilization of the stone (ureteral catheter, URS) is only indicated: in emergency cases (colic, fever, hydronephrosis) together with insertion of a double-J stent; if the stone cannot be located because it is too close (less than one finger breadth) to the spine or due to gross obesity or spinal deformation; if in situ ESWL failed. If retrograde mobilization has failed, however, we place a ureteral balloon catheter below the stone and extract the stone by antegrade ureteroscopy (forceps, ultrasonic lithotripsy). In the case of failure open surgery has to be done. Figure 5 shows our overall experience with

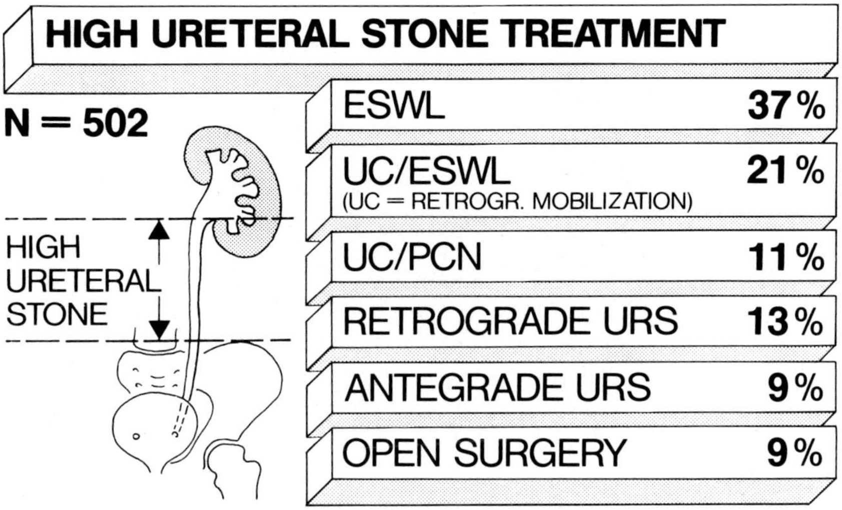

Fig. 5. The different treatment modalities for upper ureteric stones in 408 patients treated from October 1983 through August 1985 at the Urologic Clinic of Katharinenhospital, Stuttgart. It has to be emphasized that in the last 6 months retrograde URS and UC/PCN have not been used as routine techniques for retrieval of upper ureteral calculi. Within this specific period (July 1985 to January 1986) open surgery could be reduced below 2%.

the treatment of upper ureteric calculi since October 1983. It has to be emphasized that retrograde ureteroscopy and retrograde mobilization followed by percutaneous stone removal (UC/PCN) nowadays are no more standard procedures. Moreover, the rate of open surgery could be reduced below 2% (July 1985 to January 1986).

Combination ESWL–PCN

Borderline Stones. Concrements of more than 2.5 cm we define as 'borderline stones' at our department because there is an ongoing discussion whether ESWL or PCN is preferable in these cases [21]. The arguments for ESWL are: it is noninvasive and as a consequence has the lowest rate of severe complications compared to all other methods. In our whole series there has been no nephrectomy and no mortality. On the other hand, problems with passage of fragments after ESWL directly correlate with the

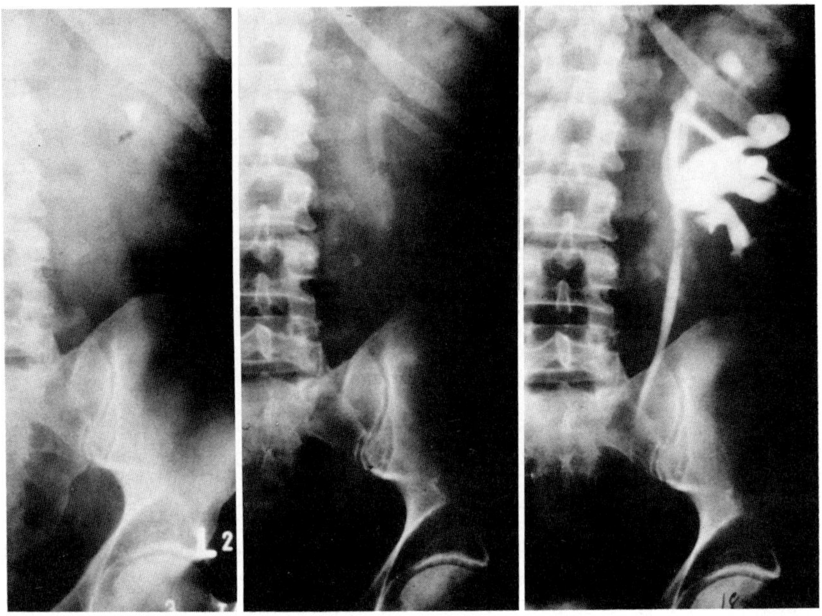

Fig. 6. Indications of PCN. Caliceal stone with severe infundibular stenosis. Stone has been disintegrated following ESWL; however, stone gravel did not pass (right). Therefore, the superior calix was punctured (intracostally under ultrasonic guidance), the stone fragments were sucked out, and the caliceal neck was dilated by use of the Alken metal bougie set (left).

overall stone mass. This leads to an increasing rate of ureteral obstruction due to the formation of prevesical 'steinstrasse'. This results in a higher number of ancillary measures following ESWL (table II). In a retrospective study we have evaluated two groups of patients who underwent ESWL monotherapy (table II). Those with kidney stones up to 2 cm which were called *easy stones* and those with a larger size which we called *problem stones*. We observed a significant difference between the two groups with regard to pain, fever, auxiliary measures and hospital stay [8, 9, 13].

In the case of *borderline stones* PCN guarantees a better retrieval of the stone fragments. Moreover, percutaneous stone removal is indicated in the case of severe caliceal neck stenosis: ESWL achieves disintegration, but stone gravel cannot pass. Together with stone extraction endoscopic dilatation of the infundibulum can be done (fig. 6).

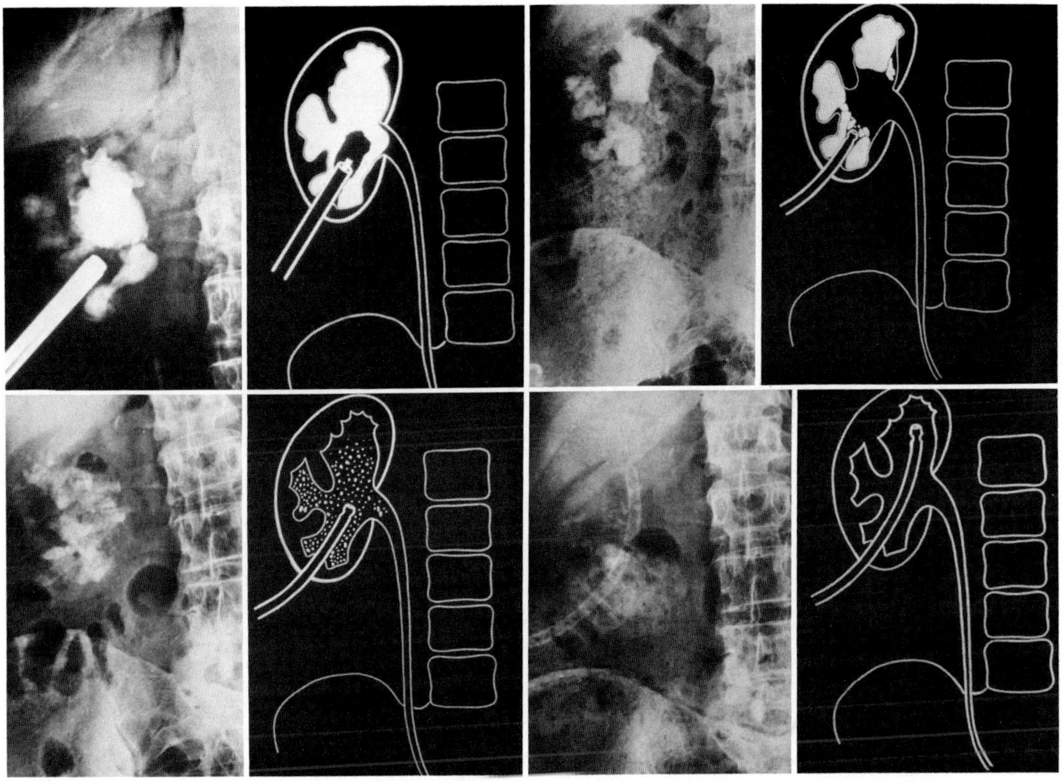

Fig. 7. Combination treatment (ESWL+PCN) in complete staghorn stone. *a* Intraoperative control during PCN shows removal of stone parts in the lower caliceal group and renal pelvis. *b* KUB prior to ESWL shows remnant stone mass in the caliceal groups whereas the pelvic stone part has been removed by PCN. *c* KUB after second ESWL session demonstrates complete disintegration of the caliceal stone parts. *d* KUB 5 days following the second ESWL documents that the patient is nearly stone-free with only some few fragments left in the lower caliceal group. The stone fragments passed either via the nephrostomy tube or via the ureter without any colic or pain for the patient.

Staghorn Calculi (Partial, Complete). Larger calculi up to partial and complete staghorn stones are treated with percutaneous nephrolithotomy as the first step. Any residual particles are then disintegrated by shock waves in a second or third session after 4 days (fig. 7). Our experience in the treatment of staghorn calculi has shown that by combination of both techniques disadvantages, namely the technical difficulties with increasing complication rate in PCN and the increased rate of side effects and aux-

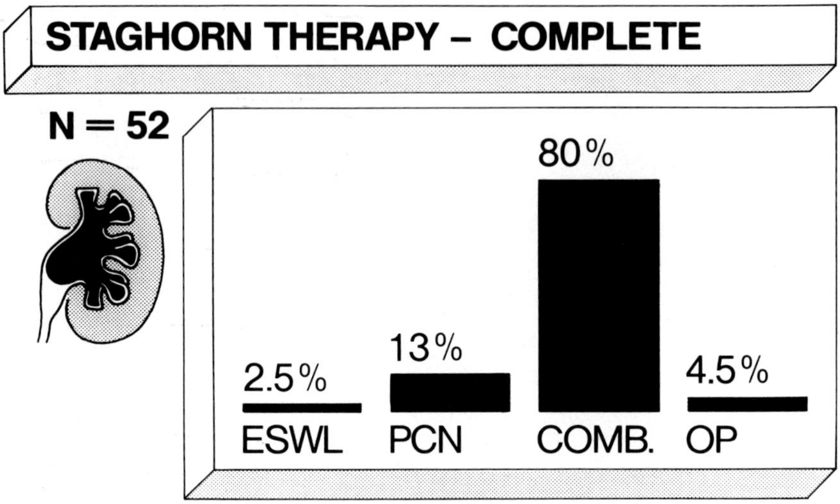

Fig. 8. Treatment modalities in 52 complete staghorn stones (October 1983 to August 1985).

iliary measures due to problems with stone passage after ESWL, can be overcome [9, 12, 19, 20]. So this combination has become the method of choice in complicated stone disease at our department and we now have treated more than 300 cases (fig. 8).

What Is Left for Open Surgery?

In the case of renal calculi associated with UPJ stenosis, pyeloplasty should be done with removal of the stone. Moreover, large stones with narrow collecting system, stenosis of the infundibula and large peripheral and central stone mass should be treated by open surgery.

Conclusion

In conclusion ESWL proved to be a safe and reproducible technique for the treatment of upper urinary stones. Three months following the treatment 75% of patients are completely stone-free, and only 5% need re-treatment because of the residual fragments. In combination with the new endo-urological techniques, such as percutaneous nephrolithotomy and ureterorenoscopy, more than 95% of the patients can be treated without the need of open surgery. Even cases of recurrent stone formation ('stone cancer') seem to be treatable, which could not be achieved before despite major improvements of surgical technique [26].

References

1 Alken, P.; Hardeman, S.; Wilbert, D.; Thürhoff, J.; Jacobi, G.H.: Extracorporeal shock wave lithotripsy (ESWL): alternatives and adjuvant procedures. Wld J. Urol. *3:* 48–52 (1985).

2 Chaussy, C.; Schmiedt, E.; Jocham, D.; Schiller, J.; Brandl, H.; Liedl, B.: Extracorporeal shock wave lithotripsy (ESWL) for treatment of urolithiatis. Urology *23:* 59–66 (1984).

3 Chaussy, C.; Schmiedt, E.; Jocham, D.; Brendel, W.; Forssmann, B.; Wather, V.: First clinical experience with extracorporeally induced destruction of kidney stones by shock waves. J. Urol. *127:* 417–420 (1982).

4 Chaussy, C.; Fuchs, G.: Erfahrungen mit der extracorporalen Stosswellenlithotripsie nach 5 Jahren klinischer Anwendung. Urologe A *24:* 305–309 (1985).

5 Eisenberger, F.; Schmiedt, E.; Chaussy, C.; Wanner, K.; Forssmann, B.; Hepp, W.; Pielsticker, K.; Brendel, W.: Berührungsfreie Harnsteinzertrümmerung. Stand der Forschung. Dt. Ärzteblatt *74:* 1–5 (1977).

6 Eisenberger, F.; Chaussy, C.; Wanner, K.: Extrakorporale Anwendung von hochenergetischen Stosswellen – ein neuer Aspekt in der Behandlung des Harnsteinleidens. Akt. Urol. *8:* 3–15 (1977).

7 Eisenberger, F.; Fuchs, G.; Miller, K.: Erfahrungen mit der berührungsfreien Nierensteintherapie (ESWL). Ärzteblatt Baden-Württemberg *12* (1983).

8 Eisenberger, F.; Fuchs, F.; Miller, K.; Rassweiler, J.: Non-invasive renal stone therapy with extracorporeal shock wave lithotripsy (ESWL); in Heuck, Donner, Radiology today, vol. 3, pp. 161–167 (Springer, Berlin 1985).

9 Eisenberger, F.; Fuchs, G.; Miller, K.; Rassweiler, J.: Extracorporeal shock wave lithotripsy and endourology – an ideal combination for the treatment of kidney stones. Wld. J. Urol. *3:* 41–47 (1985).

10 Eisenberger, F.; Gumpinger, R.; Miller, K.; Horbaschek, H.; Skeblitz, H.: Stereoröntgen in der Endourologie. Urologe A *24:* 342–345 (1985).

11 Forssmann, B.; Hepp, W.: Stosswellen in der Medizin. Med. unserer Zeit *4:* 10–14 (1980).

12 Fuchs, G.; Miller, K.; Rassweiler, J.: Alternatives to open surgery for renal calculi: percutaneous nephrolithotomy and extracorporeal shock wave lithotripsy; in Schilling, Klinische und experimentelle Urologie, vol. VIII, pp. 153–177 (Zuckschwerdt, München 1984).

13 Gumpinger, R.; Miller, K.; Fuchs, G.; Eisenberger, F.: Antegrade ureteroscopy for stone removal. Eur. Urol. *11:* 199–202 (1985).

14 Häusler, E.; Kiefer, W.: Anregung von Stosswellen in Flüssigkeiten durch Hochgeschwindigkeitstropfen. Verh. DPG G 786 (1971).

15 Hepp, W.: Survey of the development of shock wave lithotripsy (Dornier Medical Systems, September 1984).

16 Marshall, F.; Makofiki, R.; Mark, F.; Weisskopf, F.; Leo, F.; Guier, W.; Sanders, R.; Massey, J.T.: Shock wave destruction of renal calculi: new technical modifications. J. Urol. *133 A:* 118 (1985).

17 Meyer, W.H.; Klosterhalfen, H.; Becker, H.; Schulte am Esch, J.; Koch, E.: Effektivitätssteigerung der extracorporalen Stosswellenlithotripsie (ESWL) durch high-frequency-jet-ventilation (HFJV). Akt. Urol. *16:* 252–254 (1985).

18 Miller, K.; Fuchs, G.; Rassweiler, J.; Eisenberger, F.: Financial analysis: personnel planning and organizational requirements for the instillation of a kidney lithotripter in an urological department. Eur. Urol. *10:* 212–215 (1984).

19 Miller, K.; Fuchs, G.; Bub, P.; Rassweiler, J.; Eisenberger, F.: Kombination von perkutaner Nephrolithotomie (PCN) und extracorporaler Stosswellenlithotripsie (ESWL) – eine neue Möglichkeit zur Behandlung von Nierenausgusssteinen. Akt. Urol. *15:* 317–321 (1984).

20 Miller, K.; Fuchs, G.; Rassweiler, J.; Eisenberger, F.: Treatment of ureteral stone disease: the role of ESWL and endourology. Wld J. Urol. *3:* 53–57 (1985).

21 Miller, K.; Gumpinger, R.; Fuchs, G.; Rassweiler, J.; Eisenberger, F.: Antegrade Ureteroskopie – das Ende der offenen Chirurgie beim hohen Harnleiterstein. Akt. Urol. *16:* 291–293 (1985).

22 Rassweiler, J.; Buck, J.; Miller, K.; Fuchs, G.: Computertomographische Steindichtemessungen zur Steinanalyse vor extrakorporaler Stosswellenlithoripsie (ESWL). Akt. Urol. *16:* 30–35 (1985).

23 Rassweiler, J.; Miller, K.; Fuchs, G.; Eisenberger, F.: Kosten und Nutzen der berührungsfreien Nierensteinlithotripsie. Lebensversicherungsmedizin *37:* 80–85 (1985).

24 Rassweiler, J.: ESWL – first choice therapy for ureteral calculi. Panam. Congr. Urol., São Paulo 1986.

25 Schmiedt, E.; Chaussy, C.: Die extrakorporale Stosswellenlithotripsie von Nieren- und Harnleitersteinen. Dt. Ärzteblatt *82:* 247–252 (1985).

26 Smith, M.J.; Boyle, N.H.: Anatrophic nephrotomy and plastic calyraphy. J. Urol. *99:* 521 (1968).

F. Eisenberger, MD, Department of Urology, Katharinenhospital Stuttgart, Kriegsbergstrasse 60, D–7000 Stuttgart 1 (FRG)

Contr. Nephrol., vol. 58, pp. 253–257 (Karger, Basel 1987)

Endoscopic and Extracorporeal Lithotripsy: The Italian Experience in a Polycentric Survey

S. Rocca Rossetti, G. Muto, B. Morelli

Istituto di Nefro-Urologia, Cattedra di Urologia, Divisione Urologica Universitaria, Torino, Italia

Ultrasonic percutaneous lithotripsy and shock wave treatment of renal calculosis are well-known therapies currently used in Italy as well as elsewhere, so that a detailed description will not be made so far. All the most advanced Italian urological centers began their experiences on modern therapy of renal calculosis adopting the percutaneous technique [1–3], the shock wave technology [4–7] not being available in Italy until late 1984; in fact percutaneous lithotripsy was employed since 1982 [8]. The number of patients who underwent percutaneous lithotripsy has been strongly reduced during the last year because of the ever more frequent use of extracorporeal shock wave lithotripsy (ESWL).

Until March 1986, there were in Italy 7 centers using extracorporeal treatment for renal calculosis, and all reported a 70% effectiveness of shock wave therapy on a basis of non-selected patients. The shock wave equipment may also be used in the treatment of uppertract ureteric calculosis with the help of a ureteric catheter (inserting the calculus up in the renal pelvis) or even without it. Contrarily, lowertract ureteric calculosis must undergo operative ureteroscopy, due to the difficulty to precisely locate the stones in this area; this is the sole alternative to surgery. In the experience of Rocca Rossetti's team, surgical therapy was reserved for long-standing stones located in the ureter, when serious edema and/or hydronephrosis had developed.

Table I. Percutaneous therapy with ultrasound in the management of renal calculosis. Polycentric experience: number of treated patients and rate of complete resolution

	Number	%
Bologna	181	87.2
Genova	197	91.8
Milano	104	83.6
Napoli	83	90.4
Padova	190	82.6
Palermo	142	88.8
Roma	39	90.0
Torino	230	83.4
Total	1,066	87.2

Table II. Percutaneous therapy with ultrasound in the management of renal calculosis. Polycentric experience: calculosis

	Simple, %	Multiple, %	Staghorn stone, %	Ureteral, %
Bologna	74.5	17.1	5.5	2.5
Genova	76.6	10.6	7.1	5.6
Milano	64.0	27.3	5.7	9.5
Napoli	71.0	12.0	17.0	0
Padova	49.1	22.9	19.5	8.5
Palermo	76.7	17.6	2.8	2.8
Roma	100.0	0	0	0
Torino	71.4	19.5	7.4	2.7
Total	72.4	15.9	8.0	3.9

Percutaneous Therapy of Renal Calculosis

A report from a few Italian urological centers, considering a 3-year study and 1,066 patients treated, showed a complete success of this therapy in 87.2% cases (table I). Three kinds of calculosis were considered: simple, multiple and staghorn stones. Ureteric calculosis was included in this report, as long as the stone was inserted in the renal pelvis.

Over the above-mentioned report, 72.4% cases were simple calculosis, 15.9% were multiple, 8% were staghorn stones, 3.9% were

Table III. Percutaneous therapy with ultrasound in the management of renal calculosis. Polycentric experience: complications

	Hemorrhage, %	Infections, %	Operative lesions, %	Mortality, %
Bologna	3.3	–	–	–
Genova	2.8	8.0	0	0
Milano	3.8	1.9	0	0
Napoli	6.0	2.4	2.4	0
Padova	2.6	2.6	3.7	0
Palermo	2.8	3.5	4.2	0.7
Roma	0	2.3	0	0
Torino	2.7	0.4	1.0	0
Total	3.0	3.0	1.0	0.1

ureteric (table II). Such results were subsequently modified when shock wave treatment was preferred for simple calculosis, leaving complicated cases to the percutaneous treatment. Complications occurred at the following rates: hemorrhage 3%, infections 3%, operative lesions 1%, overall mortality 0.1% (table III).

Extracorporeal Shock Wave Treatment of Renal Calculosis

The report from 6 out of 7 centers showed an average 77.9% complete success (total expulsion of fragments) in 2,749 patients: after a 3-month follow-up they still appeared stone-free (table IV). Repeated treatment was necessary on an overall 3.4–12%, depending on the kind of calculi (table V). Associated therapy, sometimes necessary, was percutaneous, ureteric catheterization, nephrostomy, endoscopic withdrawal, surgery (table VI). Most frequent complications were: infections 8.1%, perirenal bruise 0.7% (table VII).

Final Considerations

It is fully evident, when considering the above-mentioned percentages, that there are clearly more cases treated with ESWL than with percutaneous ultrasound lithotripsy (PUL), in spite of the fact that the ESWL appeared more recently. Shock wave treatment is simpler to execute and

Table IV. ESWL – multicentric Italian experience: number of treated patients and rate of complete resolution at 3 months

	Number	%
Firenze	572	65.6
Genova	340	79.0
Milano	780	70.8
Roma	600	84.7
Palermo	364	82.9
Torino	153	89.3
Total	2,749	77.9

Table V. ESWL – multicentric Italian experience: repeated treatments

	%
Firenze	3.4
Genova	6.0
Milano	4.8
Roma	12.0
Torino	9.6
Total	7.1

Table VI. ESWL – multicentric Italian experience: associated therapies

	PUL %	Urethero-scopy %	Ureteric catheteri-zation %	Nephro-stomy %	Dormia %	Endoscopic withdrawal %	Surgery %
Firenze	1.2	–	12.7	1.0	–	–	9.5
Genova	0	0	2.0	4.0	3.0	5.0	0.3
Milano	0.6	0.2	11.5	0.2	2.2	0	0.1
Roma	4.1	0.5	2.6	0.5	0	0	0.3
Palermo	19.7	–	0.5	0.2	–	–	0.2
Torino	2.0	2.0	4.0	0	0.6	0.6	1.3
Total	4.6	0.6	5.5	0.9	1.4	1.4	1.9

Table VII. ESWL – multicentric Italian experience: complications

	Infections, %	Perirenal bruise, %
Firenze	7.3	0.3
Genova	15.0	–
Milano	9.5	–
Roma	8.0	–
Palermo	–	0.6
Torino	2.8	1.3

less invasive; this is the reason why it was preferred in the great majority of simple calculosis. On the contrary, multiple or complex calculosis requires a more careful approach, usually preferring PUL as the first stage, then using shock wave and nephrostomy for the final withdrawal of fragments (this combined technique accounts for a total of 4.6%).

References

1 Alken, P.; Hutschenreiter, G.R.; Günther, R.; Marberger, M.: Percutaneous stones manipulation. J. Urol. *125:* 463–566 (1981).

2 Alken, P.: Percutaneous ultrasonic destruction of renal calculi. Symposium of endourology. Urol. Clins N. Am. *9* (1982).

3 Alken, P.; Hutschenreiter, G.R.; Günther, R.: Percutaneous kidney stone removal. Eur. Urol. *8:* 304–311 (1982).

4 Chaussy, C.; Brendel, W.; Schmiedt, E.: Extracorporeally induced destruction of kidney stones by waves. Lancet *ii:* 1265–1268 (1980).

5 Chaussy, C.; Schmiedt, E.; Jocham, D.; Brendel, W.; Forssman, B.; Moser, E.: Berührungsfreie Nierensteinzertrümmerung durch Stosswellen. Erste klinische Erfahrungen. Dt. Ärzteblatt *18:* 881–886 (1981).

6 Chaussy, C.; Schmiedt, E.; Jocham, D.; Forssman, B.; Brendel, W.; Walther, V.: Therapiemöglichkeiten des Harnsteinleidens mit extracorporal erzeugten Stosswellen. Pathogenese und Klinik der Harnsteine. VIII. Fortschr. Urol. und Nephrol., vol. 17 (Steinkopff, Darmstadt 1982).

7 Chaussy, C.; Schmiedt, E.; Jocham, D.; Brendel, W.; Forssman, B.; Walther, V.: First clinical experiences with extracorporeally induced destruction of kidney stones by shock waves. J. Urol. *127:* 417–420 (1982).

8 Rocca Rossetti, S.; Muto, G.; Malcangi, U.; Ramello, A.: Attuali prospettive nel trattamento non chirurgico della calcolosi renale. Litiasi renale, pp. 281–287 (Wichtig, Milano 1985).

S. Rocca Rossetti, MD, Istituto di Nefro-Urologia, Cattedra di Urologia,
Divisione Urologica Universitaria, Corso Polonia 14, I–10126 Torino (Italy)

Contr. Nephrol., vol. 58, pp. 258–261 (Karger, Basel 1987)

Intercostal or Multiple Access in Percutaneous Lithotripsy

P. Buli, E. Tiozzi, E. Brunocilla, S. Spatafora, A. Martelli

Department of Urology, University of Bologna, Bologna, Italy

The position of the stone within the renal excretory tract can often condition the choice of the access to the kidney in percutaneous lithotripsy. If the stone is localized in the upper kidney pole (upper caliceal group) or multiple in different calices or complex (pelvis + 2 or more different calices), intercostal access above the XIIth rib or contemporary multiple access is needed.

From 1983 to present we have carried out 181 percutaneous procedures to remove renal stones of various size, number and position (table I). The success rate has been 90.6%.

In 16 patients 6 intercostal and 10 multiple access procedures were performed. Intercostal access was carried out for lithiasis of the upper caliceal group (fig. 1) or in patients with a reduced costo-iliac space, while multiple access was used for multiple or branched calculi. Multiple access was always performed at the beginning of the procedure, dilating the nephrostomy tracts in succession (fig. 2). With multiple access the rigid nephroscope with ultrasonic probe was always used; the flexible nephroscope was not needed in any case. In particular, the electrohydraulic probe was never used as we believe it can increase the possibility of residual fragments. At the end of procedure, drainage was left in one of the nephrostomy tracts for 48 h. No bleeding took place in any case and, in particular, hospitalization time and lumbar pain have been the same as for cases treated with single access.

Table I. Location of stone and results in 181 percutaneous lithotripsies

	%
Pelvic stone	98
Single caliceal stone	90
Pelvic and inferior caliceal stones	97
Pelvic and middle caliceal stones	83
Simple branched stone	90
Complex or multiple stones	65
Success rate	90.6

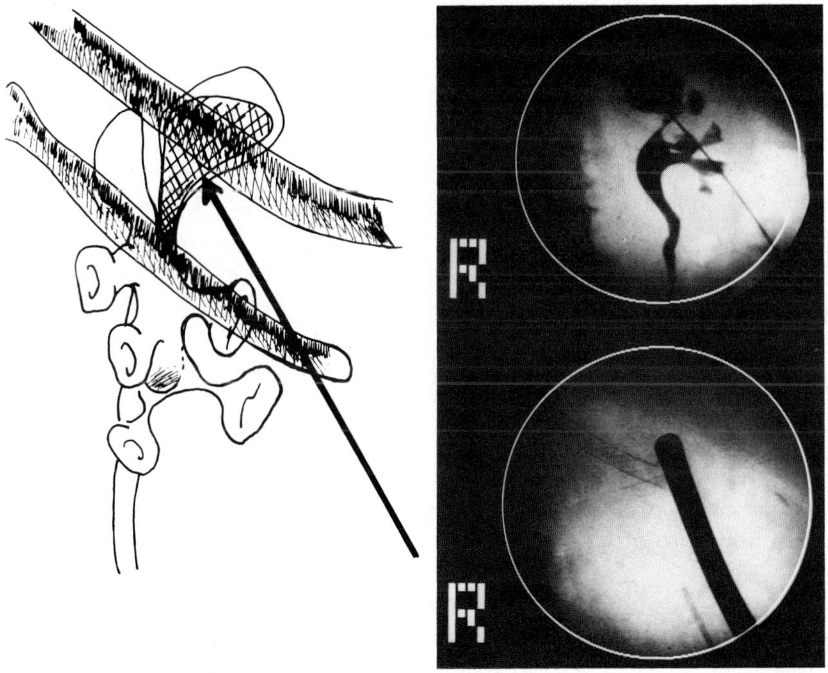

a b

Fig. 1. Intercostal approach in a right upper caliceal stone. *a* Diagrammatic representation. *b* Puncture and post-operative plain film.

a, b

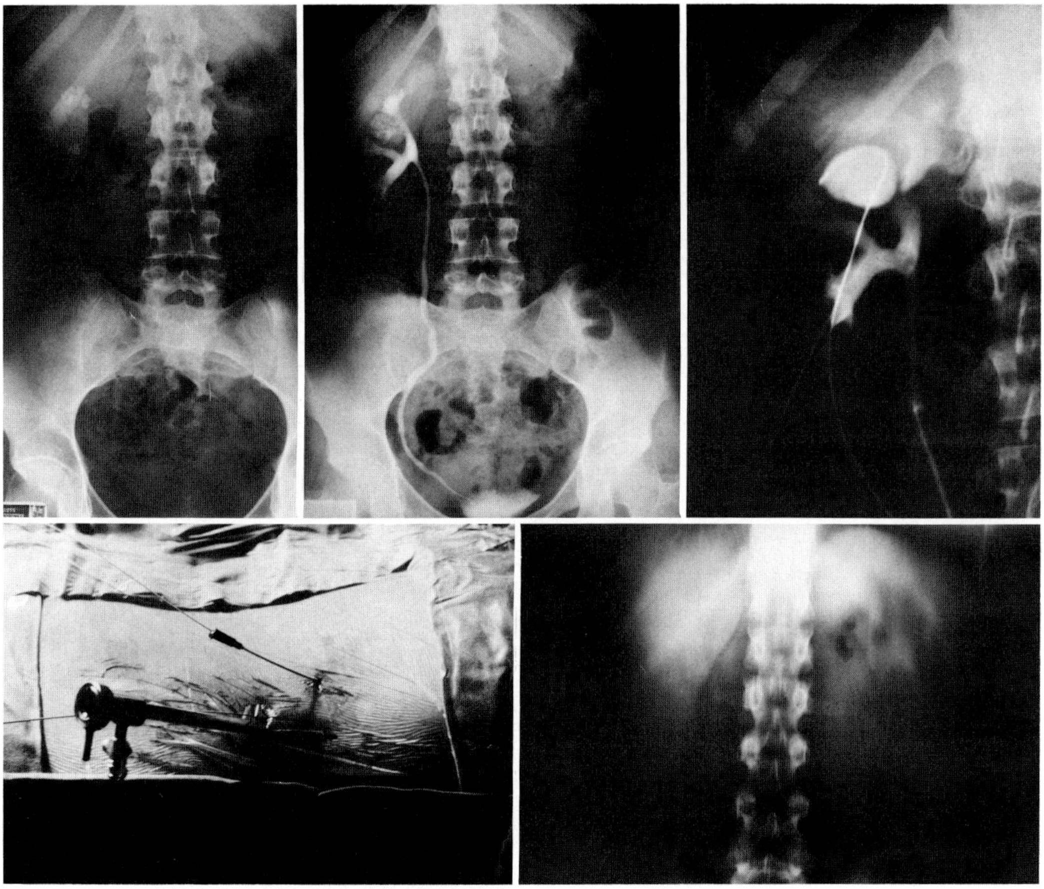

c

d

e

Fig. 2a–e. Pelvic and multiple caliceal stones in a solitary left kidney in a 22 year old woman before, during and after lithotripsy.

Conclusions

The use of intercostal and multiple access has widened the field of percutaneous lithotripsy (table II). It must be pointed out that intercostal access needs to be performed while the patient is breathing out, keeping sufficiently far from the lower edge of XI (intercostal artery) and the upper edge of XII (periosteum).

Table II. Results related with single and multiple approach

	Multiple or complex stones	Positive results %
Single approach	14	50
Multiple approach	10	80
Mean		65

Multiple access (generally 2) allows one to have a good threedimensional vision of renal cavities, so that only the rigid nephroscope is necessary. Consequently, the ultrasonic probe with suction can also be used, which significantly lowers the possibility of residual fragments, in comparison with the electrohydraulic probe. The latter is used only for small single fragments in secondary calices where removal with forceps can be difficult. The nearly total absence of complications depends on the correct performance of the method.

P. Buli, MD, Department of Urology, Via Massarenti 9, I–40138 Bologna (Italy)

Contr. Nephrol., vol. 58, pp. 262–265 (Karger, Basel 1987)

Indications and Limits of Percutaneous Nephrolithotripsy and Extracorporeal Shock Wave Lithotripsy Combined Treatment

F. Di Silverio, M. Gallucci, G. Alpi, A. Cassanelli, C. Molinari, G. P. Ricciuti, D. Fini

Università degli Studi di Roma 'La Sapienza', Patologia Urologica, Roma, Italia

The complete staghorn stone represents one of the most important problems for the urologist regarding technical difficulties and the high incidence of recurrences. Since 1976 urinary stone disease management has undergone a complete change: open surgery has been replaced by percutaneous nephrolithotripsy (PCN) before and extracorporeal shock wave lithotripsy (ESWL) now in the treatment of an increasing number of urinary stones [1–20].

Both new techniques are considered inadequate to treat one-size staghorn stones larger than 5 cm. Eisenberger and associates [21–24] suggest in these cases a combination therapy PCN+ESWL. We show our experience in 18 cases treated from March to December 1985.

Materials and Methods

Eighteen complete staghorn stones larger than 5 cm were treated by PCN + ESWL combined therapy. The age of the patients (9 male and 9 female) ranged from 18 to 76 years, with a mean of 43.4. 8 patients had a history of operations for recurrent stone disease. 14 patients had an urinary tract infection.

The first step of combined therapy is the treatment by PCN using always a transparenchymal peripheral access to the lower calyx of the collecting system. The ESWL followed after a minimum of one week. 14 patients were submitted to one PCN and 4 to two PCN. The patients underwent ESWL one time in 8 cases, two times in 9 cases and four times in 1 case. General anesthesia was performed in all sessions of combination therapy. All patients received antibiotic therapy.

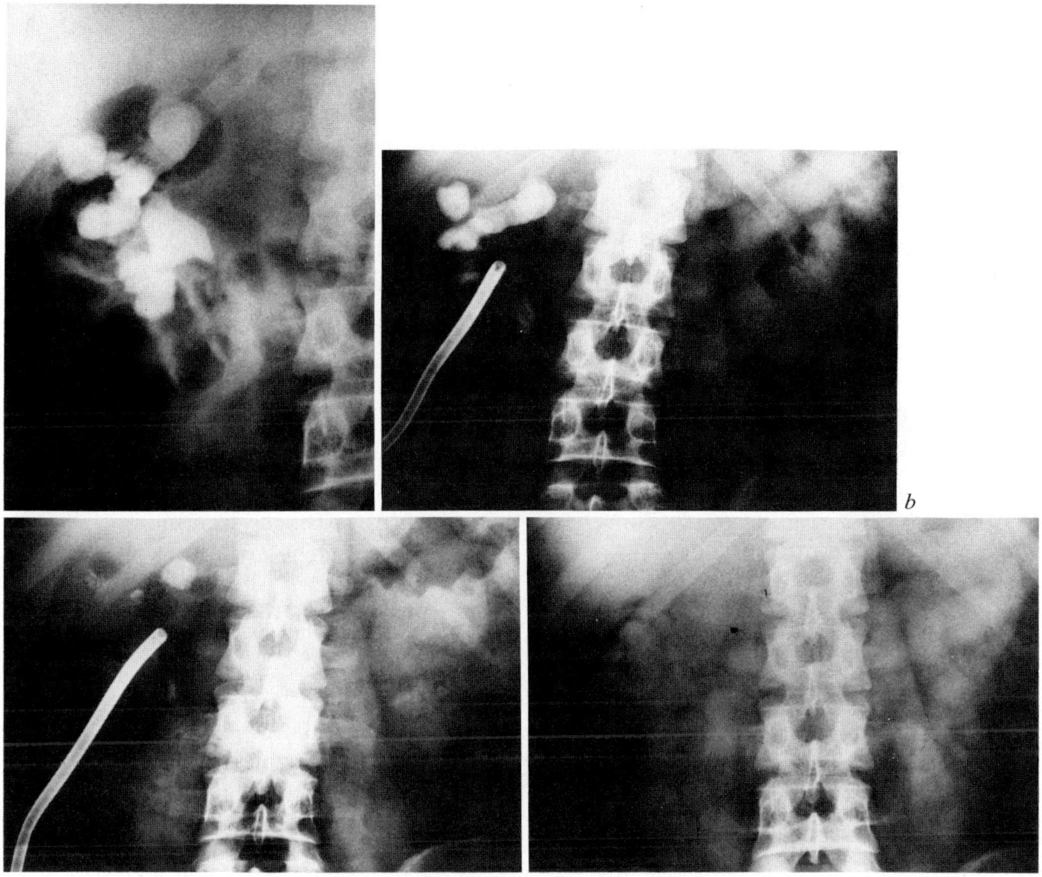

a b c d

Fig. 1. Plain X-ray. *a* Right staghorn stone; *b* after PCN; *c* after second ESWL treatment; *d* final result after combined treatment.

Results

Thirteen patients are completely stone-free, 4 with fragments < 1 cm and 1 with a fragment > 1 cm.

The complications were: 3 intraoperative hemorrhages treated by blood transfusion, and 1 perirenal hematoma treated firstly by blood transfusion therapy and secondly by surgical operation.

There was sepsis in 2 patients who needed uretheropyeloscopic ultrasound lithotripsy to get the ureter patent from obstruction.

Discussion and Conclusions

The combination therapy PCN + ESWL in the one-size staghorn stones larger than 5 cm shows good results (fig. 1), considering 15–20% of residual stones reported also in the best series of open surgery-treated staghorn stones.

The goal of PCN is to get stone-free the lower calyx and the pelvis, and to give the possibility of fragment elimination after ESWL treatment through the ureter or the nephrostomy catheter.

The PCN + ESWL combination, in our results, is an excellent and safe technique to solve the staghorn stones problem alternatively to open surgery, and we think that further improvement will be achieved with increasing experience.

The long time of realization, the multiple anesthesias, the high costs in comparison to open surgery in Italy ($ 4,934 vs $ 3,780 on the average) are the limitations. However, the staghorn stones treatment by PCN + ESWL combination is an advanced technical solution well accepted by the patients.

References

1 Fernström, I.; Johannson, B.: Percutaneous pyelolithotomy: a new extraction technique. Scand. J. Urol. *10:* 257–259 (1976).
2 Kurth, K.H.; Hohenfeller, R.; Altwein, J.E.: Ultrasound litholapaxy of a staghorn calculus. J. Urol. *117:* 242–243 (1977).
3 Wickham, J.E.A.; Kellet, M.J.: Percutaneous nephrolithotomy. Br. med. J. *283:* 1571–1573 (1981).
4 Alken, P.; Hutschenreiter, R.; Günther, M.; Marberger, M.: Percutaneous stone manipulation. J. Urol. *125:* 463–466 (1981).
5 Ball, T.P.; Endoscopic and percutaneous manipulation in stone disease. Urol. Clins. N. Am. *8:* 277–298 (1981).
6 Castaneda-Zuniga, W.R.; Miller, R.P.; Amplatz, K.: Percutaneous removal of kidney stones. Urol. Clins. N. Am. *9:* 113–119 (1982).
7 Segura, J.W.; Patterson, D.E.; LeRoy, A.J.; McGough, P.F.; Barret, D.M.: Percutaneous removal of kidney stones. Preliminary report. Mayo Clin. Proc. *57:* 615–619 (1982).
8 Marberger, M.; Stackl, W.; Hruby, W.: Percutaneous litholapaxy of renal stones. Eur. Urol. 236 (1982).
9 Clayman, R.V.; Surya, V.; Miller, R.P.; Castaneda-Zuniga, W.R.; Amplatz, K.; Lange, P.H.: Percutaneous nephrolithotomy. An approach to branched and staghorn renal calculi. J. Am. med. Ass. *250:* 73–75 (1983).
10 Whitfield, H.N.: Percutaneous nephrolithotomy. Br. J. Urol. *55:* 609–612 (1983).

11 Chaussy, C.; Eisenberger, F.; Wanner, K.; Forssmann, B.: Extracorporale Anwendung von hochenergetischen Stosswellen. Ein neuer Aspekt in der Behandlung des Harnsteinleidens. Akt. Urol. *9:* 95 (1978).

12 Chaussy, C.; Brendel, W.; Schmiedt, E.: Extracorporeally induced destruction of kidney stones by shock waves. Lancet *i:* 1265–1268 (1980).

13 Chaussy, C.; Schmiedt, E.; Jocham, D.; Forssmann, B.; Brendel, W.; Walther, V.: First clinical experience with extracorporeally induced destruction of kidney stones by shock waves. J. Urol. *127:* 417–420 (1982).

14 Di Silverio, F.; Gallucci, M.; Cerulli, C.; Alpi, G.; Molinari, C.; Cassanelli, A.; Fini, D.; Ricciuti, G.P.: Litotrissia extracorporea con onde d'urto: prime esperienze. Urologia *53:* 101–106 (1986).

15 Gallucci, M.; Cerulli, C.; Alpi, G.; Cassanelli, A.; Molinari, C.; Fini, D.; Ricciuti, G.P.; Di Silverio, F.: La calcolosi renale a stampo con onde d'urto: esperienza su sette casi. Urologia *53:* 107–110 (1986).

16 Di Silverio, F.; Gallucci, M.; Cerulli, C.; Alpi, G.; Cassanelli, A.; Fini, D.; Ricciuti, G.P.: Osservazioni e risultati dei primi 140 trattamenti con lithotripter. Giornate di Radiourologia, Palermo 1985; in Momenti di radiourologica, pp. 239–244 (Acta Medica, Rome 1986).

17 Di Silverio, F.; Gallucci, M.; Cerulli, C.; Alpi, G.; Molinari, C.: Importanza della preparazione e posizione del malato nel lithotripter. Giornate di Radiourologia, Palermo 1985; in Momenti di radiourologica, pp. 235–238 (Acta Medica, Rome 1986).

18 Di Silverio, F.; Gallucci, M.; Cerulli, C.; Alpi, G.; Ricciuti, G.P.; Molinari, C.; Cassanelli, A.; Fini, D.; Giacobini, S.: ESWL nella calcolosi renale: nostra esperienza. Convegno Soc. di Urologia Centro Meridionale e delle Isole, Capri 1985 (in press).

19 Di Silverio, F.; Gallucci, M.; Cerulli, C.; Alpi, G.; Molinari, C.; Cassanelli, A.; Ricciuti, G.P.; Fini, D.: Calcolosi ureterale con ESWL: possibilità e limiti. Convegno della Soc. di Urologia Centro Meridionale e delle Isole, Capri 1985 (in press).

20 Di Silverio, F.; Gallucci, M.; Cerulli, C.; Alpi, G.; Cassanelli, A.; Ricciuti, G.P.; Molinari, C.; Fini, D.; Giacobini, S.: Valutazione morfologica e funzionale del rene dopo trattamento con ESWL. Convegno della Soc. di Urologia Centro Meriodionale e delle Isole, Capri 1985 (in press).

21 Fuchs, G.; Miller, K.; Rassweiler, J.: Alternatives to open surgery for renal calculi: percutaneous nephrolithotomy and extracorporeal shock wave lithotripsy; in Schilling, Klinische und experimentelle Urologie (Zuckschwerdt, München 1984).

22 Miller, K.; Fuchs, G.; Bub, P.; Rassweiler, J.; Eisenberger, F.: Kombination von perkutaner Nephrolithotomie (PCN) und extracorporaler Stosswellenlithotripsie (ESWL) – eine neue Möglichkeit zur Behandlung von Nierenausgusssteinen. Akt. Urol. *15:* 317 (1984).

23 Fuchs, G.; Miller, K.; Rassweiler, J.; Eisenberger, F.: Extracorporeal shock-wave lithotripsy: one-year experience with the Dornier lithotripter. Eur. Urol. *11:* 145–149 (1985).

24 Fuchs, G.; Miller, K.; Eisenberger, .; Bub, P.; Rassweiler, J.: The advantages of the combination of PCN and ESWL in the treatment of staghorn calculi. Proc. 9th Int. Symp. Boltzmann Stiftung, Vienna 1985.

Michele Gallucci, MD, via Asmara 72, I–00199 Roma (Italy)

Contr. Nephrol., vol. 58, pp. 266–269 (Karger, Basel 1987)

The Role of ESWL in the Treatment of Radiolucent or Scarcely Radiopaque Renal Stones

Cesare Selli, Marco Carini, Carlo Fiorelli

Department of Urology, University of Florence, Florence, Italy

Uric acid stones are characteristically frequent in the Mediterranean area, and according to epidemiological studies in Italy they are found in pure and mixed form in 26.4% of patients presenting with stones of the upper urinary tract [4]. Medical treatment, based on dietary purine restriction, alkalinization and allopurinol, is still the basic therapeutic choice for pure uric acid stones, with a reported dissolution rate of about 90%. Successful dissolution requires strict patient compliance regarding drug intake, hydration and dietary restrictions. Until recently surgical treatment was reserved only to failures after prolonged medical therapy and to obstructive, infected, mixed and staghorn stones. Obstructive calculi required aggressive treatment because hydronephrosis prevented successful hydration and alkalinization. Infected radiolucent calculi represented a surgical indication because alkalinization enhances bacterial virulence; likewise the presence of calcification virtually negates all attempts at medical dissolution. Staghorn uric acid stones were often operated since their dissolution would have been too time-consuming and demanding for the patient. All these situations of surgical domain have been recently totally subverted by the advent of percutaneous ultrasound lithotripsy (PUL) and extracorporeal shock wave lithotripsy (ESWL).

Contrast-negative stones have been considered to represent a contraindication to ESWL by the forerunners of the technique because they could not be readily visualized on X-ray monitors during treatment, and therefore could not be accurately centered for shock wave discharge. It was also feared that radiolucent ureteral fragments could have caused problems following treatment [1, 3]. For these reasons PUL has been proposed as a valid alternative, since it allows removal of all concrements in one session [2]. Due to the relatively high incidence of uric acid stones in Italy, we initially faced the need to treat with ESWL cases with strict surgical indications, and later on due to the good results, also in those patients who were reluctant to undergo prolonged medical therapy and expressed their choice for non-invasive stone destruction.

Patients and Methods

During a 12-month period we treated with ESWL 572 reno-ureteral units and 53 (9.5%) were contrast-negative: 46 radiolucent and 7 scarcely radiopaque. Chemical analysis of the expelled concrements revealed pure uric acid in 3, mixed stones with a predominance of uric acid in 49 cases and cystine in 1. There were 15 staghorn stones (6 total, 5 partial), 21 pyelic, 7 caliceal, 7 multiple and 7 ureteral. In order to visualize the upper urinary tract a ureteral catheter was placed before immersing the patient in the water in 46 cases, and retrograde pyelograms were obtained by injecting under strict sterile conditions a 60% solution of iodamide whenever it appeared necessary during fluoroscopic monitoring of the effects of treatment. Endoscopic introduction of the catheter in the upper tract was not possible due to various anatomical reasons in 7 cases, and contrast medium was administered intravenously (60–120 ml of 60% iodamine).

ESWL treatment was performed in the usual manner, delivering between 500 and 3,500 shock waves (mean 1,930). Two cases had repeated treatments. Patients were placed on vigorous alkalinization with intravenous sodium bicarbonate and Ringer lactate from the beginning of ESWL throughout the hospitalization period. Once at home patients with uric acid stones were prescribed oral alkali, allopurinol 300 mg OD, abundant fluid intake and a diet restricted in purines; the patient with cystinuria had mercaptopropynil glycine and alkalinization. Patients were followed with daily sonograms during hospitalization, and monthly after discharge. IVP was obtained in 5 cases only.

Results

Successful stone fragmentation during ESWL treatment was observed in all cases with fluoroscopic monitoring (fig. 1). The average hospitalization period was 3.2 days; 9 patients presented severe colics requiring i.v. antispasmodics and 6 had fever, presumably related to the endoscopic maneuvers. Sonographic control was performed between 1 month and 5 months after treatment in 46 out of 53 patients. 23 were studied after one month: 12 were completely stone-free, 8 presented only dust, while 3 had fragments still visible, with some dilatation in two. Controls after 2–5 months in 23 patients revealed 17 completely stone-free and 6 with dust. The overall results are therefore 63% free, 30% with dust and 7% with fragments.

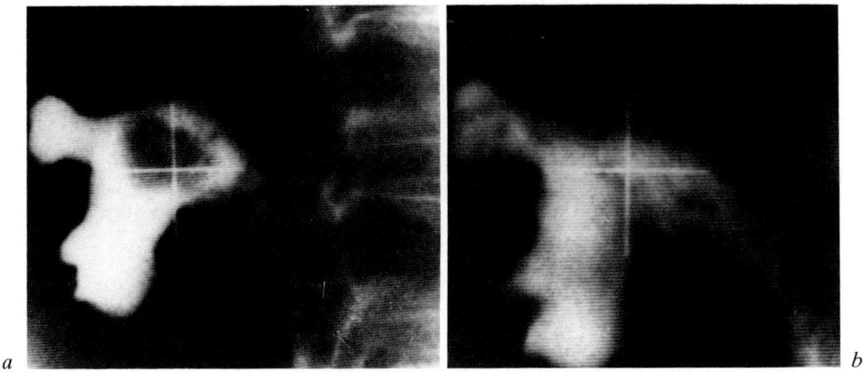

Fig. 1. *a* Visualization of a renal pelvic radiolucent stone on the TV monitor of a Dornier lithotripter with retrograde pyelography. *b* Effect of ESWL.

Discussion

Radiolucent and scarcely radiopaque stones no longer represent a contraindication to ESWL, since they can be adequately visualized on X-ray monitors with the help of contrast medium, which can be either infused directly with a ureteral catheter or be secreted by the kidney when injected intravenously. In our experience retrograde pyelography is by far the more satisfactory way to visualize contrast-negative stones, since it provides immediate delineation of the excretory tract and allows a graduation of the amount of intrapyelic contrast under fluoroscopic monitoring according to different stages of stone fragmentation. It is our policy to inject 5 ml of 60% iodamide solution at the beginning of stone localization and subsequently further variable amounts, whenever more detailed opacification is considered necessary. If an excessive amount of contrast medium is believed to mask fragments requiring further treatment, it is usually easy to aspirate the ureteral catheter until optimal image adjustment is found. Various anatomical conditions, such as ureteral strictures, BPH with median lobe, mucosal folds and incomplete ureteral duplication prevented in some cases successful catheterization of the ureter. In these patients we used to intravenous pyelography, which is less satisfactory because the time lag for optimal visualization is much longer and fine adjustments of intrapyelic contrast medium are not possible, particularly at the final stages of stone fragmentation. The initial fear of obstructive complications due to impacted radiolucent fragments in the ureter so far has not materialized in our experience. Daily sonographic controls and post-treatment clinical course did not differ significantly from those of patients with radiopaque stones of similar size. The favorable results observed may be in part explained by the fact that concrements originated by ESWL present a contact surface with alkalinized urine much greater than the original stone (fragment surface = $\sqrt[3]{n}$ × original surface, where n = number of fragments). Therefore, the process of chemical dissolution produced by an increase in urine pH and in urine volume is greatly accelerated.

References

1 Chaussy, C.; Schmiedt, E.; Jocham, D.; Brendel, W.; Forssman, B.; Walther, V.: First clinical experience with extracorporeally induced destruction of kidney stones by shock waves. J. Urol. *127:* 417–420 (1982).

2 Eisenberger, F.; Fuchs, G.; Miller, K.; Bub, P.; Rassweiler, J.: Extracorporeal shock wave lithotripsy and endourology: an ideal combination for the treatment of kidney stones. Wld J. Urol. *3:* 41–47 (1985).

3 Fuchs, G.; Miller, K.; Rassweiler, J.; Eisenberger, F.: Extracorporeal shock wave lithotripsy: one-year experience with the Dornier lithotripter. Eur. Urol. *11:* 145–149 (1985).

4 Miano, L.; Paradiso-Galatioto, G.; Cusumano, G.; Ferrone, G.; Goldoni, S.: La calcolosi renale oggi. Indici statistico-epidemiologici. Atti Soc. ital. Urol. *1:* 9 (1980).

C. Selli, MD, Clinica Urologica, viale Pieraccini 18, I–50139 Florence (Italy)

Contr. Nephrol., vol. 58, pp. 270–273 (Karger, Basel 1987)

The Percutaneous Treatment of the Cast, Branched and Staghorn Renal Stones

P. Tombolini, A. Mandressi, M. Ruoppolo, G. Dormia, A. Trinchieri, G. Zanetti, E. Montanari, E. Pisani

Institute of Urology, University of Milan, Milan, Italy

The acquisition of new techniques, such as extracorporeal shock wave lithotripsy (ESWL) and percutaneous litholapaxy, brought about an absolute improvement in the management of kidney stones. However, to perform the complete clearance of the cast, branched and staghorn renal stones by percutaneous procedure, some technical problems, due to the feature of the stones, ought to be solved. First of all the protraction of the procedure due to the width of the branched stones, then the hardness of some cast stones due to their chemical structure, finally the ramifications into the peripheral calices of staghorn stones.

Patients and Methods

From January to November 1985 we treated by percutaneous litholapaxy 24 patients (12 male, 12 female, ranged between 12 and 72 years, average 42.6) with complex renal stones (table I). On the day of hospitalization the patients had a complete blood count, urine analysis and culture. The renal function was normal in all the patients but one, who had it impaired because of bilateral staghorn stones (serum creatinine 4.3 mg/dl). Before the ureteral catheter was positioned, the patients were given an antibiotic i. v. (monobactam).

The collecting system was then outlined by retrograde pyelography. The percutaneous track was always performed in general anesthesia together with the management of the stones. The dilation, by Alken telescopic dilators [1], was made under fluoroscopic control, then the nephroscopy was carried out by inserting into the sheath a 24.5-Ch nephroscope. A variety of instruments was used for viewing and managing the stones, but the favoured methods were to use ultrasonic lithotripsy (USL), electrohydraulic lithotripsy (EHL) by 9- and 5-Ch probes, the flexible nephroscope 14.5 Ch (flex. N.) and mechanical means (MM) (table II). At the end of the procedure a nephrostomic tube (22 Ch) was placed. A nephrostomogram was obtained 3 days postoperatively. Nephrostomy was removed as soon as the urinary tract was working well.

Table I. Complex renal stones and their chemical analysis (24 patients)

5	struvite staghorn stones
15	branched pyelocaliceal stones (1 carbonate apatite, 4 apatite, 10 mixed oxalate-apatite)
4	pelvic cast stones (2 oxalate monohydrate, 1 uric acid, 1 cystine)

Table II. Methods of litholapaxy used in 36 percutaneous procedures (24 patients, 8 by one-step and 14 by two-step treatment)

	Cases
USL + flex. N. + EHL 5-Ch and 9-Ch + MM	10
USL + EHL 9-Ch	10
EHL 9-Ch + MM	1
USL + MM	1
USL only	14

Abbreviations given in 'Patients and Methods'.

Results

Hospitalization for stone extraction ranged from 3 to 25 days. The mean time of intrarenal manipulation was 90 min. 19 (80%) of the 24 patients had a complete clearance of the stones. 3 (12%) had some small fragments left but they remained asymptomatic, so no further treatment has been undertaken. In 2 cases (8%) the percutaneous procedure failed because of the lack of space for the dilation due to a complete casting of the inferior calices: so the patients underwent open surgery. 14 patients (58%) needed a two-step procedure: 11 because of the large size of the stones, 3 because of the bleeding during the first treatment. One patient (4%) had two percutaneous tracks (the second one through the superior calix) to completely remove the stones. The patient having renal function impaired had an improvement of the renal function (serum creatinine 3.1 mg/dl); the patients having normal renal function did not show any alteration of serum creatinine. The complications that occurred during and after the treatment are indicated in table III.

Table III. Significant complications in percutaneous procedure of complex stones (24 patients)

	Patients	%
Fever without urinary sepsis	3	12
Excessive intraoperative bleeding (procedure stopped)	3	12
Extravasation	1	4

Discussion

Considering our experience the percutaneous treatment of the complex stones is possible if a good preoperative planning is done [2]. A study of the stones and renal cavities is essential because the assaulted calix must be the one which more clearly allows the best approach to the whole collecting system. In fact it might be necessary to reinsert the nephroscope to remove residual fragments detected by the postoperative X-ray film [2]. Moreover, we have to consider the possibility or necessity to sting not only the inferior-posterior calix, but also other calices to obtain the complete clearance of the stones.

The problem represented by the length of time needed to disrupt the branched stones, which directly depends on their hardness and width [3], can be solved by using EHL. The EHL made by a 9-Ch probe through the rigid nephroscope makes shorter the operation whatever the width and hardness of the stones. Generally we prefer the rigid instruments, which give a better view than the flexible nephroscope [4], but the EHL made by a 5-Ch probe through the flexible nephroscope gives the possibility to get and destroy the stones nestled in the most peripherical calices; the fragments then can be washed out. To avoid high pressure in the collecting system it would be better to stop the procedure when it lasts too long. In fact the increment of pressure might damage the renal interstice expecially when there is a pre-existing infection [1]. The stopped procedure can be completed in a second step after 3–4 days with local anesthesia.

When heavy bleeding occurs, the procedure is stopped, a nephrostomic tube is placed into the percutaneous track and a continuous washing of the renal cavities is started through the ureteral catheter. The procedure can be carried out again when the bleeding ceases. The extravasation has been controlled by giving the patient diuretics. If the renal stones are infected it is very important to give prophylactic antibiotics before and after any manipulation [4], to avoid any septic reflux. In conclusion the percutaneous nephrolithotomy made by EHL is a safe procedure that lets one manage percutaneously the cast, branched and staghorn renal calculi and keeps the morbidity low with a quicker return to work [5]. Only the complete filling by the stone of small posterior renal calices is a bar to carry out the percutaneous procedure. Percutaneous litholapaxy and ESWL, which are now mutually dependent [6], make this pathology less serious for the patients.

References

1 Alken, P.; Hutschenreiter, F.; Günther, R.; Marberger, M.: Percutaneous stone manipulation. J. Urol. *125:* 463–466 (1981).

2 Segura, J.W.; Patterson, D. E.; LeRoy, A.J.; Williams, H. J., Jr.; Barrett, D.M.; Benson, R.C., Jr.; May, G.R.; Bender, C.E.: Percutaneous removal of kidney stones: review of 1,000 cases. J. Urol. *134:* 1077 (1985).

3 Segura, J.W.; Patterson, D.E.; LeRoy, A.J.; May, G.R.; Smith, L.H.: Percutaneous lithotripsy. J. Urol. *130:* 1051 (1983).

4 Wickham, J.E.A.; Kellett, M.J.; Miller, R.A.: Elective percutaneous nephrolithotomy in 50 patients: an analysis of the technique, results and complications. J. Urol. *129:* 904 (1983).

5 White, E.C.; Smith, A. D.: Percutaneous stone extraction from 200 patients. J. Urol. *132:* 437 (1984).

6 Whitfield, H.N.; Mills, V.A.: Percutaneous nephrolithotomy. Br. J. Urol. *57:* 603 (1985).

Alberto Mandressi, MD, Istituto di Urologia dell'Università,
via della Commenda 15, I–20122 Milano (Italy)

Contr. Nephrol., vol. 58, pp. 274–277 (Karger, Basel 1987)

Cystine Lithiasis: Combined Extracorporeal and Litholytic Treatment

P. Rigatti, F. Francesca, F. Ronchi, V. Di Girolamo, M. Grasso, R. Colombo, M. Maffezzini

Ospedale Raffaele, Divisione di Urologia, Milano, Italia

Cystine lithiasis is among the less frequent urinary lithiases (0.5–3%) [6, 9]. Yet it appears to be a quite relevant pathology because of the high frequency of recurrencies, the young age of the patients affected and the important therapeutic problems involved. This is the reason why we suggest a combined protocol of treatment, which assures good results and can be repeated with no restriction in the case of recurrencies. Such combined treatment consists of extracorporeal shock wave lithotripsy (ESWL) [1] associated with chemolysis in situ. ESWL is known to be the most effective and least traumatic treatment of urinary lithiasis [1]; therefore, it now represents the treatment of choice in 80–90% of all lithiases of the urinary tract. ESWL alone is not the ideal treatment of cystine lithiasis because the shock waves are less effective on the 'elastic' structure of this kind of stone. A high number of waves in more than one treatment are usually required.

Patients and Methods

426 patients have been treated during these first 9 months of experience with ESWL. Only 7 patients, 4 women and 3 men, age 17–45 years, were affected by cystine lithiasis. One patient had a solitary surgical kidney; 2 were affected by bilateral lithiasis; one had previously undergone right kidney autotransplantation after 3 pyelo-cysto-neostomies for recurrent lithiasis, performed to easily remove other possible recurrencies. Pure cystine was detected in 5 cases, and mixed stones in 2 cases (carbonate apatite).

Nine kidneys, from 7 patients, underwent ESWL treatment. Only 4 kidneys required one treatment: they belonged to 2 patients with bilateral lithiasis, the first with pure cystine stones, the second with mixed lithiasis.

One patient, with solitary kidney and mixed lithiasis, required two treatments; 2 patients required three treatments, one patient four treatments and one patient required 5 treatments. No further therapy was needed in the patient with solitary kidney that underwent two ESWL treatments; while the other 4 patients that required more than one ESWL treatment had local alkalinization between one ESWL treatment and the other due to the size and number of the stones. The litholytic solution used was tromethamine, a buffer solution, pH 8.2, effective both in vitro and in vivo [2, 5, 7]. In 2 cases the solution was introduced in the renal pelvis by means of a transureteral catheter (angiographic pigtail); in the others it was introduced through a percutaneous nephrostomy; and in both by slow drop infusion of about 500 ml/24 h, according to the patient's endurance (pain caused by the stretching of the renal pelvis) and urinary pH. The urinary pH was checked daily and kept around 8. A urine culture was made every other day.

Results

As shown in table I, 4 of the 9 kidneys treated in this study were completely cleared from stones; the other 4 showed a significant reduction of number and size of the stones, while only one case required surgery. The combined ESWL + chemolysis in situ treatment cleared the kidney in one case, reduced significantly size and number of the stones in 2 cases and failed in one.

Discussion and Conclusion

The ESWL represents a valid alternative to traditional or percutaneous surgery in the treatment of cystine lithiasis [4, 5]. However, due to the peculiar structural characteristics of these stones, ESWL alone does not always succeed in cleaning the kidney. In the most severe lithiasis (big stones and staghorn), we suggest to associate ESWL with local alkalinization with different solutions, by a transureteral angiographic pigtail or a percutaneous nephrostomy.

In our division, 4 cases have been treated with ESWL + local alkalinization with tromethamine. The theory that ESWL causes an enlargement of the surface of the stone in contact with the litholytic solution, is supported not only by the experimental data of Schmeller et al. [5] but also, we believe, by clinical practice. Someone may object that hospitalization required for this kind of treatment (42 days on the mean) is longer than that required for litholysis alone (25–37 days) [3, 8].

However, we must point out the huge size and number of the stones treated in this study, data not always reported by other authors. Side effects

Table I. Cystine lithiasis – casuistry

Patient	Sex	Kidneys	Stones		ESWL therapy			Result
			size, cm	n	treatments	shock, n	chemolysis	
S.L. mixed	M	1	1.5 × 1	3	2	4,000	–	cleared
V.L.	M	2	3 × 2	1	4	9,850	yes	surgery
F.G.	F	3	2.5 × 1	4[a]	3	6,500	yes	1 stone (0.5 × 0.5)
F.A.	F	4	5.5 × 3	1	3	7,000	yes	2 stones (1.5 × 1.5) (0.3 × 0.3)
G.S. mixed	M	5 right	4 × 0.5	8[b]	1	2,150	–	cleared
		6 left	2 × 0.5	4	1	1,850	–	2 fragments
C.S.	F	7 right	3.6 × 3	3	1	2,000	–	cleared
		8 left	1.8 × 1	2	1	1,300	–	1 stone 1 × 1
C.G.	F	9 left	5.8 × 4.3	2	5	8,100	yes	cleared
		10 right	surgery: autotransplant					cleared

[a] After reductive percutaneous surgery.
[b] After reductive surgery.

were of little relevance: no complications due to ESWL; only two mild urinary tract infections due to litholytic therapy. Therefore we may conclude that this combined shock wave + litholysis in situ treatment can improve the prognosis of patients affected by cystine lithiasis.

References

1 Chaussy, C.; Schmiedt, E.; Jocham, D.: Extracorporeal shock wave lithotripsy. New aspects in the treatment of kidney stone disease (Karger, Basel 1982).

2 Dretler, S.; Pfister, R.; Newhouse, J.; Prien, E.: Percutaneous catheter dissolution of cystine calculi. J. Urol. *131:* 216–219 (1984).

3 Hayase, Y.; Fukatsu, H.; Segawa, A.: The dissolution of cystine stones by irrigated tiopronin solution. J. Urol. *124:* 775–778 (1980).

4 Kersting, H.; Chaussy, C.; Jocham, D.; Liesl, B.: Modern strategy of cystine calculus treatment. Helv. chir. Acta *52:* 485–488 (1985).

5 Schmeller, N.; Kersting, H.; Schüller, J.; Chaussy, C.; Schmiedt, E.: Combination of chemolysis and shock wave lithotripsy in the treatment of cystine renal calculi. J. Urol. *131:* 434–438 (1984).

6 Tizzani, A.; Frea, B.; Linari, F.: La litiasi cistinica – attuali orientamenti terapeutici. Minerva Urol. *33:* 253–258 (1981).

7 Tseng, C.; Talwalkar, Y.; Tank, E.; Hatch, T.; Alexander, S.: Dissolution of cystine calculi by pelviocalicea irrigation with tromethamine-E. J. Urol. *128:* 1281–1284 (1982).

8 Weirich, W.; Frohneberg, D.; Ackermann, D.; Alken, P.: Practical experiences with antegrade local chemolysis of struvite/apatite, uric acid and cystine calculi in the kidney. Urologe *23:* 95–98 (1984).

9 Williams, G.; Chaudary, M.; Castro, J.: Cystine stones. Urology *16:* 339–342 (1980).

P. Rigatti, MD, S. Raffaele Hospital, Divisione di Urologia, via Olgettina 60,
I–20132 Milano (Italy)

Contr. Nephrol., vol. 58, pp. 278–284 (Karger, Basel 1987)

Non-Invasive Treatment of Renal and Ureteral Lithiasis: Relationship with the Site and Nature of the Stone

P. Puppo, E. Belgrano, F. Germinale, P. Bottino, C. Caviglia, L. Giuliani

Department of Urology, University of Genova, Italy

The introduction of new non-invasive technologies has changed in a radical way the old philosophies concerning the management of renal and ureteral stones [1, 4, 6, 9, 11, 12]. Nowadays the stone patients are more and more addressed toward well-equipped and trained stone centers, where the new technologies, too expensive for a wide-spread use, can reach the best cost-benefit ratio [7, 8].

In October 1985, the first shock-wave lithotripter in Italy purchased by the National Health Service was installed in a purpose-built stone center of the Urological Clinic of the University of Genoa, where since 1970 more than 3,000 open operations for stones had been carried out and where in 1983 the percutaneous techniques (PCN) had been introduced in the routine management of renal and ureteral stones [3], followed in 1984 by operative ureterorenoscopy (URS).

Up to March 15th, 1986, our experience of non-invasive treatment is based on 340 cases of extracorporeal shock wave lithotripsy (ESWL), 220 cases of PCN and 44 cases of URS. As far as the related percentages are concerned, figure 1 shows that PCN (together with URS) did never replace completely open surgery (OS), because of the poor availability of endourological radiological equipment. On the contrary, ESWL greatly increased the number of stone patients treated and, in the first period, it practically cancelled out PCN and OS. Today, in view of the considerations that we are presenting in this paper, PCN and OS are regaining a well-defined place in our practice. Once the new techniques have been mastered, the real problem of a stone center consists in establishing the correct indica-

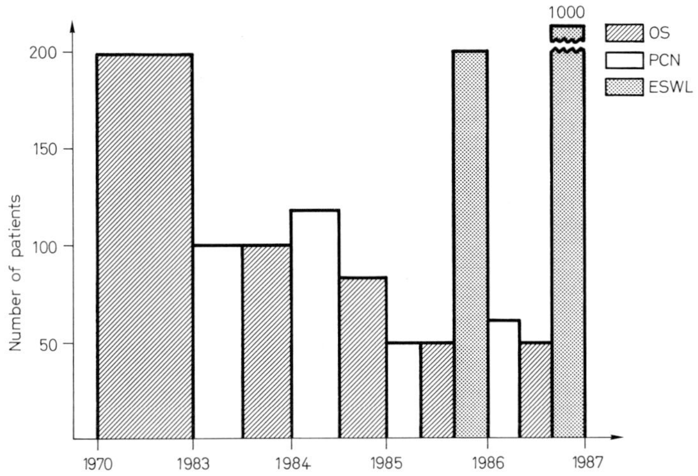

Fig. 1. Surgical and non-invasive treatment for renal stones in the last 15 years in the Department of Urology of the University of Genova.

tions for each patient. In the case of renal stone we have three cards to play alternatively (ESWL, PCN and OS), five in the case of ureteral stone, i.e. ESWL, PCN, OS, URS and simple transurethral extraction (TUE) by sling or basket. In most cases ESWL is the card preferred by the patient and his physician, so that the problem of the correct indication should be investigated starting from this technique, evaluating its results and trying to establish some criteria for electing a patient for ESWL on the basis of the characteristics of the stone and of the patient himself.

Patients and Methods

340 patients underwent ESWL since October 1985, of whom 206 were males and 134 females. The youngest patient was 13 years old and the oldest was 78, with a mean age of 44 years. 18 patients underwent two sessions of ESWL. 165 out of 340 patients have been followed until complete stone clearance or up to 3 months after treatment. The following parameters were considered for these 165 patients: number and location of stones (table I); size of the stones, measured by one (or two) diameters (table I); nature of the stones, as determined by X-ray refractometry (table I); urine culture; number of shock waves required; complication rate (table I); incidence of adjunctive treatment (table I); time required for the complete passage of stone fragments (table I). All these data were recorded on a Digital P 350 computer and carefully analyzed with respect to their correlations.

Table I. Parameters considered for the computerized study

Stone position, n (%)		*Stone size, n (%)*		*Nature of stones, %*	
Pyelic	42 (25)	10 mm	58 (35)	Oxalate	62
Caliceal	46 (28)	10–20 mm	56 (34)	Phosphate	34
Multiples	30 (18)	20–30 mm	36 (22)	Cystine	4
PU junction	16 (10)	30 mm	15 (9)		
Incl. staghorn	11 (7)				
Compl. staghorn	6 (4)				
Ureteral	14 (8)				
Free of stones, n (%)		*Complications, %*		*Adjunctive treatments, %*	
1–15 days	91 (55)	Ureteral obstr.	8	Perc. nephrostomy	4
15–30 days	32 (18)	Fever	13	Meatotomy	5
30–60 days	29 (17)	Sepsis	2	Basket extraction	3
60–90 days	13 (10)			Stenting	2

Results

The number of shock waves required and the time between ESWL and the first stone-free X-ray controls (clearance time) were assumed as discriminating parameters. The nature of the stones was matched with these parameters but only a slight positive correlation was found. In other words, oxalate stones are more resistant than phosphate to ESWL. Neither cystine stones showed different features. Surprisingly, the size of a stone did not seem to influence significantly the number of shock waves and the clearance time. We expected some positive correlation between stone size and clearance time, but in this case too no statistically significant data could be checked.

In order to revise the feasibility of stone size measurement, stone size was controlled in 6 patients with large stones by echography and computerized tomographic (CT) scanning. Notwithstanding the small number of cases, CT seems to offer a better evaluation of the real stone volume (fig. 2), even if some problem is produced by breathing movements; echography can be useful only in spherical or oval-shaped stones. The complication rate did not differ according to the nature of the stone, neither to the site or to the size.

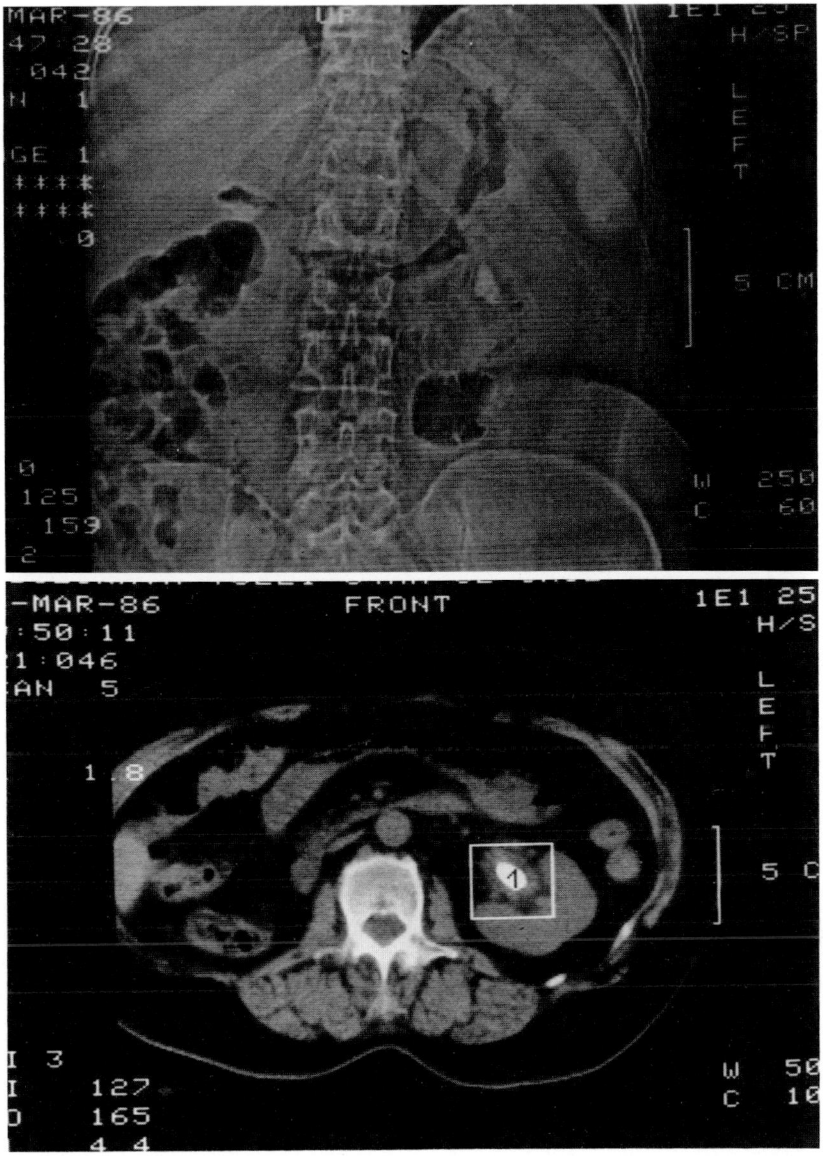

Fig. 2. CT shows the real volume (1.8 cm^3) of the stone.

Discussion

ESWL is the less invasive treatment of renal and ureteral stones, so that it should be considered as the first-choice treatment [17]. In our experience ESWL gave good results, with 79% of stone-free patients within 3 months and 10% free of symptoms. Conversely, it is undebatable that for the remaining 11% ESWL has not been the right therapy and correct preoperative planning should have avoided wasting of time and money. Besides, the results of the patients free of symptoms but with fragments cannot be considered as fully satisfactory.

PCN can offer a more invasive but faster method of stone removal and should be always proposed as an alternative to ESWL [11, 14, 15]. Besides, radiolucent stones cannot be treated with the actually available extracorporeal lithotripter and should be operated on percutaneously. In staghorn stones, especially if not operated on previously, open surgery can still represent the best solution.

As a matter of fact, there is no definite criterion in large renal stone for deciding which card to play (ESW, PCN or OS?). Our statistical study is based only on 165 patients, so that a definite statement cannot be drawn, but we have the serious impression of a certain degree of serendipity in our results. Considered that serendipity cannot be accepted as an indication and that the theoretical basis of the stone treatment should be outlined and followed, we are now developing a working hypothesis on an index for stone treatment (IST). This can be summed as follows:

$$\frac{\text{SV (stone volume)} \times \text{UTI (urinary tract infection)}}{\text{CUT (compliance of urinary tract)} \times \text{PC (patient cooperation)}}.$$

The stone volume is difficult to observe preoperatively because our informations are generally bidimensional. Alken et al. [2] suggested a stone diameter of 2 cm as a discrimination between ESWL and PCN, but it is largely insufficient, because the percentage of spherical stones is very low. Also in our series the bidimensional evaluation of the measurement revealed as not suitable. Probably a threedimensional evaluation, as supplied by CT scanning, can give more feasible indication, provided that a discriminant volume should be fixed and routine CT scanning of large stone should be available. In IST we should consider the nature of the stone but up to now there is evidence but no value for different behaviors, even if cystine stones are commonly defined as the hardest ones.

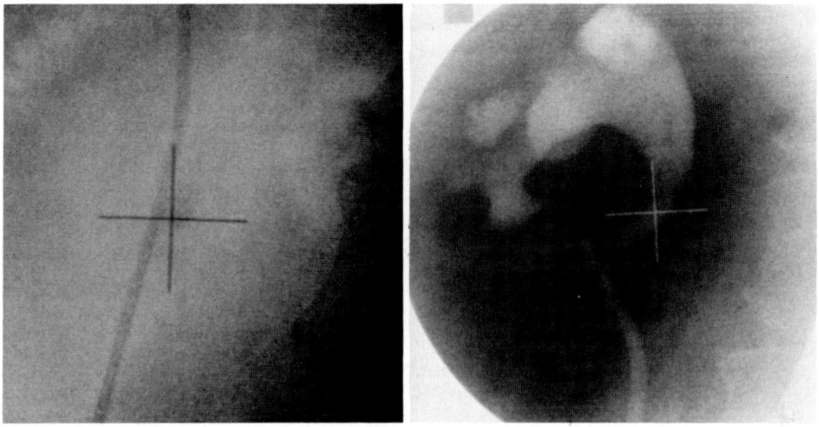

Fig. 3. A right ureteral stone. Intraoperative view with the ureteral catheter.

The presence of significant UTI can worsen the prognosis after ESWL treatment, so that it can be rightly included in IST. PCN or OS have a minor problem with UTI because they always provide a good external urinary drainage [9, 11]. The compliance of the urinary tract is the most difficult parameter to be evaluated, because routine IVP gives certainly too little informations [10]. The cooperation of the patient is mandatory to the good result of ESWL, because not all patients enjoy this kind of therapy. Presently, we are not able to give any definite value to the IST, but we are persuaded that every effort in defining it could be extremely helpful for the good policy of every stone center. At last we have to discuss the indications for ureteral calculi, where the problem is completely different being only a question of level. Besides, the possibilities of choice are five (ESWL, PCN, TUE, URS and OS). As many authors agree, the ureteral stones above the iliac crest should be first treated with ESWL and secondly, in the case of failure, with PCN or OS. Below the iliac crest, TUE and URS come into play, while open surgery should be always available as second-choice treatment.

Contrary to the first reports [16], ESWL of ureteral stone, especially if performed under the guide of an ureteral catheter (fig. 3), has given very good results in our experience, with a success rate of 85%.

In conclusion, we want to outline that the new technologies for non-invasive treatment of stones, and especially ESWL, are extremely fascinating and their results very encouraging, but the correct criteria for their best application have not yet been assessed.

References

1 Alken, P.; Hutschenreiter, C.; Günther, R.; Marberger, M.: Percutaneous stone manipulation. J. Urol. *125:* 463–466 (1981).

2 Alken, P.; Hardeman, S.; Wilbert, D.; Thüroff, J.; Jacobi, G. H.: Extracorporeal shock wave lithotripsy (ESWL): alternatives and adjuvant procedures. Wld J. Urol. *3:* 48–52 (1985).

3 Belgrano, E.; Puppo, P.; Quattrini, S.; Bottino, P.; Germinale, F.; Giuliani, L.: Il trattamento percutaneo della calcolosi renale. San Martino *2:* 85–92 (1985).

4 Chaussy, C.; Eisenberg, F.; Wanner, K.; Forssmann, B.; Hepp, W.; Schmiedt, E.; Brendel, W.: The use of shock waves for the destruction of renal calculi without direct contact. Urol. Res. *4:* 175 (1976).

5 Chaussy, C.; Schmiedt, E.; Forssmann, B.; Brendel, W.: Contact free renal stone destruction by means of shock waves. Eur. surg. Res. *11:* 36 (1979).

6 Chaussy, C.; Brendel, W.; Schmiedt, E.: Extracorporeally induced destruction of kidney stones by shock waves. Lancet *ii:* 1265 (1980).

7 Chaussy, C.: Extracorporeal shock wave lithotripsy (ESWL) for kidney stones. An alternative to surgery? Urol. Radiol. *2:* 80 (1984).

8 Clayman, R. V.; Surya, V.; Miller, R. P.; Castaneda-Zuniga, W. R.; Smith, A. D.; Hunter, D. W.; Amplatz, K.; Lange, P. H.: Percutaneous nephrolithotomy: extraction of renal and ureteral calculi from 100 patients. J. Urol. *131:* 868–871 (1984).

9 Fernström, I.; Johannson, B.: Percutaneous pyelolithotomy: a new extraction technique. Scand. J. Urol. *4:* 257–259 (1976).

10 Kaye, K. W.: Renal anatomy for endourologic stone removal. J. Urol. *130:* 1051–1054 (1983).

11 Marberger, M.; Stackl, W.; Hruby, W.: Percutaneous litholapaxy of renal calculi with ultrasound. Eur. Urol. *8:* 236 (1982).

12 Perez-Castro Ellendt, E.; Martinez-Pineiro, J. A.: Ureteral and renal endoscopy. A new approach. Eur. Urol. *8:* 117–120 (1982).

13 Puppo, P.; Belgrano, E.; Bottino, F.; Germinale, F.; Giuliani, L.: La litotrissia extracorporea ad onde shock. San Martino *2:* 95–98 (1985).

14 Reddy, P. K.; Lange, P. H.; Hulbert, J. C.; Clayman, R. V.; Breen, J. F.; Hunter, D. W.; Coleman, C. C.; Castaneda-Zuniga, W. R.; Amplatz, K.: Percutaneous removal of caliceal and other 'inaccessible' stones: results. J. Urol. *132:* 443–447 (1984).

15 Segura, J. W.; Patterson, D. E.; Leroy, A. J.; May, G. R.; Smith, L. H.: Percutaneous lithotripsy. J. Urol. *130:* 1051–1054 (1983).

16 Schmiedt, E.: Extracorporeal shock wave lithotripsy of kidney and ureteric stones. Urol. int. *39:* 193 (1984).

17 Wickam, J. E.: Extracorporeal shock wave lithotripsy: the first 50 patients treated in Britain. Br. med. J. *290:* 1188 (1985).

P. Puppo, MD, Department of Urology, University of Genova, I–16132 Genova (Italy)

Contr. Nephrol., vol. 58, pp. 285–293 (Karger, Basel 1987)

Advances in Preoperative Localization and Surgery of the Parathyroid Glands

L. Giuliani[a], *P. Puppo*[a], *U. Repetto*[a], *F. Germinale*[a], *P. Pittaluga*[a], *G. Ferlin*[b]

[a]Department of Urology, Università degli Studi di Genova;
[b]Service of Nuclear Medicine, Castelfranco Veneto, Italy

The incidence of primary hyperparathyroidism (PHP) in stone patients (2–5%) is considerable and becomes even more relevant if one considers only recurrent calcium stones (6–10%). The relative concentration of patients in well-trained stone centers, which can provide non-invasive treatment of stones, accounts for the number of parathyroid patients operated in our clinic during the last 10 years (122 cases).

Preoperative localization of abnormal parathyroid tissue may be a valid help for the surgeon reducing operative time and the need for more extensive exploration and lessening operative morbidity. PHP is most frequently related to parathyroid adenomas, but diffuse hyperplasia also frequently occurrs (10–20%); carcinoma, on the contrary, is extremely rare (no case in our series). In case of diffuse hyperplasia, total parathyroidectomy plus autotransplantation, introduced in the 1970s, is affirmed as the technique of choice [18–20].

Preoperative Localization

In the beginning of our experience, this delicate task was mainly afforded by ^{75}Se-scintigraphy (fig. 1), even if some authors had reported poor results with this method, with an overall sensitivity rate of only 40%. Selective arteriography was then proposed, but its complication rate was too high when compared to the sensitivity (no more than 50–60%). In 1973 we began to adopt parathyroid hormone (PTH) radioimmunoassay on selectively sampled venous blood [2, 4, 10, 11] (fig. 2).

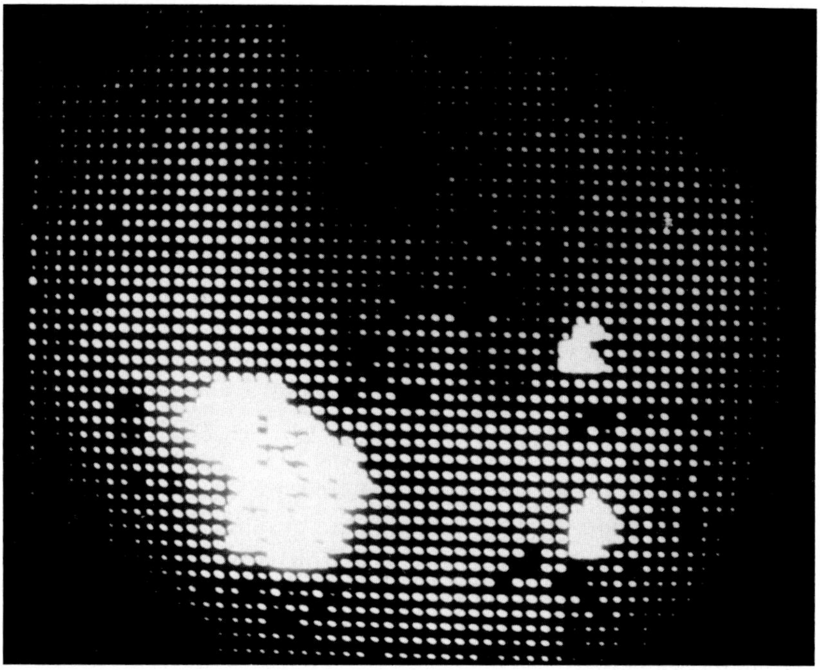

Fig. 1. False-positive results with ^{75}Se-scintigraphy scanning: presence of a right warm zone is possibly referrable to a parathyroid adenoma (at surgery left inferior adenoma).

In our hands selective PTH radioimmunoassay gave good results. The analysis of PTH concentration at the different levels of sampling suggested a correct preoperative localization in 75% of the cases. However, this technique is not always easy and requires superselective catheterization and sampling from the thyroid plexus in order to achieve satisfactory results. Therefore, it becomes time-consuming and very expensive, owing to the numerous [15–20] assays required.

That notwithstanding, we routinely performed selective PTH assay in all patients with certain or suspected PHP up to 1983, when we started a prospective trial using ultrasounds and computerized tomography (CT) scanning together.

Ultrasound alone showed a sensitivity rate of 55% with 33% of false-negative results and 11% of false-positive results. CT alone gave respectively 66, 22 and 12%. Read together, CT and ultrasounds allowed a sen-

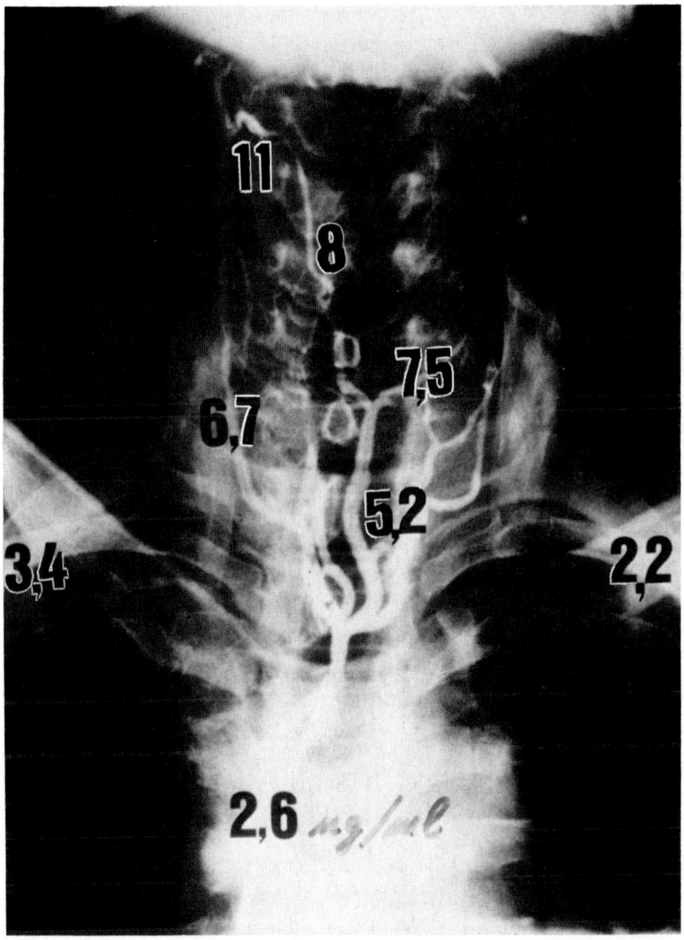

Fig. 2. Selective venous sampling and PTH radioimmunoassay: the peak of PTH concentration reveals the presence (confirmed by surgery) of a right superior adenoma.

sitivity rate of 77% with only 23% of false results. Giving CT and ultrasounds the same results as PTH-selective sampling and being non-invasive techniques, we adopted them as routine preoperative investigations in parathyroid patients. In 1985, we started a cooperation with the group of Ferlin, who introduced in 1983 the $^{99m}Tc/^{201}Tl$ subtraction double-tracer

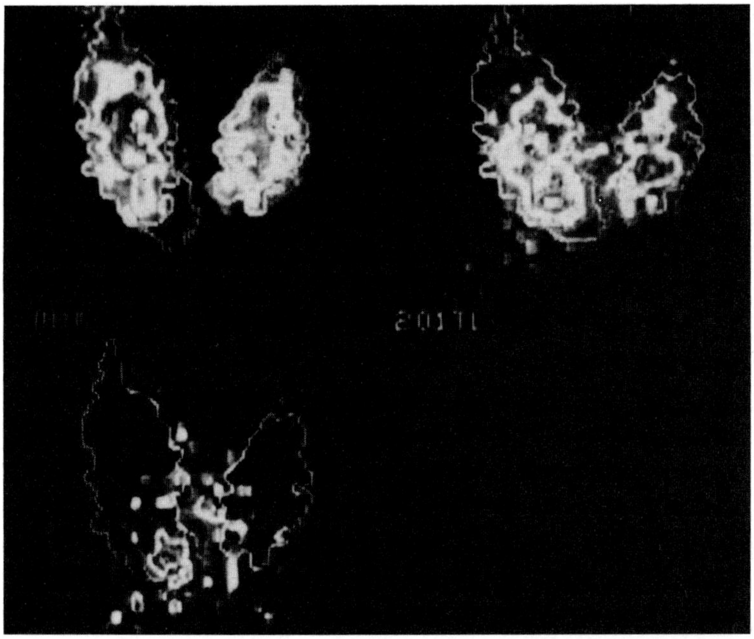

Fig. 3. Subtraction scintigraphy: right inferior parathyroid adenoma (confirmed by surgery).

scintigraphy and reported an overall success rate of 92% [5–7]. Ferlin's technique is as follows:

1 mCi of the ^{99m}Tc-pertechnetate is injected intravenously; a 50,000-count anterior image of the thyroid is obtained using a gamma camera with a pinhole collimator and connected on-line to a computer. 1 mCi of ^{201}Tl is then injected intravenously and two images per minute are obtained for the subsequent 25 min. The technetium image is then recalled from memory, and a region of interest is marked over the entire thyroid image. The thallium images are displayed and normalized to the technetium image, and the technetium views are then subtracted from the thallium images. At the end of the procedure, the abnormal parathyroid tissue can be clearly seen on the computer screen (fig. 3).

At the moment, double-tracer scintigraphy has given in our cases a 100% sensitivity and specifity rate. Probably these extremely good results are related to the selective small number of cases (9) and are subjected to a certain degree of worsening, but they are enough to make double-traced scintigraphy the first-choice technique in the preoperative assessment of parathyroid patients. Ultrasounds can be used together to better evaluate doubtful cases.

Technique of Neck Exploration

Surgery of parathyroid adenomas requires careful exploration of the neck from the thyroid cartilage down to the jugulum, performed through a transverse Kocher incision.

The subhyoid muscles should be better divaricated than divided, in order to obtain a better cosmetic result. Sharp dissection should be carried out between the deep sheath of the sternothyroidal muscle and the thyroid capsule, that is progressively dissected free from its lateral attachments in order to be easily moved upward and medially. This maneuver makes visible the posterior face of the thyroid gland. The recurrent nerve should be at least identified (or sometimes isolated) before any maneuver on the parathyroid glands.

The parathyroid glands are not easy to find owing to their small volume (normal 5 × 2 to 3 mm, weight 40 mg) and its often ectopic situation. The superior glands are generally localized behind the median portion of the correspondent thyroid lobe, adherent to the thyroid tissue, so that sometimes they are considered as intrathyroid glands. According to our experience they are not 'true' intrathyroid glands, but 'intracapsular' glands.

Once the thyroid capsule has been incised, the parathyroid glands come out and become well visible. The inferior parathyroid gland lies behind, aside or below the inferior pole of the thyroid gland. They are often deeply located into the jugular area. A transcervical thymectomy is therefore required for their complete excision. Rarely, the parathyroid glands are deeply located in the anterior or posterior mediastinum and sternotomy becomes unavoidable if an adenoma has developed from one of these glands [8].

Being an operation much more stressing than cervical exploration, it should be performed in a second operative session, possibly after repeated careful attemps to preoperative localization (fig. 4). When possible, all four parathyroid glands should be identified and isolated in order to rule out a diffuse hyperplasia. This can be suspected when at least three glands appear macroscopically increased in volume. Biopsy is very difficult, requires a very experienced pathologist and implies the risk of ischemic damages to the glands, so that the so-called microscopic hyperplasia is routinely unrecognized. Diffuse hyperplasia poses particular problems of extension of the exeresis, thus posing the risk of undertreatment (recurrence of hyperparathyroidism due to one or even half a hyperplastic gland left in place) and overtreatment (persistent hypoparathyroidism after total parathyroidectomy). Total parathyroidectomy with parathyroid autotransplantation seems to be a reasonable compromise to this problem.

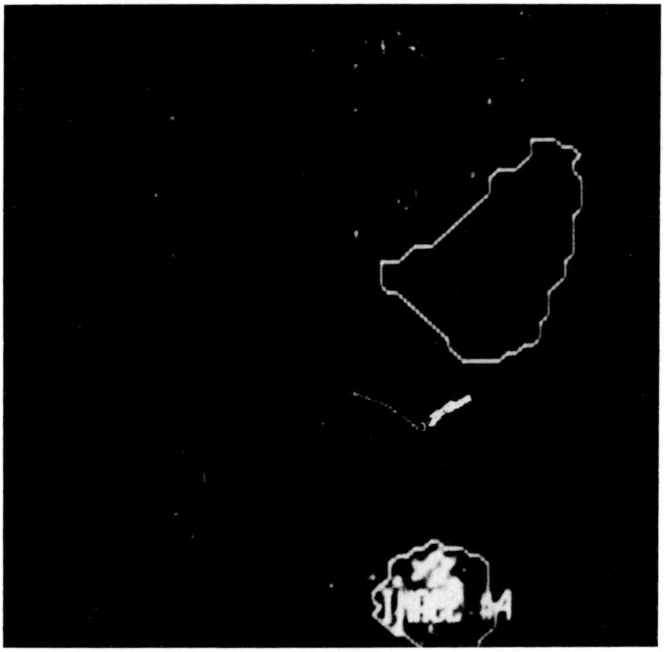

Fig. 4. Subtraction scintigraphy: mediastinal parathyroid adenoma (confirmed by surgery).

Parathyroid Autotransplantation

The indications of total parathyroidectomy with parathyroid autotransplantation are primary or secondary diffuse parathyroid hyperplasia and recurrent or persistent hyperparathyroidism. Parathyroid autotransplantation is also indicated in total thyroidectomy for carcinoma in order to prevent postoperative hypoparathyroidism. In our opinion parathyroid autotransplantation is preferable to subtotal 3/4 or 7/8 parathyroidectomy because: (1) it allows for an exact measure of the parathyroid tissue left behind; (2) the evaluation of the function of the grafted tissue is easy and sure; (3) failures can be corrected by reimplantation of frozen tissue; (4) in the case of graft hyperfunction the excess of parathyroid tissue can be removed easily under local anesthesia.

Operative Technique

All four parathyroid glands are identified and isolated and only when all four glands appear enlarged in size are they removed. Half of each gland is sent for histological examination and the remaining half is placed into a cold sterile ice bath of Waymouth's tissue culture medium. When histological confirmation arrives, one or two residual glands are carefully cleaned and then diced into small pieces measuring 1 or 2 mm in diameter. Using microsurgical instruments, 20 of these pieces are implanted intramuscularly into small beds bluntly created in the flexor muscles of the forearm. Each implantation site is closed with a 6/0 prolene interrupted suture, which prevents extrusion of the parathyroid tissue and serves as a marker.

After autotransplantation the remaining parathyroid tissue is divided into small pieces and placed into chilled vials containing 10% dimethylsulfoxide, 10% autologous serum and 80% Waymouth's medium for long-term preservation at −196 °C. This tissue could be useful in the case of failure of the autotransplantation and consequent hypoparathyroidism status. Up to date, we have one successful experience of frozen parathyroid tissue reimplantation. In the immediate postoperative period the patients are given dihydrotachysterol (3–8 mg/day) and oral calcium (3 g/day). Intravenous gluconate calcium is administered only when signs or symptoms of hypocalcemia are observed. The serum calcium concentration is determined daily. Since the 15th postoperative day, PTH secretion from the grafted tissue is determined according to the method suggested by Wells. Venous occlusion is obtained by simultaneously applying tourniquets to both arms above the elbow for 5 min and then blood samples were drawn from each antecubital vein.

Results

From June 1974 to December 1985 we operated on 122 patients for hyperparathyroidism, 52 were males and 70 females. Age ranged from 8 to 76 years. 101 (83%) patients were recurrent calcium stone formers; 11 had obstructing urolithiasis which was treated simultaneously with hyperparathyroidism due to chronic renal failure; 5 (4.1%) presented with acute hyperparathyroidism, which resolved only with emergency parathyroidectomy. Five patients (4.1%) suffered also from bone cystic disease. At neck exploration 85 single adenomas, 1 double adenoma and 36 diffuse hyperplasias (29.5%) were found. The most common orthotropic adenomas were the left inferior ones (29), followed by the right inferior (21), the left superior (15) and the right superior ones (12). Five adenomas were found in the jugulum and 5 in the anterior mediastinum. The latter ones required mediastinotomy by sternal splitting.

Diffuse hyperplasia was treated by 3/4 parathyroidectomy in 4 cases, by 7/8 parathyroidectomy in 3 cases and by total parathyroidectomy and autotransplantation to the forearm in 29 cases. The complication rate was very low, including only 3 cases of transient dysphonia and 1 case of hemorrage. The results of parathyroid surgery in stone-forming patients, evaluated in terms of prevention of stone recurrence, were satisfactory (only 1 recurrence out of 101 cases).

The results of parathyroid autotransplantation, evaluated by serum calcium values and by separate PTH radioimmunoassay, were fully satisfactory in 26 cases, uncertain in 2 cases and negative in 1 case, where hypercalcemia persisted after total parathyroidectomy. The uncertain results were so classified because of negative separate PTH assay in the presence of normal serum calcium values (fifth gland?).

Conclusion

The surgery of hyperparathyroidism cannot obviously be considered as a routine urological operation and it is not strictly necessary that every urological department include it in its program. What is needed everywhere is the awareness of the real incidence of such a disease in stone formers. Screening and therapy of hyperparathyroidism, on the contrary, is a specific job of stone centers, which should provide the treatment of the 'symptom' stone (the least invasive possible) and at the same time of the 'disease' lithiasis, by removing the causes of lithogenesis. Among the causes, hyperparathyroidism can offer the greatest satisfaction, when cured, to the urologist who, being essentially a surgeon, is extremely gratified by a radical surgical resolution.

References

1 Carmignani, G.; Belgrano, E.; Puppo, P.: L'iperparatiroidismo primitivo in urologia. Urologia *1:* 3–96 (1977).

2 Carmignani, G.; Belgrano, E.; Puppo, P.: La localizzazione pre-operatoria degli adenomi paratiroidei mediante dosaggio del PTH e cateterismo venoso selettivo. Minerva chir. *32:* 491–498 (1977).

3 Carmignani, G.; Belgrano, E.; Puppo, P.; Repetto, U.; Giusti, M.; Giordano, G.; Giuliani, L.: PTH radioimmunoassay and loading tests in the diagnosis of patients with primary hyperparathyroidism. Eur. Urol. *8:* 102–106 (1982).

4 Doppman, J.L.; Mallette, L.E.; Marx, S.J.; Monchic, J.M.; Broadus, A.; Spiegel, A.M.; Beazley, R.; Aurbach, G.D.: The localization of abnormal mediastinal parathyroid glands. Radiology *115:* 31 (1975).

5 Ferlin, G.; Conte, N.; Borsato, N.; Perelli, R.; Fioretti, P.; Gasparoni, P.; Camerani, M.: Parathyroid scintigraphy with ^{131}Cs and ^{201}Tl. J. nucl. Med. all. Sci. *25:* 119–123 (1981).

6 Ferlin, G.; Borsato, N.; Camerani, M.; Zotti, D.: Double-tracer ($^{99m}Tc/^{201}Tl$) scintigraphy and ultrasonography in the detection of enlarged parathyroids. Nucl. Med. Biol. Adv. *1:* 1269–1273 (1982).

7 Ferlin, G.; Borsato, N.; Camerani, M.; Conte, N.; Zotti, D.: New prospectives in localizing enlarged parathyroids by technetium-thallium subtraction scan. J. nucl. Med. *24:* 438–441 (1983).

8 Freeman, J.B.; Sherman, B.M.; Mason, E.E.: Transcervical thymectomy. An integral part of neck exploration for hyperparathyroidism. Archs. Surg., Chicago *11:* 359 (1976).

9 Giuliani, L.; Carmignani, G.; Belgrano, E.; Puppo, P.: I reinterventi nella chirurgia dell'iperparatiroidismo. Minerva chir. *32:* 499–506 (1977).

10 Giuliani, L.; Carmignani, G.; Belgrano, E.; Puppo, P.: Value of selective parathormone radioimmunoassay in primary hyperparathyroidism. Urology *156* (1979).

11 Giuliani, L.; Carmignani, G.; Belgrano, E.; Puppo, P.: Die selektive Parathormonbestimmung als Lokalisationsmittel der Nebenschilddrüsenadenome beim primären Hyperparathyreoidismus. Urologe *17:* 23–28 (1978).

12 Giuliani, L.; Carmignani, G.; Belgrano, E.; Puppo, P.; Cichero, A.; Repetto, U.: Surgical hyperparathyroidism in calcium stone formers. A retrospective study of 20 cases. Eur. Urol. *7:* 144–149 (1981).

13 Giuliani, L.; Carmignani, G.; Belgrano, E.; Puppo, P.; Repetto, U.: Iperparatiroidismo en urologia. Arch. esp. Urol. *35:* 27–38 (1981).

14 Giuliani, L.; Carmignani, G.; Belgrano, E.; Puppo, P.; Repetto, U.; Giusti, M.: Parathyroid autotransplantation. Eur. Urol. *7:* 335 (1981).

15 Giuliani, L.; Belgrano, E.; Puppo, P.; Repetto, U.; Pittaluga, P.: Hyperparathyroidism and obstructing urolithiasis: combined surgical approach. Acta urol. belg. *4* (1983).

16 Giuliani, L.; Carmignani, G.; Belgrano, E.; Puppo, P.; Repetto, U.; Giusti, M.; Pittaluga, P.; Trombetta, C.: Immediate and long-term results of parathyroid autotransplantation in primary and secondary hyperparathyroidism. Int. Urol. Nephrol. *16:* 91–99 (1984).

17 Giuliani, L.: Chirurgie de l'hyperparathyroidie chez les patients urologiques. A propos de 76 cas opérés. J. Urol. *89:* 521–528 (1983).

18 Giuliani, L.; Carmignani, G.; Belgrano, E.; Puppo, P.: Il nostro orientamento in tema di iperparatiroidismo. Urologia *43:* 225 (1976).

19 Heath, H.; Hodgson, S.F.; Kennedy, M.A.: Primary hyperparathyroidism; incidence morbidity and potential economic impact in a community. New Engl. J. Med.: 189–193 (1980).

20 Wells, S.A.; Gunnels, J.C.; Shelburne, J.C.: Transplantation of the parathyroid glands in man: clinical indications and results. Surgery, St. Louis *78:* 34 (1975).

L. Giuliani, MD, Department of Urology, Università degli Studi di Genova, I–16132 Genova (Italy)

Subject Index